Advances in Biomaterials 1

Advances in
Biomaterials

1

EDITED BY

Stuart M. Lee
EDITOR
SAMPE JOURNAL

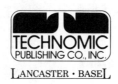

TECHNOMIC
PUBLISHING CO., INC.
LANCASTER · BASEL

Published in the Western Hemisphere by
Technomic Publishing Company, Inc.
851 New Holland Avenue
Box 3535
Lancaster, Pennsylvania 17604 U.S.A.

Distributed in the Rest of the World by
Technomic Publishing AG

Printed in the United States of America
10 9 8 7 6 5 4 3 2 1

Main entry under title:
  Advances in Biomaterials 1

A Technomic Publishing Company book
Bibliography: p.

Library of Congress Card No. 86-72347
ISBN No. 87762-504-2

TABLE OF CONTENTS

PART III: TESTING

PREFACE

The human body is a well engineered machine, but age, wear and tear, stress and injuries can result in its inability to repair itself. From ancient times man has always been intrigued with the concept of replacing broken and deteriorating parts in the body. However, it is only since the introduction of synthetic materials that tremendous strides have been made in the rise of biomaterials from plaster of Paris, the first bioceramic used in 1892, to our present unique carbon-carbon materials.

What are biomaterials? These substances can consist of ceramics, polymers, metals or their combinations and are used to augment or replace an organ, tissue or body function in a living system.

The interest in biomaterials is tied to the growth of our older population. Americans for example face 750,000 deaths annually due to heart and cardiovascular diseases as well as the permanent disability of millions. Each year we have upwards of 60,000 individuals who require a new heart, but unfortunately must compete for the only 2000 available biological hearts. The number of people requiring replacement of other body parts continues to climb, e.g., last year there were some 150,000 surgical hip replacements performed.

We can also see the need of biomaterials as tied to their demand. Recently the sales of medical grade polymeric materials has been quoted to be a staggering 3 billion dollars/year, which doesn't include ceramics or metals.

What are the prerequisites for a biomaterial? For an implant material to be successful, it must be biocompatible and also function in the human body. This has resulted in the design and screening of bio-engineered materials as compared to the earlier pragmatic selection approach. At best we can expect a compromise in matching biomaterial physical/mechanical properties with the supporting tissue. However, some of our recent substitute materials have shown remarkable properties. Polymethyl methacrylate (PMMA) reinforced glass fibers are compatible with living tissue with bending strengths of 2,000 to 15,000 kg/cm^2 which surpasses 1,800 kg/cm^2 for natural bone. In addition, the bending elasticity or toughness of PMMA bone is rated from 80,000 to 600,000 kg/cm^2 as compared to 160,000 kg/cm^2 for human bone. Carbon fibers can perform as biodegradable ligaments and consist of 10,000 to 96,000 carbon filaments, 7μm in diameter. These can serve as a support for the regeneration of natural ligaments with a strength of six times that of natural ones, while braided carbon fibers exhibit 5 to 10 times the elasticity of unidirectional fibers and have a longer fatigue life.

Biomaterials pose the same problems as other materials. They are similarly concerned with fatigue, wearout and environmental effects. In addition, we must also cope with many other problems, e.g., when some polymeric devices are implanted, body fluids can immediately begin penetration resulting in a reduction in tensile strength. Polymers can also contain a variety of organic functional groups and not be homogeneous such as a polyurethane which may have low molecular weight compounds which tend to migrate to the surface. These moieties can leach-out into the biological media resulting in an alteration of the surface structure of the material. Another more subtle change can be encountered when an orthopedic implant device is attached to the bone. This can result in a condition of a continuous remodeling state reacting to applied stresses and causing the addition or removal of bone.

In this first volume is a collection of technical papers from several sources including the session on biomaterials presented at the 30th National SAMPE Symposium and Exhibition sponsored by the Society for the Advancement of Material and Process Engineering held in Anaheim, California on March 19–21, 1985 (and published in the proceedings), the technical papers published in the *SAMPE Journal, 20* (4), 8–34 (1984), the technical papers presented at the 42nd Technical Conference of the Society of Plastics Engineers (SPE), ANTEC '85 during April 29 through May 2, in Washington, D.C., and that published in *Modern Plastics,* May 1985.

The broad spectrum of these technical papers selected for this first volume have been divided into four parts: Part I–Analysis, Part II–New Materials, Part III–Testing, and Part IV–Reliability.

In the first part on analysis the authors discuss: advanced instrumental techniques for the rapid bioassay of toxic materials, creep analysis of Delrin stents in cardiac bioprosthesis devices using finite element analysis, the potential use of electron spectroscopy for chemical analysis (ESCA) for study of biomaterial surface, an approach to the characterization of porous coatings used for implant systems, the use of gel permeation chromatography for molecular weight distribution and physical properties of biomedical plastics, the application of automation systems for the improvement of accuracy and productivity of polymer analysis and property changes of ultrahigh molecular weight polyethylene (UHMWPE) in vitro and in vivo storage.

The authors in Part II—New Materials, which is the largest part, describe the utilization of sintered powder metal coated implants as an alternative to the use of PMMA bone cement, the potential of LTI-Si carbon material orthopedic implants, the effects of mixing techniques on the properties of PMMA bone cement, epoxy resin dental adhesives and keratinized surface adhesives, high performance cycloaliphatic based thermoplastic polyurethane elastomers for medical devices, artificial skin consisting of a bilayer polymeric membrane, developing systems of monomeric hydrophilics to preformed substrates with a high oxygen and carbon dioxide transport, the use of high performance, medical grade silicone elastomers for permanent implant, the options available for the replacement of ligaments, the machining of Bioglass prosthetic devices under operating room conditions, the development of sustained release wound dressings, the replacement of phthalate esters used as PVC plasticizers shown to be toxic with citric acid esters, the development of visible light cured dental biomaterials, the status of silicone elastomeric contact lenses and the use of combination titanium alloy/alumina ceramics with UHMWPE for a total hip joint replacement.

In Part III—Testing, the technical papers analyze the method for the determination of the biostability of polyether polyurethanes under stress, biochemical and mechanical testing systems and the use of automated servohydraulics for the replication of multi-dimensional motions of biomechanical movements.

Part IV—Reliability covers the prediction of durability and the fatigue lifetime of elastomeric biomaterials and the reliability of implantable titanium feedthroughs.

The editor would like to thank the Society for the Advancement of Material and Process Engineering, The Society of Plastics Engineers and McGraw-Hill Publishing Company for their permission to reproduce their technical material.

I would also like to acknowledge the helpful and able assistance of Dr. Felix Battat for his many fruitful and lucid discussions relative to orthopedic materials from his broad viewpoint and experience as an orthopedic surgeon.

STUART M. LEE

PART I

Analysis

A Rapid Bioassay for Assessing the Toxicity of Chemicals Extracted from Medical Grade Plastics

ANTHONY A. BULICH
SmithKline Beckman Corporation
Clinical Diagnostics Division
Carlsbad, California 92008

INTRODUCTION

I N THE PAST 20 years there has been a proliferation of new man-made
materials which have found a variety of applications for medical,
dental and pharmaceutical needs. Medical devices alone comprise
10,000 to 20,000 different products which range from simple containers
to complex implantable devices. The basic structural component for
most medical devices are synthetic polymeric materials generally
defined as plastics.

Commercial plastics can contain, in addition to the basic polymer,
unreacted monomer or one of several supplementary agents or additives. These additives, such as plasticizers, antioxidants, stabilizers
or colorants are added to influence specific properties of the plastic
material. Toxic reactions to a device material may result from the
release of any of these agents directly from the material to surrounding
tissue or from fluids which are later administered through the device.
An extractable agent may provide a local toxic response or systemic injury depending upon the particular device [1].

The biological safety of biomaterials and medical devices may depend
on the relative toxicity of any extractable chemical substances.
Chemical analysis, although useful, cannot quantitate actual toxicity
of extractable substances. Extracts may contain several compounds,

Presented at ANTEC '84, The Society of Plastic Engineers, Inc. 42nd Technical Conference and Exhibition, April 30–May 3, New Orleans, LA.

3

each in relatively low concentration which, in combination, can be very toxic.

Traditional toxicity test methods, which utilize animals or cell cultures, have several disadvantages. The test procedures are time consuming, (one to five days required) expensive, and often lack standardization. The cell cultures or animal populations required for the testing must be continually maintained.

TEST METHODS—THE BIOLUMINESCENT CONCEPT

Toxicity is the propensity of a chemical or condition to cause harm to the life process. The minimum requirement for monitoring toxicity is a set of interdependent enzyme systems controlling measurable physiological parameters, and the appropriate measurement system. For a practical, real-time measurement of acute toxicity, a biological system must be selected which can provide a simple, sensitive and rapid measurement.

The bioluminescent assay system fulfills these conditions. The production of light by the organisms which constitute the bacterial reagent is a result of the total metabolic process of the cells and is a reflection of their state of health. Light, in turn, can be measured more sensitively with simple instruments than can any other physiological parameter.

Light production in these microorganisms is an expression by the cells of the total rate of which a complex set of energy-producing reactions is operating. Inhibition of any one of the multitude of enzymes involved in this process may cause a change in this rate. Thus, many different modes of action or types of toxicants can be accommodated by this bacterial test system.

BIOASSAY ORGANISMS

The bacterial reagent is the heart of the bioluminescent toxicity analyzer system. The reagent organism is a marine luminescent bacterium, selected from hundreds of other luminescent bacterial strains on the basis of its response to a wide spectrum of toxicants. This harmless bacterium most closely resembles *Photobacterium phosphoreum* in its characteristics.

During production of the bacterial reagent, the cells are rapidly frozen and dried under vacuum which provides maximum cell survival and long shelf life at 2–8°C. The cell culture preserved in this manner can be easily and quickly rehydrated to provide a ready to use cell suspension [3].

DESCRIPTION OF PHOTOMETER

The toxicity analyzer used is a precision photometer specially designed for use with the bacterial reagent. The analyzer is equipped with digital display which expresses sample readings in units of light output. Two sensitivity ranges are provided. The reaction chamber, located in the turret, has an adjustable temperature range of 10–25°C. A fifteen-well incubator chamber is temperature controlled to within ± 0.3°C of the selected reaction chamber temperature (see Figure 1). The actual temperature of the turret, incubator and air chambers may be read on the digital display by depressing the appropriate push-button on the front panel [2].

TEST PROCEDURE

In general, after the instrument is adjusted to the desired test temperature, the reagent is rehydrated and stored in the special well behind the turret. (The turret serves as a shutter for the light sensor.) Five to seven pairs of cuvettes are placed in the incubator block. To a single member of each pair is added 0.5 mL of the rehydrated reagent (cell suspension). Disposable plastic-tipped pipettors are used for these additions. The other member of each pair receives approximately 1.0 mL of appropriate sample dilutions (or samples to be compared) plus

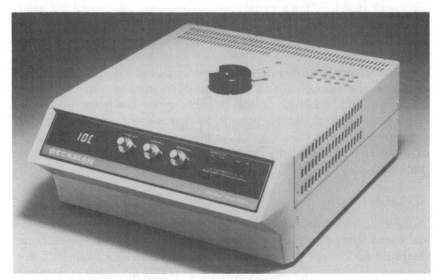

FIGURE 1. Microtox™ toxicity analyzer.

diluent in one cuvette to serve as a blank. After allowing about five minutes for the cuvettes to reach the test temperature, initial readings (relative to the blank) are taken for each of the cell suspensions. After the desired reaction time (15 minutes for most applications) final readings are taken for each cuvette. The blank is used to correct the sample readings for time-dependent drift in light output [2].

COMPARISON OF BIOLUMINESCENT ASSAY WITH THE TISSUE CULTURE TEST

The bioluminescent test was used by several medical device manufacturers to assess the toxicity of extracts prepared from a variety of biomaterials and medical devices. Extracts from the same medical devices or biomaterials were concurrently tested using the standard cytotoxicity test procedure [4]. Four grams of test material was suspended in 20 mL of MEM culture medium and extracted for 24 hours at 37°C. Cell cultures (L-929 mouse fibroblast) were exposed to the extract while incubated in a CO_2 incubator at 37°C. The cells were microscopically examined for death or damage at 24 and 48 hours.

Four grams of test material were also extracted in 20 mL of 2% saline for 24 hours at 37°C. Two percent NaCl is the normal test solution (diluent) used for the bioluminescent system and is required for osmotic stabilization of the bacterial reagent. Ten μl aliquots of the bacterial suspension were transferred to each test cuvette containing 0.5 mL of diluent. Extracts of the appropriate controls were also tested. Exposure time for each sample was 15 minutes at 15°C. Those samples which caused a light loss 50% greater than the negative control were scored toxic.

Extracts from 107 different samples were tested with the bioluminescent and the tissue culture procedure. The results which are summarized in Table 1 show greater sensitivity for the bacterial test for six of the samples. 100 samples (93%) scored identically by both procedures. Additional studies are in progress comparing the luminescent assay with tissue culture and other commonly used toxicity test methods.

APPLICATIONS

Important features of the bioluminescent assay system include the speed and simplicity of the test procedure. 20 to 40 sample extracts can be tested within one hour. Furthermore, additional characterization of any sample can easily be accomplished. Serial dilutions of a special sample can be tested to determine dose response characteristics and

Table 1. Comparison of bioluminescent and tissue culture toxicity data.

Response Category	Number of Samples
Microtox (−) Tissue Culture (−)	44
Microtox (+) Tissue Culture (+)	56
Microtox (+) Tissue Culture (−)	6
Microtox (−) Tissue Culture (+)	1

(−) = non-toxic; (+) = toxic.

minimum inhibitory concentrations of the extract.

The high precision, (coefficient of variation is 10 to 12%) which has been demonstrated with the bacterial bioluminescent system, is useful for optimizing sample extraction procedures. Sample extracts from a controlled series of extraction times and temperatures can be tested to establish leaching rates or suitable extraction time/temperatures from specific materials or products.

Manufacturers and users of medical grade resins must assure the safety of these materials prior to inventory commitment. The bioluminescent test represents a simple and reliable tool to screen new resin lots for possible toxic contamination. After product molding, representative sample extracts can be assessed for possible toxic contamination from manufacturing or sterilization processes.

Laboratories interested in developing new improved biomaterials can easily screen new biochemicals or chemical constituents for relative toxicity. Chemical analyses, although useful for quantifying extracted chemical species, cannot quantify toxicity of individual chemicals or additive or synergistic effects of chemical mixtures.

CONCLUSIONS

Motivated by the need for a rapid, low cost, simple standardized toxicity test, Beckman Instruments developed an advanced instrumental approach to toxicity testing. This toxicity testing system, called Microtox™, uses a specially selected strain of luminescent bacteria as the test organism [3].

REFERENCES

1. J. Autian, *Adv. Modern Toxicology, I*, 119 (1977).
2. Beckman Instruments, Inc., "Microtox System Operating Manual," *Beckman Manual 015-555879*, Beckman Instruments, Inc., Carlsbad, California (1982).
3. A. A. Bulich, M. W. Greene, and D. L. Isenberg, "Reliability of the Bacterial

Luminescence Assay for Determination of the Toxicity of Pure Compounds and Complex Effluents," ASTM STP 737, D. R. Branson and K. L. Dickson, Eds., American Society for Testing and Materials, pp. 338–347 (1981).

4. Health Industry Manufacturers Association, "Guidelines for the Preclinical Safety Evaluation of Materials Used in Medical Devices," Washington, D.C. (1983).

Creep Analysis of Delrin Stents for Cardiac Bioprosthesis Devices

E. MILLER AND C. B. GILPIN
California State University
Long Beach, California

INTRODUCTION

NATURAL HEART VALVES are being replaced by a wide variety of commercially available prosthetic devices. The two major design configurations currently in use are the lateral flow and the central flow types. A lateral flow valve contains a centralized valve mechanism such as a ball, disk or flapper valve, and is usually produced with metallic load bearing members. Central flow valves are modelled on the basic anatomy of the human trileaflet aortic valve by employing a porcine valve sewn to an artificial support or stent. The term bioprosthesis is frequently employed to separate the purely mechanical valves from those with biologically originated leaflets. The bioprosthesis porcine valve is comprised of three tissue leaflets sutured onto a frame with three posts to support the leaflets. The leaflets are usually strengthened by immersion in a gluteraldehyde solution. The frames (stents) have been manufactured of metal and a variety of polymers. They are covered with a light Dacron outer cloth cover, which includes the sewing ring for attachment during implantation. The covering also presents excessive contact of the stent material with the blood to lower the probability of thromboembolism occurring.

The blood flow path in the lateral flow valve is forced around the central valve mechanism, producing greater turbulence and shearing forces on the blood than in the central flow type of valve which more closely approaches the configuration of the normal heart [1]. The homo-

---

Presented at ANTEC '84, the Society of Plastics Engineers 42nd Technical Conference and Exhibition, April 30–May 3, New Orleans, LA.

graft central flow valve has the distinct advantage that fewer throm-
boembolic episodes have been noted with these valves than with lateral
flow valves, and those incidents reported are less severe. In addition,
hemolysis is the subclinical [2], and the necessity for long-term anti-
coagulant therapy is minimized.

Flow of blood through the heart, and the mechanics of blood flow
through heart valves has been studied extensively [3]. The blood flow
generates forces on the leaflets, which during the opening and closing
of the valve are transferred to the stent support posts, and in turn to
the arterial wall. The ultimate lifetime of the implanted device is controlled by three factors:

1. Degradation of the leaflets. Early porcine xenografts were fixed in
   formaldehyde. These were relatively weak, and failed in less than
   one year. The gluteraldehyde fixed leaflets are significantly
   stronger. Accelerated tests of valves containing leaflets have been
   performed [4], as well as evaluation of implanted valves. The expected lifetime of these leaflets is between five to ten years.
2. Detachment. The forces generated by the blood flow through the
   heart and valve have been observed to be sufficient in some cases to
   cause buttress detachment of the arterial wall which eventually required replacement of the implant. To reduce the stress transferred
   to the arterial wall, Reiss et al [5] designed and utilized flexible
   polymeric stents. Flexible stents have been manufactured from
   polypropylene and acetal copolymer.
3. Stent Post Creep. Pohlner observed that in vitro flow studies the
   polypropylene flexible stents exhibited stent post deflection of up to
   1.2 mm (.047 inch), and acetal copolymer post deflections of 0.68 mm
   (.027 inch). These values can be compared to maximum deflections
   of 0.29 mm (.011 inch) for the relatively inflexible Hancock valves
   under the same pressure. Measurements on stents recovered from
   implants of the valves with flexible stents in dogs indicated that significant inward post bending had occured in a five month period, in
   agreement with the vitro studies. These large creep deformations
   seriously affected the flow characteristics of the valves.

Failure is dependent on the forces generated by the blood flow on the
device, and is also dependent on the mechanical properties of the
assembly. The first failure mode (leaflet failure) is independent of the
other two modes. Leaflet failure is a function of leaflet strength and
compliance, which in turn are functions of the fixation process, and the
state of stress within the tissue at the time of fixation.

The other two failure modes are related to the mechanical properties of the polymeric materials comprising the stent assembly and are strongly interrelated. Detachment is a result of stress transfer to the supporting walls, and is related to the flexibility and visco-elastic properties of the stent and cover assembly. The more flexible the stent, the less stress transfer. Unfortunately, the greater the flexibility, the greater the tendency to inward deflection of the stent posts and degradation of the flow characteristics of the valve. Correct compromise between these two competing design considerations requires an adequate understanding of the behavior of the stent under the long term varying loads that occur as a result of the blood flow in the heart.

The design and analysis of the behavior of such a complex structural part can best be performed utilizing finite element analysis. The objective of this investigation therefore was to study the behavior of the stent as predicted by the finite element program NASTRAN, one of the most widely used and powerful programs. The finite element program was used to predict the behavior of the stent under constant load over an extended time period. Experimental creep data was also obtained under constant load for stents to permit comparison with the computed deformation. Since long term extrapolation of material creep data is required for the analysis, some results on such extrapolation are also reported.

EXPERIMENTAL TEST PROCEDURES

a. Static Creep of Solid Samples

Dogbone shaped creep specimens of various grades of Dow polyacetal were prepared by injection molding with material flow along the length of the specimen from a single gate at one end of the specimen. All specimens had a 5 cm long reduced section with a nominal cross section of 0.3 cm by 1.3 cm. Specimens were placed in ATS creep frames and loaded in tension by weights affixed directly to the bottom grip. The extension was determined by LVDT type extensometers.

b. Static Creep of Stents

To measure static stent post deflection at body temperature, 27 mm stents were mounted on a cylindrical fixture which fit inside the stent up to the sewing ring. This prevented deformation of the stent sewing ring area during loading. Loads were applied to the LR post by hooking thin wires through the stent covering at the point where the porcine valve would be attached to the post. Small weights were then attached to the wires, and the assembly placed inside the furnace, which was equipped with a sight port. Deflection of the posts were measured periodically by observing a fiduciary mark on the hanger wire with a cathetometer.

c. Dynamic Creep of Stents

Dynamic tests on stent frames and cloth covered stents were performed by placing the stent on the flat bed of an MTS fatigue machine, and applying the load vertically by a conical head with a 60 degree apex angle being forced over the stent posts, bending them inward. The ram was driven $a^{\cdot}1$ Hz under load control at a stress ration R (maximum/minimum stress) = 0.1.

FINITE ELEMENT ANALYSIS

The finite element method is the standard procedure for the analysis of complex structures. The structure is divided into small (finite) pieces such as bars, rods, panels, etc. The displacements and stresses of each element are represented by matrices of equations. These are then synthesized into large overall structural matrices and the solution of the model is obtained by the use of system equilibrium equations. The general solution is found by evaluation of the potential energy of the individual elements. The unknown displacements are obtained by using the principle of minimum potential energy, which states that for stable equilibrium, the displacement configuration that satisfies internal compatibility and boundary conditions also produces a minimum potential energy.

a. Overall Procedure for Finite Element Analysis

The finite element procedure was utilized to determine the deflection of the stent posts under static loading conditions as a function of time. Since the modulus of the polymeric stent varies with stress level and time, the following procedure was utilized:

1. To determine deflections with time, the creep modulus of the material was evaluated at various time intervals and stress levels.
2. From the symmetry of the construction of the stent and of the loading, the segment that represented the whole part was selected. This model is shown in Figure 1. A finite element model of this segment, in conformance with NASTRAN formats was then prepared and checked for geometry and solution problems.
3. This model was then run utilizing the static elastic modulus. The

output was studied for the magnitude and variation of stress and deformation throughout the model. The magnitude of the deformation was used to determine the type of analysis necessary for the runs simulating the behavior at long creep times. This evaluation indicated that a nonlinear analysis was required.

4. From this initial stress pattern, creep modulus values were modified to conform to the stress value for the individual elements, and a new NASTRAN stress pattern obtained for the model at the first time interval studied.

5. This stress pattern was used to modify the creep moduli for incorporation into the model for the next time sequence. This procedure was repeated until all the specified time intervals were analyzed.

b. Creep Modulus Selection

Creep modulii and stress-strain data utilized in these computations were obtained from the Delrin Handbook. The Handbook presents data at temperatures of 23°C, 45°C, 85°C and 100°C. These plots cover stress levels up to 3000 psi and times of exposures of from 1 to 10000 hours. There are several techniques available for interpolating between these temperatures to obtain modulii at intermediate temperatures which are discussed later. However, it was decided to utilize the creep data as published, and evaluate the stent model at 45°C. This

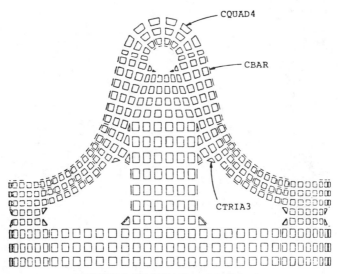

FIGURE 1. NASTRAN model of stent.

permitted use of shorter times to obtain indications of the total deflection of the stent.

Creep data is usually represented by plots of the sample strain under constant load as a function of time. The creep modulus was computed from these graphs at the selected time of 1, 10, 100, 1000, and 10000 hours as the applied stress/total creep strain at the selected time.

Table 1 shows the creep strain and creep modulus values. It can be seen that for Delrin at 23°C, the creep modulus is independent of the stress level, and the material can be considered linear viscoelastic with good accuracy over the stress level applied in loading the stent. Plots of log E (creep modulus in psi) vs log t (time in hours) show a linear relationship, and the modulus can be accurately represented by the equation:

$$E = 409275 \ t^{-0.088} \tag{1}$$

For analysis at room temperature, one modulus may therefore be chosen for all the elements. Results computed at 45° C are listed in Table 2. It can be seen that at this temperature the creep modulus at any selected time varies significantly with stress within the stress

Table 1. Creep strain and modulus: at ambient temperature of 23°C (73°F).

Stress (psi)	Time in Hours				
	1	10	100	1,000	10,000
Creep Strain, in./in.					
1,000	0.25	0.30	0.355	0.43	0.58
1,500	0.375	0.45	0.55	0.65	0.875
2,000	0.50	0.60	0.71	0.86	1.15
Creep Modulus, psi: From Creep Curves					
1,000	400,000	333,330	281,690	232,558	172,414
1,500	400,000	333,330	272,730	230,770	171,424
2,000	400,000	333,330	281,690	232,560	173,913
Creep Modulus, psi: Arithmetic Mean					
All	400,000	333,330	278,705	231,960	172,585
Creep Modulus, psi: Least Squares Fit					
All	409,275	333,585	271,895	221,610	180,625

Table 2. Creep strain and modulus: at ambient temperature of 45°C (113°F).

Stress (psi)	Time in Hours				
	1	10	100	1,000	10,000
	Creep Strain, in./in.				
1,000	0.36	0.47	0.56	0.65	0.75
1,500	0.56	0.75	0.88	1.10	1.325
2,000	0.775	1.025	1.20	1.55	1.90
	Creep Modulus, psi: From Creep Curves				
1,000	277,780	212,765	178,570	153,845	133,330
1,500	267,860	200,000	170,455	136,365	113,210
2,000	258,065	195,125	166,670	129,030	105,265
	Creep Modulus, psi: Least Squares Fit				
1,000	264,700	221,270	184,960	154,615	129,245
1,500	258,645	209,540	169,755	137,530	111,415
2,000	252,975	202,875	162,695	130,475	104,635

range of 6.9 MPa to 13.8 MPa (1000 to 2000 psi). Delrin therefore does not correspond well to a linear viscoelastic material at elevated temperatures, and the creep modulus for different elements must be chosen to correspond to the stress level within that element. For a selected value of applied stress, the modulus was modelled utilizing an equation of form identical to that of Eq. (1):

$$E = A \, t^n \tag{2}$$

The constants A and n were evaluated by least squares analysis of the creep data at 45°C, and are shown in Table 3. The numerical values of the creep modulus obtained from these equations are also listed in Table 2.

Table 3. Creep modulus equation constants for different stress levels at 45°C ambient temperature.

Stress Level, psi	A	B
1,000	264,700	−.0778
1,500	258,645	−.0914
2,000	252,975	−.0959

In order to introduce the appropriate creep modulus into the NASTRAN finite element program, at the end of each run stress patterns were mapped for the model. The elements were grouped into selected stress ranges and assigned the creep modulus value at the midpoint of that range. For example, the elements which are stressed between 6.9 MPa and 10.3 MPa (1000 and 1499 psi) at any given time interval were given the modulus equivalent to the 8.6 MPa (1250 psi) stress value. Figure 2 is a plot of the modulus vs time at 45°C, and shows the stress ranges chosen and the modulus values assigned to each range for different total creep times.

c. Stent Description

The stent modelled was the Hancock II mitral stent, 33 mm (1.3 inch) nominal diameter. It consists of 3 commisures. They are labelled right, left and noncoronary and have a peripheral angular spread of 135, 120, and 105 degrees respectively. Except for this variation in the angular orientation and in some minor details such as 1.6 mm (.063 inch) holes or slots, the stent can be divided into three identical subdivisions. This symmetry of construction along with the loading severity determines the critical segment for modeling.

As described by Wright et al (4), the peak load on the stent arises from the back pressure of 120 mm Hg across the valve while in the

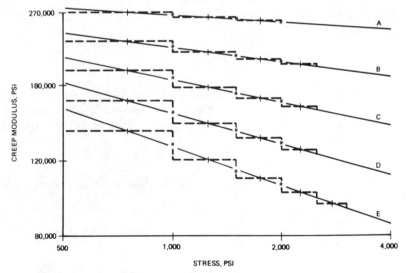

FIGURE 2. Creep modulus vs stress.

Table 4. Angular spread of each post of the Delrin stent.

Post. No.	Commissure Supported	Angular Spread (degrees)
1	Left and right	1/2 (120 + 135) = 127.50°
2	Right and noncoronary	1/2 (135 + 105) = 120.0
3	Noncoronary and left	1/2 (105 + 120) = 112.50

closed position. The load acts at three points along the coaptive ridges and from there it is distributed among the three posts. Each of the posts span one half of each adjacent commissure. The load transferred to each post is therefore in proportion to the angular spread of the commissure it supports as given in Table IV.

Since the pressure is uniform on the surface of the stent, it is obvious that the maximum load will be carried by Post Number 1. Hence the stent model was prepared in this study for Post Number 1, as illustrated in Figure 1.

d. Modeling Input

The mathematical modeling data required consists of the following items:

1. Model geometry: The circumferential dimension of the model is 33 mm (1.3 inch), the maximum height at the post being 21.6 mm (0.852 inch). The circumference was divided into 34 divisions and the post centerline into 21 parts. The average spacing of the grid points mesh is thus 1 mm × 1 mm (0.040 inch by 0.40 inch). The total number of grids in the model is 451, one point at the center of the cylindrical axis being a reference point for loading only.

2. Elements required: The elements used for modeling were three hundred sixty CQUAD4 (quadrilateral plate, membrane, and bending elements), eighteen CTRIA3 (triangular plate, membrane, and bending elements), and one hundred fifty two CBAR (simple beam elements). The CBARS with minimal section properties of the order of 10^{-7} units were added to stabilize the mathematical model and to remove any ill-conditioning of the matrices.

   Model geometry and structural continuity were checked by suitable plots and shrink views. Shrinks plots (Figure 1) help ensure continuity by separating any overlapping elements.

3. Material properties: For time zero analysis, the flexural modulus was specified as $E_c = 3.1 \times 10^3$ MPa (450,000 psi). This value corresponds to the creep modulus at a time exposure of about 4 seconds

at an ambient temperature of 45°C and stress level of 6.9 MPa (1,000 psi). For subsequent creep analyses, creep modulus values computed as described previously were employed. The value of Poisson's ratio was 0.35 and was considered constant for all conditions.

4. Element properties: The thickness of all panel elements was fixed at 0.86 mm (0.034 inch). Material specification entries also specified that all panels had out of plane bending stiffness.

5. Boundary conditions: with the assignment of out of plane bending capability to all panels, all grid points have 6 degrees of freedom (DOF), 3 of which are translational and the other 3 DOF are rotational. However, the base of the stent was assumed to be fixed in all directions.

6. Loading conditions: Load on the stent from the valve was considered to be applied as a point load at the apex of the stent post at an angle of 30° to the post axis. This load was resolved into a component of 1.72 N (0.386 lb) along the x-axis perpendicular to the stent post axis and 2.97 N (0.668 lb) along the axis of the stent post.

7. Nonlinear solution use: the criteria for large deflection analysis is determined by the relationship between the part thickness and displacement. When displacement tends to be of the order of the thickness, then midplane stretching occurs and a nonlinear solution is preferred. In the current problem, at time zero with $E = 450,000$ psi, the maximum displacement is 0.5 mm (0.019 inch). At a creep interval of one hour, the linear displacement increased to 0.81 mm (0.032 inch). At higher creep intervals, as the value of E goes down, the displacement tends to be of the order of 2 to 3 times the thickness. Hence, a geometric nonlinear solution was utilized.

EXPERIMENTAL RESULTS

a. Creep Data Extrapolation

Extrapolation of creep data for times in excess of five years is necessary to predict the behavior of the devices over their expected lifetimes. Figure 3 shows the results of creep tests on polyacetal at 37°C and 55°C for times up to 9000 hours (1 year) at the stress levels of 6.9, 13.8, 20.7 MPa (1000, 2000 and 3000 psi). While many mathematical representations of creep data have been proposed, the most general and precise expression has been shown to be [6]:

$$e = e_0 + a\, t^n \qquad\qquad (3)$$

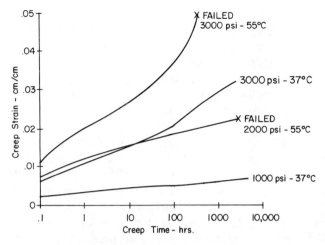

FIGURE 3. Creep Delrin samples.

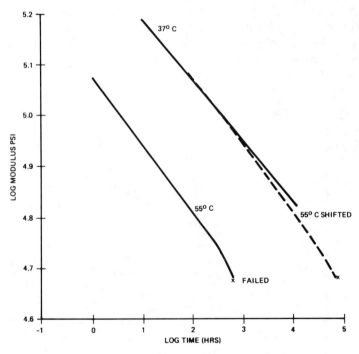

FIGURE 4. Modulus of Delrin vs time. WFL transformation between 55°C and 37°C.

where e is strain, t is the time, and e_0, a, n are functions of stress. The constant e_0 can frequently be neglected compared to the other terms. This equation predicts a straight line on a log-log plot of strain vs time. Similarly, the modulus should decrease with time according to the same type of equation. In Figure 4, the modulus is plotted. It can be seen that the modulus does not decay as rapidly as predicted by an exponential type decay. For extrapolation purpose, therefore, this equation will predict higher creep rates and lower moduli values than actually observed. This type of equation therefore predicts conservative values for design use. At 55°C, both samples of Delrin tested at 6.9 MPa (1000 psi) and 2.7 MPA (3000 psi) exhibited sudden brittle failure at 4365 and 501 hours respectively. Data on pipe samples in water indicate similar creep rupture failure times.

Another method for extrapolation that is frequently employed is that of the WFL time-temperature transformation. Figure 4 shows a plot of the log modulus of polyacetal at 37°C and 55°C vs log time. The WFL superposition by horizontal shifting is also shown in the figure. Exact superposition does not occur. For the superposition to be applicable, the molecular deformation processes occurring at the two temperatures must be identical: this is apparently not true for this polymer. However, the superposition also predicts greater creep than is experimentally observed, which also produces a safe design result.

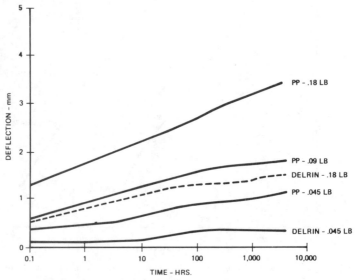

FIGURE 5. Deflection of cloth covered stents under load.

Table 5. Constants for creep of Delrin 27 mm stents at 37°C.

Load	A	B	Deflection at 10000 hrs
.176 lb	.880	.171	1.7 mm
.088 lb	.380	.100	0.9
.044 lb	.281	.038	0.5

b. Creep of Stents

Figure 5 shows the deflection of the stent posts of covered 27 mm stents of Delrin under constant load at 37°C. This load was applied perpendicularly to the stent post axis, and corresponds to the component along the x-axis in the finite elemental model of the stent. These tests were initiated well before the finite element model was finalized, and the load applied to these models was less than that utilized for the finite element analysis. The tests were performed for a total of 15500 hours (1.77 year). The creep of the stent post can best be represented by an equation of the form:

$$D = A + B \log t \tag{4}$$

the value of A and B represent the deflection of the tip (D in mm) as function of time (t in hours) of the Delrin stents under various loads as given in Table 5.

The predicted deflection at 10000 hours is also given. Deflection of polypropylene stents are also shown for comparison. The greater stiffness of Delrin stents is apparant.

c. Effect of Varying Loading On Stent

The deflection of covered and uncovered Delrin stents under cyclic loading are given in Table 6. A load ratio $R = 0.1$ was utilized to assure that the load ram maintained contact with the stent throughout the cycle to avoid any relative movement between the stent and the platen faces. The deflection was recorded at maximum and minimum loads. Delrin is a relatively stiff polymer, and the deflection increases only slightly with increasing cycling, for both the covered and uncovered stents. However, the covered stents deflected much less than the bare stents initially; and the deflection increases at a greater rate with increasing cycling for the bare stents. The deflections could be expressed by equation 4 above; the Dacron covering offers significant resistance to deformation. The resistance probably is strongly depen-

Table 6. Maximum deflection of Delrin stents under varying
loading of R = 0.1.

Load	A	B	Max. Load (lb)
27 mitral covered	0.830	0.028	.95
27 mitral bare	1.69	0.034	1.48
33 miral bare	2.95	0.106	1.48

Deflection = A + B log N.
N = No. of cycles.

dent on the tightness of sewing of the Dacron since these stents covering were hand sewn, their tightness probably varied significantly
between valve assemblies.

FINITE ELEMENT MODELLING

For any given element the stress levels from the previous run were
used to determine the range midpoint. The moduli values for the particular stress range was then selected from Figure 2 for the next itera-
tion. The stress patterns were symmetric about the centerline of the
model studied. The maximum displacement and stress outputs for the
various time intervals are given in Table 7. The maximum displacement at the tip of the stent post is plotted in Figure 6. The creep displacement, defined as the difference between the total displacement
and initial displacement is also shown in the Table 7.

As expected, the maximum stress occurs at the root of the stent post
at all time values. As creep occurs, the stent post bends inward, and the
component of the load tending to cause handling increases further, increasing the stress levels within the stent. The stress at the base of the
post increases from 13.5 MPa (1965 psi) in compression at the initial
time to 20.9 MPa (3051 psi) in compression at 10000 hours. The stress
at the critical section at the base of the post is due to the component of
the load normal to the stent surface, the component along the axis of
the post contributing negligibly to the creep of the post. The primary
stress distribution can be attributed to the out of plane bending as a
result of the load normal to the post.

However, secondary bending of the narrow strip around the slot in
this stent causes high stress concentrations in this area. The variation
of stress through the thickness and along the width of the narrow strip
suggests a combined action of the axial and bending curvature of this
region also contributes to the complexity of the stress patterns. Due to

the large stress variation over the entire surface of the stent, the use of the maximum stress only as the criteria for predicting creep effects, as proposed by Wright et al [4] would produce very conservative results.

The stress can be seen to increase with increasing time, from 13.4 MPa (1950 psi) to 21 MPa (3050 psi) in compression, in the period from the initial loading to 10000 hours due to bending of the stent post. The deflection at the tip of the stent post increases in the same time period increases from 1 mm (0.041 inch) to 4 mm (0.162 inch).

One objective of the study was to permit prediction of the inward creep of the end of the stent posts. The creep rate for simple tensile and flexural specimens can be described by the power function type of equation discussed in the first section of this paper. The same type of creep expression should be valid for the entire structure. To test this type of analysis, the log(creep displacement at the tip) is plotted in Figure 6 vs log(time). The data can be represented accurately by a straight line in

Table 7. Geometric nonlinearity solution: output summary.

Time in Hours				
1	10	100	1,000	10,000
Maximum Compressive Principal Stress, psi				
−2107	−2167	−2292	−2540	−3051
Maximum Tensile Principal Stress, psi				
−1597	−1694	−1849	−2138	−2785
Maximum Displacement at Tip, in.				
0.0410	0.0532	0.0714	0.1012	0.1624
Creep Displacement at Tip, in.				
0.0197	0.0319	0.0501	0.0799	0.1411
Least Squares Fit: Maximum Compressive Principal Stress, psi				
−2012	−2202	−2409	−2635	−2883
Least Squares Fit: Maximum Tensile Principal Stress, psi				
−1506	−1723	−1972	−2255	−2580
Least Squares Fit: Creep Displacement at Tip, in.				
0.0194	0.0315	0.0513	0.0834	0.1355

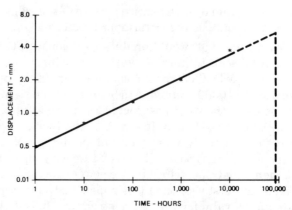

FIGURE 6. Computed displacement of stent post from NASTRAN model.

this graph, and the equation representing the creep deflection of the stent tip is:

$$\text{Deflection} = 0.48 \ t^{.22}$$

where t is in hours and deflection in mm.

This equation can be utilized to extrapolate data to longer times, assuming that secondary creep or creep rupture does not occur. The extrapolation to a ten year lifetime yields a creep displacement at the tip of 5 mm. Uniform bending of the stent post occurs with no buckling or folding at either the hole or slot.

This deflection was computed at 45°C. Experimental data obtained at 37°C under a constant load of 0.78 N (0.176 lb) was described above. The load was applied perpendicular to the stent post: this corresponds to the x-component. The finite element model was developed for a load of 1.7 N (0.386 lb) along the x-axis, which corresponds to a maximum stress of 13.8 MPa (2000 psi). The finite element model was computed at 45°C, while the experimental data was obtained at 37°C. To adjust the computed data for comparison with the experimental data, the experimental deflection data was multiplied by the ratio of moduli for the difference in temperature and stress.

$$\text{Deflection at } 0.380 \text{ lb, } 45°\text{C}$$

$$= (\text{Deflection, 176 lb, 37°C}) \left[\frac{0.386 \text{ lb}}{0.176 \text{ lb}} \right] \left[\frac{^E370C}{^E450C} \right] \left[\frac{^E3000 \text{ psi}}{^E1000 \text{ psi}} \right]$$

The ratio of moduli was obtained from the data of Table 1 to 3. The results of these computations are shown in Figure 7.

The predicted deflection at 10000 hours from the finite element program is 4, and from the experimental data is 5 mm.

Comparison with the creep data for covered stent indicate that the finite element model predicts less initial deformation, and a greater increase with time than experimentally observed. The Dacron covering apparantly significantly stiffens the stent for long time deformation.

There were significant differences between the two types of stents which preclude exact comparison. The stent analyzed by finite element procedures was 33 mm in diameter, and uncovered. The stents experimentally investigated were covered 27 mm stents. It would be expected that the smaller 27 mm stents would distort to a smaller extent, and that the cloth covering would also increase the resistance for deformation. The similar values obtained for both the experimental and calculated values suggests that the finite element procedure may not adequately take into account the variation of modulus with stress levels in the model. This total deflection extrapolated to 10 years is quite small, and indicates that Delrin is a very satisfactory material for extended use.

As a result of the deformation and change in shape of the stent, the maximum stresses increased with time. To permit extrapolation of

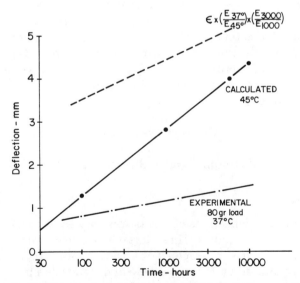

FIGURE 7. Comparison of calculated and measured deflections, normalized to 45°C.

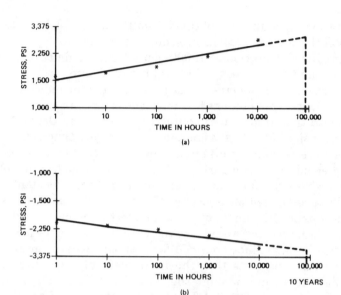

FIGURE 8. Variation of stress with time under constant load due to stent post deflection.

these stresses to longer times, the maximum tensile and compressive stresses were also plotted on a log-log plot vs time in Figure 8. The graph indicates that the compressive stress conforms very closely to a power law dependence on time. However, the tensile stress appears to increase more rapidly with time, possibly due to the local stress variations around the cutouts in the stent. However, reasonable extrapolation of both tensile and compressive stresses can be obtained using a power law type of expression. The equation for the maximum stresses (in psi) in the stent as a function of time (in hours) can be computed from the equations:

$$\text{Maximum Compressive Stress} = -2010 \ t^{0.04}$$

$$\text{Maximum Tensile Stress} = 1500 \ t^{0.06}$$

CONCLUSIONS

Significant post deflections of stents were observed to have occurred *in vitro* and *in vivo* studies. These large creep deformations seriously affected the valve flow characteristics. Device failure is dependent on the forces generated by the blood flow and its mechanical properties. The design and analysis of this complex structural device was performed utilizing finite element analysis (NASTRAN). The creep modulus for Delrin at 23°C was shown to be independent of the stress level. A stent model was prepared employing the generated data. Extrapolation of total deflection data to ten years for Delrin was found to be very small and indicated that it was satisfactory for extended use. It was also found that until the compressive stress conformed very closely to a power law dependence on time.

ACKNOWLEDGEMENTS

The authors would like to thank Mr. S. K. Bajaj who performed the Finite Element Analysis and Mr. C. Leontiev for creep studies.

REFERENCES

1. V. J. Ferans, T. C. Spray, M. E. Billingham, and W. C. Roberts, *Am. J. Cardial.*, *41*, 1159 (1978).
2. M. H. Yacoub, M. Kothari, D. Keeling, M. Patterson, and D. N. Ross, *Thorax*, *24*, 283 (1969).
3. B. J. Bellhouse and L. Talbot, *J. Fluid Mech.*, *35*, 721 (1969).
4. J. T. M. Wright, C. E. Eberhardt, M. L. Gibbs, T. Gaut, and C. B. Gilpin, "Hancock II," *Proceedings Second International Symposium on Cardiac Bioprosthesis*, Rome (May 1982).
5. R. L. Reis, W. D. Hancock, J. W. Yarbrough, D. L. Glabcy, and A. G. Morrow, *J. Thorac. Cardiovasc. Surg.*, *62*, 683 (1971).
6. T. L. Sterrett and E. Miller, *Proc. SPE Annual Meeting*, New Orleans, p. 495 (1984).

ESCA: Biomedical Studies

BUDDY D. RATNER
Center for Bioengineering and Department of Chemical Engineering
University of Washington
Seattle, WA 98195

ABSTRACT

Electron spectroscopy for chemical analysis (ESCA) is perhaps the most valuable single technique available for the analysis of the surfaces of materials intended for biomedical studies. This paper will consider why surface analysis is important for these systems, why ESCA can be used to obtain information of value and how ESCA has been applied to biomedical problems.

1. INTRODUCTION

SYNTHETIC MATERIALS USED for medical applications (biomaterials) represents a multibillion dollar industry in the United States. Yet, little is known about how biomaterials function in a biological environment or how they can be improved. Since biological interactions occur primarily at the surfaces of synthetic materials that are free of cytotoxic leachable components, studying the surface of such materials has the potential to advance our understanding of the performance of biomaterials.

Surface analysis methods have their primary utility in biomaterials science in five areas:

1. Unknown identification—The surface region of a solid is almost invariably different in composition from that in the bulk of the material. Two reasons for this are the enhanced surface chemical reactivity due to accessibility of a surface to reactants, and a ther-

Reprinted from Vol. 30 SAMPE Proceedings, courtesy of Society for the Advancement of Material and Process Engineering, Covina, CA U.S.A.

modynamic driving force to minimize interfacial energy. In addition, for biomedical applications, surfaces are often consciously modified to achieve new properties. Finally, manufacturers of biomedical devices are rarely as candid (or as cognizant) about the precise nature of their product as fundamental researchers would prefer. For these reasons, the ability to specifically analyze and identify the nature of a surface region is particularly important.

2. Contamination detection—Surfaces are readily contaminated with substances that are plentiful in our environment. Silicones and hydrocarbons are two common examples of materials that rapidly deposit upon surfaces. Surface analysis tools are useful, and often irreplaceable, since they allow the detection of the minute amounts of contaminant material that one often finds at interfaces and they provide a means to develop protocols to clean the surface or optimize preparative techniques to minimize contamination.

3. Reproducibility Assurance—Since surfaces are so readily contaminated, one must always be concerned in biomedical studies about the ability to achieve the same surface from one day to the next. In addition, a manufacturer of a biomedical implant device must attempt to insure that the device will perform identically each time a physician uses it. ESCA and other surface analysis tools can help to achive this important reproducibility assurance between experiments and between batches of devices or materials.

4. Quality Control—If an affinity chromatography column is to be prepared, a cell culture substrate modified, a polymer film deposited on a glass surface, or any of a large variety of other preparations involving small amounts of material used to alter surfaces, one would like to have a direct (non-biological) means to assay to quality of the preparation. Using surface analysis tools questions such as "is the glass plate completely covered by the polymer?" or "has the correct amount of ligand been attached to the surface of the affinity column?" can be answered. Often, surface analysis methods are the only tools available to unambiguously address these questions.

5. Surface Property/Biological Response Correlation—Biological assays for evaluating the responses of biological systems to various types of surfaces and interfaces are often expensive and time consuming. It would certainly be desirable to be able to perform a relatively straightforward physical measurement and get information that might hint at the biological reaction that could occur. The potential of surface analysis to predict biological responses and prescreen surfaces for performance in biological or medical applications has been suggested by a number of studies.

INFORMATION OBTAINED FROM THE ESCA TECHNIQUE

ESCA has the potential to provide more useful information about biomaterials system than any other method because of its high information content, its strong surface localization and its advanced state of development. In particular, from ESCA, the following specific types of information can be obtained:

1. All elements present in the surface region (except *H* and *He*).
2. Semiquantitative analysis of those elements found in the surface.
3. Molecular bonding environment and oxidation state for most atoms in a surface.
4. Differentiation of aromatic and aliphatic structures (in some cases).
5. Suggestions concerning the nature of bonding interactions at accessible interfaces.
6. Surface electrical properties and surface charging.
7. Non-destructive depth profiling (composition as a function of depth into the surface).
8. Destructive depth profiling of inorganic materials using ion etching or *RF* plasma methods.
9. Identification of specific organic functional groups based upon binding energy shifts and chemical derivitization studies.
10. Fingerprint identification of materials by using valence band or molecular orbital spectra.

GENERAL DESCRIPTION OF THE ESCA TECHNIQUE

When matter is bombarded by electromagnetic radiation (photons), low energy electrons are emitted by a process often called photoionization. The energy with which these electrons are ejected from the core orbital levels of atoms is related to the atomic and molecular environment from which they emerge. The ESCA experiment consists of measuring the numbers of electrons emitted as specific energies after low energy X-ray bombardment. A plot of electron energy versus number of electrons emitted is the usual manner in which ESCA data is collected and presented. Electron energy can be expressed either in terms of the kinetic energy (KE) actually measured in the ESCA instrument for the photoemitted electron, or as the binding energy (BE) with which that electron was held within its parent atom. The relationship between the binding energy and the kinetic energy is:

$$BE = h\nu - KE - \phi \qquad (1)$$

where $h\nu$ is the characteristic energy of the X-ray line used for excitation and ϕ is the work function of the spectrometer (a parameter independently determined for each spectrometer and used as a constant).

The x-rays used to induce the photoionization process have an excellent ability to penetrate into matter (typical penetration depths are of the order of microns).

However, the photoelectrons emitted from the sample have a very short penetration distance in matter. Only the electrons emitted from the surface region (perhaps the uppermost 10–20 atomic layers) that do not become involved in collisions will contribute to the photoemission signal that is used analytically. This phenomenon accounts for the utility of ESCA as a surface analysis method.

LITERATURE SURVEY

ESCA has found many applications in the study of biomaterials and the interactions of biological systems with synthetic surfaces. A partial listing of ESCA applications in biomaterial sciences is presented in Table 1.

CONCLUSIONS

ESCA has shown the potential to be an extremely valuable tool in the study of biomaterials and biological problems. The application of the method to problems in biology is new, however. Consequently, techniques are first being developed, and new applications are being discovered. The National ESCA and Surface Analysis Center for Biomedical Problems (NESAC/BIO) at the University of Washington has been established by the National Institutes of Health with its primary

Table 1. Some ESCA applications in the Biomedical Sciences.

	Reference #
Polyurethanes	1–6
Contamination detection	7,8
Hydrogels	9,10
Cell Culture Substrates	11,12
Proteins and Biomolecules at Interfaces	13–16
Dental Applications	17,18
Orthopedic Applications	19,20
Blood Compatibility studies	4,6,21
General References	22,23

goals being to introduce this method to the biomedical research community and to make ESCA services and expertise available to biomedical researchers. Through this Center, and other research groups attempting to apply ESCA to medical problems, major advances are anticipated.

ACKNOWLEDGEMENT

The authors acknowledge support of NIH grants RR01296 and HL25951 during the preparation of this manuscript and for some of the studies described herein.

REFERENCES

1. B. D. Ratner, *Photon, Electron, and Ion Probes of Polymer Structure and Properties,* ACS Symposium Series, D. W., Dwight, T. J., Fabish, and H. R., Thomas, Eds., Vol. 162, p. 371, American Chemical Society, Washington, DC (1981).

2. B. D. Ratner, *Physicochemical Aspects of Polymer Surfaces,* K. L., Mittal, Ed., Vol. 2, p. 969, Plenum Publishing Corp., New York (1983).

3. R. W. Paynter, B. D. Ratner, and H. R. Thomas, *Polymers as Biomaterials,* S. W., Shalaby, A. S., Hoffman, T. A., Horbett, and B. D., Ratner, Eds., Plenum Publishing Co., New York (1985).

4. V. Sa Da Costa, D. Brier-Russel, E. W. Salzman, and E. W. Merrill, *J. Coll. Interf. Sci., 80,* 445 (1981).

5. S. W. Graham and D. M. Hercules, *J. Biomed. Mater. Res., 15,* 465 (1981).

6. M. D. Lelah, L. K. Lambrecht, B. R. Young, and S. L. Cooper, *J. Biomed. Mater. Res., 17,* 1 (1983).

7. B. D. Ratner, *Arch. Ophthal., 101,* 1434 (1983).

8. B. Ratner, in "Treatise on Clean Surface Technology," K. L., Mittal, Ed., Plenum Press, New York (1985).

9. B. D. Ratner, P. K. Weathersby, A. S. Hoffman, M. A. Kelly, and L. H. Scharpen, *J. Appl. Polym. Sci., 22,* 643 (1978).

10. D. R. Miller and N. A. Peppas, *ACS Polym. Prepr., 24,* 12 (1983).

11. B. D. Ratner, J. J. Rosen, A. S. Hoffman, and L. H. Scharpen, in *Surface Contamination,* K. L., Mittal, Ed., Vol. 2, p. 669, Plenum Publishing Corp., New York (1979).

12. J. D. Andrade, G. K. Iwamoto, and B. McNeill, *Characterization of Metal and Polymer Surface,* L. H., Lee, Ed., Vol. 2, p. 133. Academic Press, New York (1977).

13. P. Ferruti, R. Barbucci, N. Danzo, A. Torrisi, O. Puglisi, S. Pignataro, and P. Spartano, *Biomaterials, 3,* 33 (1982).

14. M. C. Jaurand, P. Baillif, J. H. Thomassin, L. Magne, and J. C. Touray, *J. Coll. Interf. Sci., 95,* 1 (1985).

15. R. W. Paynter and B. D. Ratner, in *Surface and Interfacial Aspects of Biomedical Polymers,* J. D., Andrade, Ed., Vol. 2, Plenum, New York (1985).
16. R. W. Paynter, B. D. Ratner, T. A. Horbett, and H. R. Thomas, *J. Coll. Interf. Sci., 101,* 233 (1984).
17. H. Ohno, Y. Kanzawa, and Y. Yamane, *Dent. Mater. J., 2,* 59 (1983).
18. R. L. Bowen, *J. Dent. Res., 57,* 551 (1978).
19. J. Hoffman, R. Michel, R. Holm, and J. Zilkens, *Surf. Interf. Anal., 3,* 110 (1981).
20. K. Merritt, R. S. Wortman, M. Millard, and S. A. Brown, *Biomat., Med. Dev., Art. Org., 11,* 115 (1983).
21. S. R. Hanson, L. A. Harker, B. D. Ratner, and A. S. Hoffman, *Biomaterials 1980, Advances in Biomaterials,* G. D., Winter, D. F., Gibbons, and H., Plenk, Jr., Eds., Vol. 3, p. 519, John Wiley and Sons, Chichester, England (1982).
22. M. M. Millard, *Contemp. Top. Anal. Clin. Chem., 3,* 1 (1978).
23. B. D. Ratner, *Ann. Biomed. Eng., 11,* 313 (1983).

Characterization of Porous Coatings

TODD S. SMITH
Biomaterials Laboratory
Depuy, Inc.
Warsaw, Indiana

ABSTRACT

Bone tissue ingrowth into the porous coating of an orthopaedic implant is an attractive alternative to bone cement as a means for implant fixation. Various porous coated implant systems are presently undergoing clinical investigations. The competitive nature of the orthopaedic industry invites comparison between these systems. Of particular interest are the differences between the coatings, as the bone to porous coating interface is the key to the long-term performance of the implant system. Although porous ingrowth fixation has been in existence for 15 years, little work has been published to fully characterize these coatings. Presented is a system for characterizing these coatings. Particular emphasis is placed on a method for the quantification of the morphological characteristics. The Porocoat® AML® system will serve as the model for this study.

INTRODUCTION

CONVENTIONAL TREATMENT FOR joint disease such as arthritis is the surgical reconstruction of the joint using prosthetic joint replacement devices. Such devices are typically attached to the skeletal members comprising the joint using polymethylmethacrylate bone cement. Implant loosening remains the major mode of long-term failure of the arthroplasty [1].

Bone cement has been implicated as the major contributor to implant loosening due to its brittle nature and its poor interfacial relationship

Reprinted from Vol. 30 SAMPE Proceedings, courtesy of Society for the Advancement of Material and Process Engineering, Covina, CA U.S.A.

with the metallic implant [2]. The need for an alternative method for implant attachment is desirable. As such, the use of porous coated implants is receiving an enthusiastic response. Several porous systems both polymeric and metallic are presently being clinically investigated.

While all these systems are porous, each is morphologically unique. As such the morphological features of the porous coating as it behaves as a dynamic interface between living tissue and implant will have significant ramifications on the long-term performance of the arthroplasty. It therefore becomes necessary to physically characterize these systems in as quantitative a manner as possible.

Several methods have been commonly used to characterize porous coatings. These include visual examinations, scanning, microscopy, and mercury porosimetry. While visual examinations using a stereo microscope or SEM gives one a good feeling of the three dimensional nature of a porous coating, they lack the facility necessary to quantify it. Mercury porosimetry yields quantitative information but its value is limited at best.

Listed below in outline form are the parameters considered necessary to fully characterize porous coatings as they exist today. These coatings fall into the general categories; those produced from *fibers* and those produced from *powders*. The method outlined below can be easily applied to both types of coatings, produced from either metallic or polymeric materials.

Outline: Physical Characterization of Porous Coatings
 I. Material and Method of Manufacture
   A. Materials comprising the coating
   B. Material comprising the substrate
   C. Method of fabrication of the coating substrate
 II. Shape of coating material
   A. Powder or fiber diameter and length
   B. Spherical or aspherical powder; woven, kinked etc. fibers
 III. Coating thickness
 IV. Coating Morphology
   A. Average volume porosity
   B. Average pore size
   C. Pore size range
   D. Volume porosity and pore size gradients through coating
   E. Specific surface area
 V. Mechanical characteristics
   A. Shear strength

B. Tensile strength
C. Fatigue strength
  1. Shear
  2. Tension
D. Coating Modulus

For the purposes of this study, a powder metal system will serve as an illustration of the characterization method. This coating was developed in the early 70's by Robert Pilliar. It has been widely studied in both animal and man and is commercially marketed on the Porocoat® AML® implant system.

By way of verbal description, the coating consists of a random non-close packed array of equal size metal spheres forming a three dimensional network of interconnected pores. Unfortunately this description fits other powder metal coatings as well. Using the above outline one can define it in a quantitative manner such that it cannot be mistaken for any other system. This appears below with the exception of mechanical characteristics. Mechanical performance is important but the methods of testing are not well established.

Porocoat® Porous Coating

  I. A. Powder—ASTM F-75 Cobalt Chromium Molybdenum alloy
    B. Substrate—same as powder above
    C. High temperature inert atmosphere sintering
 II. A. −60 + 80 mesh powder
    B. Spherical shape, produced by PREP* processing
III. Coating thickness—3/4 to 1mm
IV. Coating Morphology
    A. Average volume porosity—40%
    B. Average pore size—250 microns
    C. Pore size range—10 to 1000 microns
    D. Average pore size gradient: substrate—100 microns; outer boundary—500 microns. Volume porosity gradient: substrate—20%; outer boundary—90%
    E. Specific surface area—5× uncoated surface

Determination of items I through III is relatively straightforward. Section IV on coating morphology is very important and warrants detailed discussion.

---

*Nuclear Metals, Inc., Concord, MA.

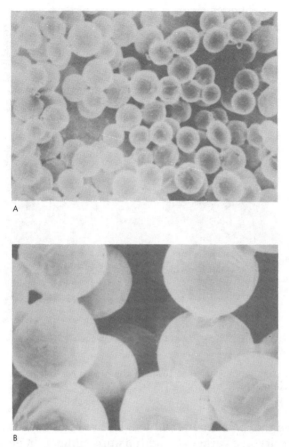

FIGURE 1. Scanning electron micrograph (*A*, low mag. *B*, high mag.) of the Porocoat® porous coating. Metal spheres are approximately 250 microns in diameter.

As one can see by examination of the SEM micrograph in Figure 1 there is much open space in this porous coating into which bone tissue may grow, especially toward its outer surface. Yet a precise definition of a pore remains elusive in part due to the different methods of manufacture and the variously shaped powders or fibers forming the boundaries of the pore space. For our purpose a pore will be defined as any space or interstice formed by three or more sinter bonded spheres. The pore is idealized as spherically shaped and quantified with a diameter measurement.

The morphological parameters can be quantified using stereologic techniques [3] in conjunction with conventional metallographic

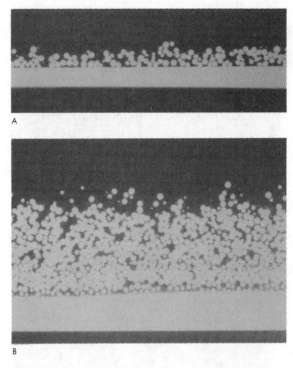

FIGURE 2. Metallographic sections through the porous coating *A*, perpendicular sections; *B*, 14° oblique section.

methods. Manual point count methods [4] can be used to assess average volume porosity in a rather straightforward manner. In either case the porous coated product is sectioned through the porous coating either perpendicular to the substrate or at an oblique angle and metallographically mounted and polished as shown in Figure 2. The oblique view has advantages. It artificially spreads the thickness (a cosine function of the angle of obliqinty) making point counting considerably easier, especially on this coatings, without changing the results. At an angle of zero degrees, one must exercise the rigor of repeated parallel sectioning down through the coating. This is unnecessarily tedious. Using either the line intercept method or conventional point counting a very precise determination of the area fractions of the porosity and solid powder areas will result. The area fraction is equal to the volume fraction or in this case the volume porosity. Computerized phase contrast image analysis can perform this function with greater ease in much less time.

A difficulty that arises in both methods is in determining the outer coating boundary. In the case of an illdefined boundary, one must carefully consider that outer boundary beyond which the coating has no direct mechanical interaction with bone tissue. An example of this is shown in Figure 3. Observe in Figure 4 the rapid rise in pore and volume porosity as the outer boundary is approached.

Many powder coatings such as Porocoat do not have a uniform porosity. It therefore is necessary to characterize gradients in volume porosity. In this case line intercept methods are superior to manual point counting unless you have resorted to using the successive parallel sectioning technique. Computerized lineal analysis [5] again facilitates this measurement with a high degree of precision. The angle of the section is of no consequence here, except that the lower angle oblique sections will require fewer metallographic sections for a given level of statistical significance.

For pore size range and average pore size determinations, past researchers have made very cursory measurements from metallographic sections or SEM micrographs of coatings. This highly subjective method can be quite inaccurate. Manual methods using line intercept techniques would be too rigorous to be considered here. Again, computerized lineal analysis via phase contrast afforded by a reflected light microscope and image analyzer greatly facilitates these determinations. Selected field measurements can be made to determine the total number of pores and the pore size distribution. Depending upon the image analyzer used each pore may be classified by its projected area, perimeter, length, width, longest dimension, etc. For our

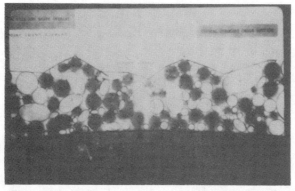

FIGURE 3. Backlit negative of micrograph of a metallographic section of a porous coating with outer boundary indicated used with point count overlay.

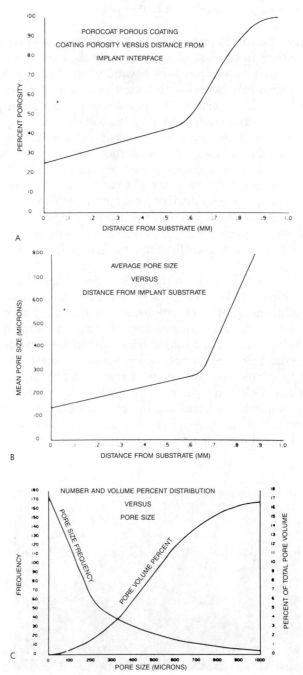

FIGURE 4. (A) Volume porosity gradient through the porous coating. (B) Average pore size gradient through the porous coating. (C) pore size frequency (left curve and left axis), and pore volume size versus percent of total porosity (right axis).

purpose the pore boundary is determined and converted to a pore diameter for recording purposes. From this data average pore size, pore size range and volume porosity are easily determined. By restricting the analyzed field to specific distances from the substrate the uniformity of the coating can be assessed. Plots made from this type of data appear in Figure 4. 4a is a plot of the volume porosity gradient. The volume porosity at the substrate is 20% and varies linearly to 60% near the outer boundary of the coating. Linearity breaks down at the coating outer boundary. The average pore size gradient shows a similar trend, increasing with distance from the substrate, Figure 4b. This result is not surprising in that it is obvious upon observing the cross sectional micrographs that the larger pores are at the coating surface. Figure 4c shows a plot of the pore size and frequency distribution on the left hand axis. It is observed that the smaller pores predominate in numbers. Interestingly, if these values are converted to pore volumes a much different trend is observed. Using the right hand axis in 4c the pores larger than 250 microns dominate the porous structure. I suggest that this is a better way to characterize the surface because the function of the coating as a dynamic interface with bone tissue is dependent upon the *quantity* of bone tissue infiltrating that surface. Taking this analysis one step further, the average pore size can be computed by dividing the total pore volume by the total pores measured rather than average pore size determined from the average diameter measured directly from the metallographic sections. This results in an average pore size increase from 200 microns to 300 microns. Therefore, when stating pore size, the method of determination needs to be explicitly stated.

CONCLUSIONS

Many different porous coated implant systems are being developed for biological fixation, however, presently there is no standard for physically characterizing these coatings. It is recognized that the performance of a porous coated system is greatly dependent upon the morphology of the coating; the important parameters being, but not limited to, volume porosity, pore size and the gradients of these two parameters. A format has been presented to classify and characterize porous coatings. Further, it has been demonstrated that a computerized varient of the lineal analysis stereologic technique can be used in conjunction with image analysis microscopy to facilitate the precise determination of the critical parameters of a porous coating. The accurate quantification of these morphological features is important in assessing the long-term clinical performance of the different porous coated systems.

REFERENCES

1. J. R. Moreland, T. A. Green, L. Mai, and H. C. Amstutz, "Aseptic Loosening of Total Hip Replacement: Incidence and Significance," *The Hip: Proceedings of the Eighth Open Scientific Meeting of the Hip Society,* St. Louis, Mo., pp. 281–291 (1980).
2. F. A. Weber, and J. Charnley, *J. of Bone and Joint Surgery, 57-B (3),*297, (1975).
3. E. E. Underwood, *Quantitative Stereology,* Addison Wesley Publishing Co., Reading, Mass. (1970).
4. ASTM Specification E-562. "Determining Volume Fraction by Systematic Manual Point Count," ASTM, Philadelphia, PA (1976).
5. I. E. Milliard and J. W. Cohn, *Transactions of the Metallurgical Society of AIME-TSSAA, 22,* 344 (1961).

Gel Permeation Chromatography as a Quality Control Tool in the Medical Plastics Industry

JOHN P. HELFRICH AND EDWARD C. CONRAD
Millipore Corporation
Waters Chromatography Division
Milford, MA 01757

INTRODUCTION

SYNTHETIC POLYMERS OR resins used in medical device manufacturing are enjoying a prominent position among the more traditional biomaterials such as metals and ceramics. Polymers, usually thermoplastics and elastomers, have experienced phenomenal growth over the last 5 years primarily because of the newer methods of purity characterization, as well as the introduction of newer synthetic hybrid plastics—copolymers. Recent estimates put the sales of medical grade plastics, both intraporporeally and paracorporeally, at over $3 billion and the market continues to grow at a significant and steady rate.

The ultimate goal in any medical plastics fabrication facility is to produce a high quality product having the correct physical and chemical properties and minimize scrap and downtime. The quality and consistency of the incoming raw materials are of significant importance in determining the processability and ultimately the end-use performance of the desired product.

Because of the nature of the polymerization process, every polymer of resin contains a distribution of molecules ranging in size and complexity from small, simple monomeric molecules to partially-polymerized structures (oligomers) to large, highly polymerized

Presented at ANTEC '85, The Society of Plastics Engineers, Inc. 43rd Annual Technical Conference, April 29–May 2, Washington, D.C., U.S.A.

molecules. Gel Permeation Chromatography (GPC), is an analytical technique which characterizes synthetic (or natural) polymers according to their size in solution and provides a "fingerprint," the molecular weight distribution. It analyzes not only the polymeric portion (polymer oligomer and monomer), but also most of the additives used in plastic compounds (plasticizers, impact modifiers, antioxidants, slip agents, etc.) and low-level impurities.

MOLECULAR WEIGHT DISTRIBUTION

In recent years, a number of industries have begun to apply gel permeation chromatography (GPC) a separation technique developed in the early 1960's to solve manufacturing problems. GPC analysis gives medical plastics fabricators valuable information about a resin. The use of this information allows an analyst to provide a rapid assessment of the physical and chemical properties of incoming resins obtained from various sources.

The analyst also can monitor the amounts of additives required to achieve proper resin performance characteristics. In addition, process-control personnel can monitor a production process and make changes to accommodate differences in resin lots. Quality assurance people also can analyze failed products to determine whether improper processing conditions might have caused the failures.

Classical tests like melt index and viscosity used to check the specifications of polymer or resin only measure an average, or bulk, characteristic. The results suffer from the same limitation of any test based on an average; they tell nothing about the distribution that makes up the average. That two batches of resin have the same melt index is an indication that their viscosity-average molecular weights are the same. Their molecular-weight distribution (MWD)—the number of molecules of various molecular weights that make up that average can be significantly different (See Figure 1).

Molecular-weight distribution is one of the fundamental characteristics of a polymer and has a direct influence on its properties (See Figure 2). Subtle variations in MWD affect processing properties like viscosity, reactivity, and cure rates. Mechanical properties also can vary considerable with MWD. Among them: tensile and impact strength, elastic modulus, hardness, coefficient of friction, stress–crack resistance, elasticity, and adhesive tract and bond strength. Knowing the MWD of a polymer or compound provides valuable insight for predicting its properties.

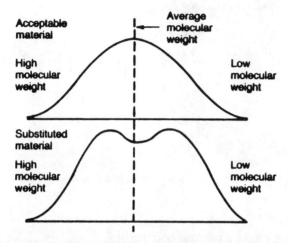

Acceptable material

High molecular weight

Average molecular weight

Low molecular weight

Substituted material

High molecular weight

Low molecular weight

- The marked differences in the molecular weight distributions of these samples would not be shown by traditional techniques.

- These equivalent average molecular weight materials will process differently and produce product with different properties.

FIGURE 1. Molecular weight distribution vs. average molecular weight.

Tensile Strength
Modulus of Elasticity
  (Before Crosslinking)
Relaxation Times of
  Elastomers
Melt Viscosity
Brittleness
Hardness
Flex Life

Softening Temperature
Elongation at Tensile Break
Impact Strength
Tear Strength
Low Temperature Toughness
Resistance to Environmental
  Stress Cracking
Drawability
Coefficient of Friction

FIGURE 2. Molecular weight distribution correlates to resin properties.

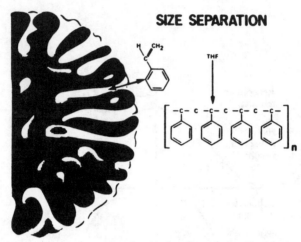

FIGURE 3. GPC is a separation of molecules based on their effective size in solution.

GEL PERMEATION CHROMATOGRAPHY

Gel permeation chromatography (GPC) is the physical separation of molecules (molecular chains) by their effective molecular size (hydrodynamic volume) in a specified solvent. In GPC a polymer sample is forced through a column (7.8mm ID $\times$ 30cm) which contains a packing material with pores of various sizes. Different components of the polymer are then separated by molecular size. For example, if two samples

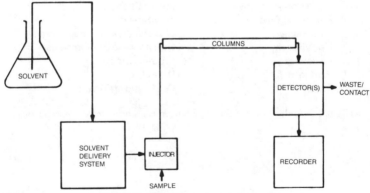

FIGURE 4. GPC system components.

(a 200,000 MW polystyrene and styrene monomer) are injected onto a GPC column the following will happen. The styrene monomer, a small molecule, will be able to permeate both the large and small pores of the GPC packing material. However, the polystyrene sample, which is larger in molecular size, will not be able to permeate the small pores of the column and therefore will elute from the column before the monomer (See Figure 3). The result is the MWD of a polymer in decreasing molecular weight.

The MWD of polymers are obtained using a gel permeation are obtained using a gel permeation chromatograph as depicted in Figure 4. In a GPC system a carrier solvent (e.g. toluene) is forced through the system using a solvent delivery module (PUMP) through an injector, a set of GPC columns, and a detector(s). A polymer sample is dissolved into the solvent and is introduced to the system via an injector. The sample is carried (as mentioned above) and elutes into a detector. The output of the detector is usually monitored with a recorder or data reduction system (computer).

INCOMING RESIN LOT QUALITY CONTROL

Figures 5 and 6 are examples of significant differences in the MWD's of resins obtained by alternate suppliers.

In the case of the polyethylene resins (Figure 5), a medical plastic fabricator obtained materials from three sources all meeting melt index and viscosity specifications. The material from vendor 1, could not be processed while those from vendor 2 and 3 required separate molding conditions (temperature, pressure, etc.). GPC revealed obvious changes in the materials MWD.

In an attempt to qualify a secondary supplier of polyvinyl chloride (PVC) resin for intravenous filters one medical device manufacturer employed GPC as a technique to insure adequate processability and proper product performance. The PVC formulation in addition to having the usual FDA sanctioned additives and impact modifiers had to possess the correct MDW to satisfy a critical stress-cracking test required by the manufacturer. Three suppliers of medical grade PVC were chosen each providing the usual physical properties data such as tensile, melt index, impact resistance, etc. to meet the molding criteria for the device. In addition to the usual incoming product tests for quality assurance, the resin was tested by GPC to compare its MWD to the control sample prepared in the same way.

An overlay of the MWD fingerprints of the two suppliers compared to

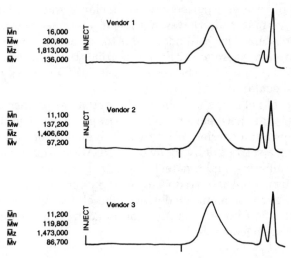

$\bar{M}n$	16,000
$\bar{M}w$	200,800
$\bar{M}z$	1,813,000
$\bar{M}v$	136,000

Vendor 1

$\bar{M}n$	11,100
$\bar{M}w$	137,200
$\bar{M}z$	1,406,600
$\bar{M}v$	97,200

Vendor 2

$\bar{M}n$	11,200
$\bar{M}w$	119,800
$\bar{M}z$	1,473,000
$\bar{M}v$	86,700

Vendor 3

FIGURE 5. Incoming Resin Lots (equivalent polyethylene resins for medical plastic products).

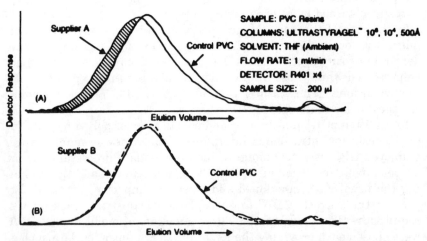

SAMPLE: PVC Resins
COLUMNS: ULTRASTYRAGEL™ 10^6, 10^4, 500Å
SOLVENT: THF (Ambient)
FLOW RATE: 1 ml/min
DETECTOR: R401 x4
SAMPLE SIZE: 200 µl

FIGURE 6. Molecular Weight Distribution (MWD) of PVC resin from different suppliers (medical device PVC resin).

the control sample showed a subtle but very distinctive shift toward the high molecular region of the polymer (see Figure 6). When small evaluation lots of resin were injection molded, conditions had to be altered to compensate for "short shots," or incompletely filled mold cavities. Even with altered processing conditions, the final medical device exhibited high rates of stress cracking only a third supplier was able to provide a resin with the right balance of physical properties and correct MWD to match the control. Gel permeation chromatography with its small sample requirements is now a part of this manufacturer's incoming materials qualification program.

PRODUCT STABILITY

Polyproplyene and polyethylene containers, packaging materials and disposable syringes are used in large quantities by the pharmaceutical and medical industries. Prior to use, these products must be sterilized. Typically, this sterilization has been accomplished by using gamma radiation from a cobalt 60 isotope. However, if the radiation exceeds certain tolerance limits, both polypropylene and polyethylene will degrade (see Figure 7).

In the case of polypropylene, excess radiation causes breakdown of the larger polymer molecules with the result that the materials have lower molecular weight. These measurable changes can be directly correlated to an alteration of the final products physical properties.

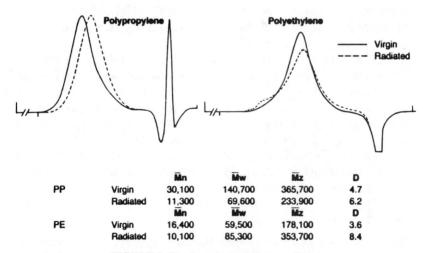

		$\bar{M}n$	$\bar{M}w$	$\bar{M}z$	D
PP	Virgin	30,100	140,700	365,700	4.7
	Radiated	11,300	69,600	233,900	6.2
		$\bar{M}n$	$\bar{M}w$	$\bar{M}z$	D
PE	Virgin	16,400	59,500	178,100	3.6
	Radiated	10,100	85,300	353,700	8.4

FIGURE 7. Final product, radiation effects.

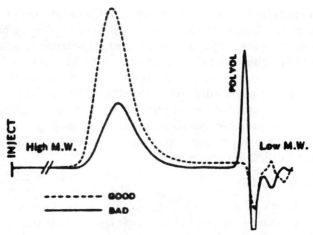

FIGURE 8. Product development, polyurethane intraaortic balloon.

Similarly, when polyethylene products are subjected to excessive gamma radiation, the materials again degrade but in a very different manner. The polymer first fragments and then recombines. If excessive recombination takes place, the polyethylene becomes brittle and, thus, unusable.

TOXIC LEACHABLES

In accordance with FDA legislation materials used in the medical plastics industry must be of significant purity specifications with respect to toxic leachables. In addition, traceability of raw materials with respect to proper documentation of quality is needed for Good Manufacturing Practice (GMP) compliance.

A manufacturer of an intraaortic balloon was GPC as a means to qualify vendors of polyurethane based on the polymeric MWD as well as additives which could be toxic in the final product. Figure 8 shows the GPC data on two batches of polyurethane whose specification was based on viscosity. Upon processing, the "bad" batch had poor end-use properties. GPC data indicated a low molecular material later identified as a polyol which was added to bring the material into the stated viscosity specification but would cause both processing and leaching problems in the final product.

CONCLUSIONS

Gel permeation chromatography (GPC) by supplying a fingerprint of the molecular weight distribution of a polymer can provide much more information than one point test such as melt index, viscosity, or other physical measurements. Exact composition of resins and plastics can be determined rapidly and correlated to differing processing conditions and functional end use properties. In critical materials such as biomedical plastics, GPC can now add an extra measure of confidence insuring against manufacturing problems due to lot variability, product failure, leaching of toxic impurities, and ultimately product liability.

Recent Advances in Medical Plastics Analysis

LECON WOO, CRAIG SANDFORD, AND ROBERT WALTER
Travenol Laboratories, Box 490
Round Lake, IL 60073

INTRODUCTION

THE MEDICAL PLASTICS industry demands the highest performance at the lowest possible cost while maintaining the absolute safety standard for the end user. To simultaneously meet these requirements constitutes a foremost challenge to the material specialist. The issue of safety goes far beyond the traditional toxicological and sterility standards. Devices can fail mechanically during high speed impact, or under a combination of chemical and mechanical stresses. Failure under use, regardless of origin, is a disastrous outcome to be avoided at all cost.

Yet in the recent past, we have faced increasing pressure from government and health care providers to limit or lower the cost. Hospital stays are shortened, single use disposable devices are subjected to multiple use. Short term devices are pressed to perform longer term functions. This adds a considerable burden to the already formidable challenge to the manufacturer. Clearly, innovative and more productive measures must be adopted for profitability or even survival in this new environment. Design and devices based on fundamental knowledge of materials is a proven method for effective engineering. By eliminating much trial and error, quality products with short development cycles can be realized. In the meantime, understanding of materials is accumulated for an ever widening sphere of applicability. Much of our knowledge is derived from polymer analysis. Thus, we focus this paper on techniques to improve accuracy and productivity of polymer analysis.

Presented at ANTEC '85, The Society of Plastics Engineers, Inc. 43rd Annual Technical Conference, April 29–May 2, Washington, D.C., U.S.A.

BACKGROUND

Over the last few years, we have seen a mass invasion of microcomputers to analytical instrumentation. As a result, we now have these capabilities:

1. automatic calibration, linearization of transducers.
2. digital manipulation and storage of data.
3. standard formatted report generation.
4. rapid and accelerating obsolescence of equipment.

A summary comparison of three generations of instruments is given in Table 1.

The rapid obsolescence of computer based equipment is due in part to the rapid advances of microelectronics technology rather than genuine fundamental advances in analytical methodology. The VLSI very large scale integrated circuit progresses by the well known Moore's Rule. In other words, device complexity and capability roughly *doubles* in a geometric progression every other year. This development creates a tremendous incentive and pressure for instrument manufacturers to upgrade their systems. In isolated instances, we have even seen vendors offering "new" systems even before software and hardware of the last systems were perfected.

Another common problem is the incompatibility among vendors. Or, in some cases, different instruments from the same vendor. Once the control program is stored in ROM, or read only memories, common system components become dedicated hardware incapable of general purpose usage.

EXPERIMENTAL CONSIDERATIONS

When we set out to construct our own laboratory automation systems, a set of goals were carefully defined:

1. computer hardware independent, or nearly so.
2. high sensitivity and long-term stability.
3. flexible reconfiguration for new applications.
4. high reliability and available long-term maintenance.
5. minimum total hardware/software (programming time) investment.
6. obsolescent resistance.

Being end users of analytical equipment, we are mainly interested in expanding total capabilities instead of competing with commercial

Table 1. Comparison of instrument capabilities.

	Analog	Digital	Microcomputer Controlled
Accuracy	0.2–2%	0.1%	0.02–0.4%
Reproducibility	0.5%	0.1%	0.1%
Long Term Drift	5–10%	1%	1%
Useful Life	5–10 yrs	10–12 yrs	3–5 yrs
Data Storage	no	no	yes
Report Generation	no	no	yes

manufacturers. We need to carefully define our application. After a series of refinements, these applications were chosen:

1. situations where no commercial source is available.
2. commercial products offering grossly inadequate performance/cost.
3. secondary processing of data where no hardware or software exists commercially.

SYSTEM INTEGRATION

We chose to integrate our system around the IEEE-488 instrument bus because of its wide acceptance and availability. Since its adoption, nearly all electronic instruments have the interface built-in or available as a low cost option. In most cases, the performance/cost ratio from these instruments is extremely high. More importantly, they offer the reliability and stability long expected from instrument manufacturers. Furthermore, compared with the life expectancy of 3–5 years for typical computers, they are built for a typical service life of between 10–15 years. During this time span, services and support are constantly available. By defining the communication protocol first, the computer assumes a secondary importance. In our experience, we have utilized a whole series of microcomputers with equal success. They include Hewlett Packard 9000 series desk top computers, and Commodore 4000 and 8000 series microcomputers. Despite minor software differences, our experiences show adapting from one computer to the other relatively simple and easy. This is due mainly to the high level commands used for IEEE-488 communication. Because of this ability to reconfigure new systems for different applications, the total investment in hardware and software development is minimized.

A schematic diagram for the system is illustrated in Figure 1. A wide range of applications and control of experiments is possible and new applications are being developed constantly. Three applications serve to demonstrate the utility of the system. (1) A temperature program-mable instrumented impact tester where in-house software enhances capability at a fraction of the commercial cost, (2) an automated multi-channel creep tester, where no commercial capability exists, (3) sec-ondary treatment and presentation of crystallization data by Avrami analysis—no commercial software currently available.

RESULTS AND DISCUSSION

(1) Instrumented Impact Testing: High speed impact performance of plastics at various service temperatures have received much attention recently (1,2,3). A low cost, flexible system was constructed around a Dynatup 8200 test frame. Impact velocity was accurately measured optically by a Hewlett Packard 5316A frequency counter. Temperature of the specimen inside the environment chamber is controlled and monitored by a Hewlett Packard 3478A digital voltmeter. The volt-meter's 100 nanovolt resolution corresponds to a temperature of about 0.002°C. In practice, temperature stability of ± 1.0°C was found to be adequate for most testings. A Biomation 8200 transient recorder con-verts the stress signal to digital form at up to 100 M Hz rate. A sche-matic for the impact system is shown in Figure 2. After conversion of load/displacement data to engineering units, the impact energy is de-termined by a numerical integration algorithm. Finally, impact results

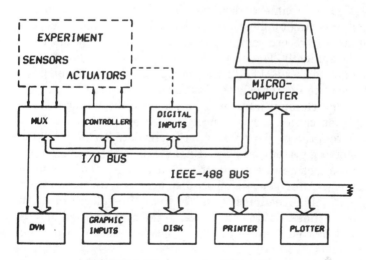

FIGURE 1. Microcomputer Automation.

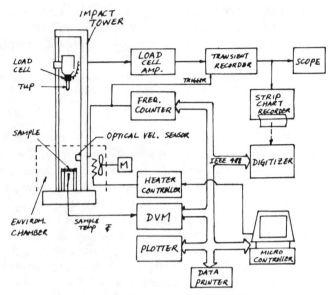

FIGURE 2. Instrumented Impact Tester.

are tabulated and stored on disk for future recall. Figure 3 shows a typical high speed impact performance of a polyolefin film.

(2) Multi Channel Automated Creep Tester: Creep, or the change of elongation with time under load, is an important polymer property with engineering applications. A multichannel tester was designed to automatically record sample length, their rate of change, and present results graphically. The unit is controlled by a Basic language program on a Commodore CBM 8032 microcomputer. The microcomputer uses a multiplexer to address six testing fixtures (Figure 4).

When the channel number is selected by the binary user port, the multiplexer connects the Linear Variable Differential Transformer (LVDT) from the proper fixture to the Hewlett Packard 7090 measurement plotting system. Via the IEEE-488 bus, the microcomputer commands the measurement unit to take a voltage reading and records it in memory. After conversion to displacement units, data are stored along with time readings (from the real time clock) in an array. At designated times, data is outputted to the disk, printed in a tabulated form and plotted (Figure 5). The process is repeated for the rest of the channels.

Advantages of the system include: (1) multichannel operation

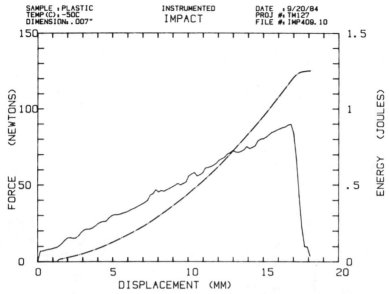

FIGURE 3. Typical high speed impact performance of a polyolefin film.

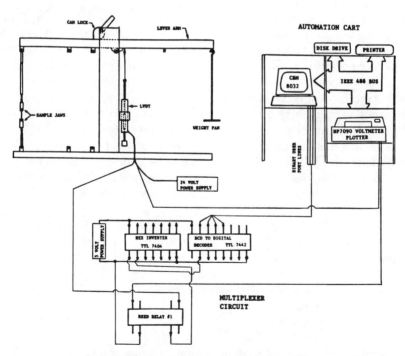

FIGURE 4. Six channel Automated Creep Tester.

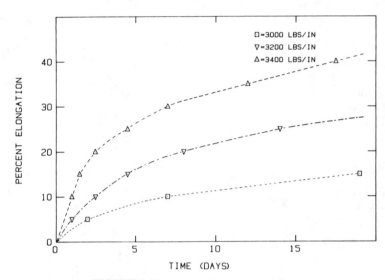

FIGURE 5. Representative creep test data.

enhances data accuracy, and data throughput, (2) minimum operator involvement, (3) automatic tabulation and graphical presentation of data. In addition, the system can be used for general purpose applications as a powerful workstation (data acquisition, general purpose plotting, word processing, etc.)

(3) Avrami Analysis of Crystallization Data: for semicrystalline polymers, crystallinity and the manner (kinetics) crystallization took place determine the ultimate physical properties of the polymer. Avrami analysis is a powerful method for treating crystallization data [4]. Briefly, the problem of crystal growth is treated analogously to a collection of randomly centered propagating spherical wave fronts. In this analysis, the development of crystallinity can be represented by,

$$1 - V^c = \exp(-Kt^n) \tag{1}$$

where

$\quad V^c$: Crystallized volume fraction at time t
$\quad K$: constant
$\quad n$: constant

Upon taking the logarithm of both sides of equation (1),

$$\log\left(-\ln(1 - V^c)\right) = \log K + n \log t \qquad (2)$$

Thus, a plot of the quantity $\log\left(-\ln(1 - V^c)\right)$ against $\log t$ yields a straight line with slope n. n, the Avrami exponent depends on the nucleation and morphology [5]. For example, spherulitic morphology and inhomogeneous nucleation yields an exponent of 3. From this analysis, one gains important insights of the kinetics of crystallization confirmable by direct morphological observations.

Since no commercial analysis software package was available, we developed one as an example of secondary processing of differential scanning calorimetry (DSC) data. In this analysis, V^c can be approximated by the partial area under the exotherm (Figure 6).

A Hewlett Packard 9111A digitizing tablet was chosen as the input device, converting the raw thermal analysis data into digital form for the computer. After unit conversions and integration by the trapezoidal rule, the resulting function is plotted on a Hewlett Packard 7470 plotter. A typical data set from a nucleated polypropylene sample is shown in Figure 7. Pronounced secondary crystallization from spherulitic to lamellar morphologies is clearly evident at about the 50% conversion

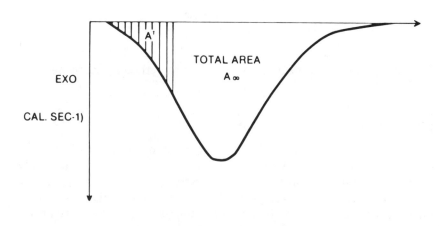

FIGURE 6. DSC Isothermal Crystallization, Avrami analysis.

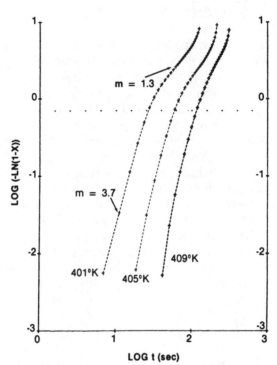

FIGURE 7. Avrami analysis nucleated pp.

line. Subsequent observations by polarizing microscopy confirmed this finding.

CONCLUSION

By our experiences and pilot examples, we have demonstrated the utilities of simple laboratory automation schemes. By using a widely accepted communication protocol, flexibility and long term service are assured. Major applications to a plastics analysis environment in a medical industry were created. These automation systems serve either as stand-alone capability or as auxillary processors to augment capabilities of commercial instruments. Since the system is based on high level language commands, and very flexible to reconfigure, obsolescent tendencies are much reduced. With the accuracy, stability, and extremely high productivity offered by these systems, we are advancing the capabilities of medical plastics analysis in meeting the challenges of the medical industry.

REFERENCES

1. G. C. Adams and T. K. Wu, *SPE ANTEC,* 185 (1981).
2. G. C. Adams and T. K. Wu, *SPE ANTEC,* 898 (1982).
3. A. J. Wnuk, T. C. Ward, and J. E. McGrath, *Poly. Eng. Sci., 21,* 313 (1981).
4. M. Avrami, *J. Chem. Physics, 7,* 1103 (1939).
5. B. Wunderlich, *Macromolecular Physics,* Vol. 2, p. 147, Academic Press, New York (1976).

Property Changes of UHMW Polyethylene During Implantation— First Hints for the Development of an Alternative Polyethylene

P. EYERER
Institut für Kunststoffprüfung und Kunststoffkunde
Universität Stuttgart
Pfaffenwaldring 32, D-7000 Stuttgart 80, West Germany

INTRODUCTION

A NECESSARY CONDITION for systematical material developments is a fundamental material analysis of retrieved implants. In recent years physical and chemical investigations have indicated severe changes of the structure of UHMWPE (1–5). Most of the changes are due to oxidative molecular chain scissions. Our aim is to develop step by step an alternative polyethylene. One of these steps is a better understanding of the in vivo aging compared with an in vitro storage. Another step is the investigation of the influence and consequences of using calcium stearate in medical UHMW PE produced by the Ruhrchemie Company or Hoechst America Company, (RCH 1000).

MATERIAL

We investigated new, retrieved and shelf stored γ-irradiated (2,5 Mrad) UHMWPE hip joint cups. Beside Hifax 1900 (Hercules-Himont, Wilmington, DE), RCH 1000 (Ruhrchemie, Oberhausen/FRG) was the most preferred material.

Presented at ANTEC '85, The Society of Plastics Engineers, Inc. 43rd Annual Technical Conference, April 29–May 2, Washington, D.C., U.S.A.

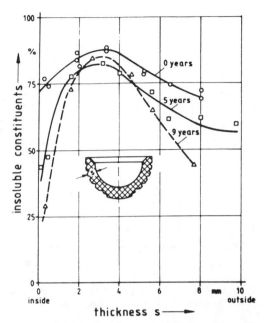

FIGURE 1. Percentage of insoluble constituents at different planes of section across the cup wall thickness. □ New, γ-irradiated not implanted cup; ○ 5 years implanted, retrieved because of loosening; △ 9 years implanted.

METHODS

Infrared spectrometry, density (column gradient) intrinsic viscosity, extraction measurements, SEM technique, EDX analysis, DSC.

RESULTS

Figure 1 shows the amount of insoluble constitutents after extraction with xylene as a function of hip cup wall thickness. The percentage of solubility increases with implantation time especially near the inner and outer surface of the cup. Because of loosened cups, both regions were in contact with the neo-synovial liquid so that oxygen (peroxide constituents of the neosynovial liquid [6] diffuses into the cup's interior and causes molecular degradation. Similar results were obtained in density measurements [4,5] Figure 2. As is shown in the 0 years curve γ-irradiation has a detrimental effect, too. Infrared extinction measurements confirm the above results, Figures 3–6. For example an increase of carbonyl group extinction is observed with in vivo application as well as with shelf storage at room temperature, Figure 3. On the other hand the aldehyde band at 1733 cm⁻¹ changes in the case of

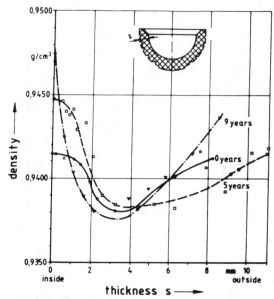

FIGURE 2. Density values of UHMWPE hip joint cups measured as a function cup wall thickness. ○ New, not implanted but γ-irradiated cup (zero years); □ 5 years implanted; △ 9 years implanted.

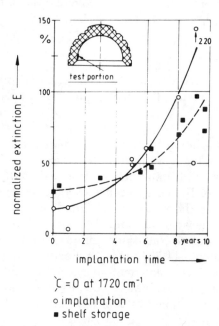

$C = O$ at $1720\ cm^{-1}$
○ implantation
■ shelf storage

FIGURE 3. Infra red extinction of carbonyl-band (CO) of UHMWPE as a function of in vivo-implantation time.

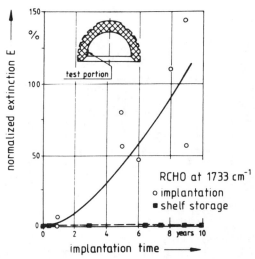

FIGURE 4. Infra red extinction of aldehyde-band (RCHO) of UHMWPE as a function of in vivo-implantation time.

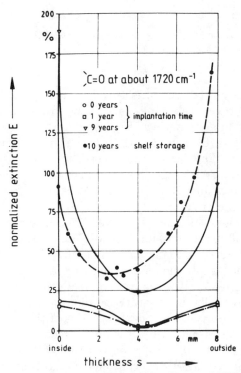

FIGURE 5. Infra red extinction of carbonyl-band (CO) of retrieved UHMWPE hip cups as a function of cup wall thickness.

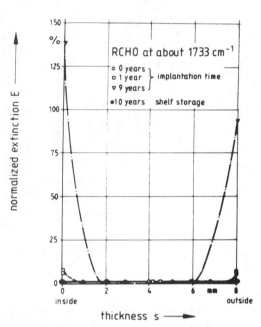

FIGURE 6. Infra red extinction of aldehyde-band (RCHO) of retrieved UHMWPE hip cups as a function of cup wall thickness.

in vivo applications but remains uninfluended by shelf storage, Figure 4. Corresponding correlations were found from microtome cuttings parallel to the hip cup surface, Figures 5 and 6. From DSC measurements Grood et al. [3] concluded that there is no difference whether the UHMWPE is implanted in vivo or exposed to air at 23°C, bovine serum or Ringer solution. Although this might be true for post crystallization our investigations show that the original chemical degradation process is sensitive to the environment.

Another problem that must be solved in order to improve the properties of RCH 1000 is the influence of calcium stearate. SEM pictures of the surface of retrieved cups as well as fracture surfaces of broken UHMPE samples show the damaging influence of calcium stearate in RCH 1000, Figure 7. EDX analysis indicate that most of the fracture centers contain calcium stearate powder particles, Figure 8. This processing aid improves the flow properties of the powder, that in our opinion, is not necessary for processing the medical UHMWPE powder. For example Hifax 1900 contains no calcium stearate. In fact, in case of the stainless high quality steels used for implants the corrosion protecting efficiency of calcium stearate is negligible. Therefore we don't see

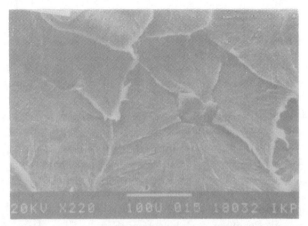

FIGURE 7. SEM picture of cold broken ($-196\,^\circ$C) UHMWPE hip cup (RCH 1000) shows calcium stearate particles in centers of the fracture structure.

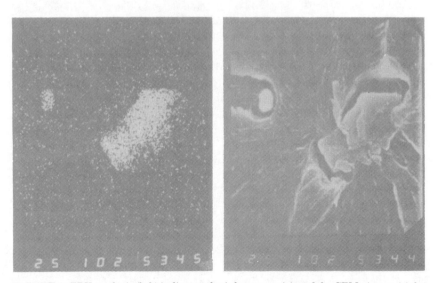

FIGURE 8. EDX-analysis (left) indicates the inhomogeneities of the SEM picture (right) as calcium stearate.

any advantage in using calcium stearate in connection with the medical application of UHMWPE but instead many disadvantages i.e. increased wear, lower strength, reduced long term properties.

CONCLUSIONS

• different aging processes between in vitro and in vivo storage show that the medium used for the simulation of in vivo conditions must be improved
• without adequate aging stabilizers γ-irradiated UHMWPE will be of limited use for in vivo long term applications (15 years and more)
• calcium stearate should not be used in medical UHMWPE

REFERENCES

1. B. S. Oppenheimer, *et al.*, *Cancer Res.*, *15*, S., 333 (1955).
2. T. W. Haas, W. Rostoker, J. Galante, and E. Y. S. Chao, *Proc. 25th Orthop. Res. Trans.*, San Francisco, p. 262 (1979).
3. E. S. Grood, R. Shastri, and C. N. Hopson, *J. Biomed. Mater. Res.*, *16*, S., 399 (1982).
4. P. Eyerer and Y. C. Ke, *J. Biomed. Mater. Res.* (1985).
5. P. Eyerer, *Biomed. Technik, 28*, S., 297 (1983).
6. H. Tschesche and H. W. Macartney, "Collagen Degradation and Mammalian Collagenase," *Int. Congr. Ser.*, *601*, *Amsterdam, Exerta Medica* (1982).

PART II

New Materials

Rationale for Biological Fixation of Prosthetic Devices

TODD S. SMITH
Biomaterials Laboratory
Depuy, Inc., Warsaw, Indiana

ABSTRACT

Biologically attached joint replacement prostheses are proving to be an attractive alternative to polymethylmethacrylate cemented implant systems. While the cemented implant systems tend to offer immediate relief of pain and rapid restoration of joint mobility, long-term results have been disappointing due to implant loosening. Sintered powder metal coatings provide implants with an effective medium for bone tissue ingrowth fixation. These implants have been used clinically for eight years with results comparable or superior to cemented implants. They are considered a conservative approach to joint arthroplasty and offer greater hope for the young, more active patients suffering from debilitating joint disease. These patients tend to have poor long-term results with cemented implant fixation. The scientific basis for biological fixation is addressed and a sintered powder metal coated implant system is described.

INTRODUCTION

JOINT DISEASES SUCH as arthritis or traumatic injury to the joints result in 150,000 surgical joint replacement procedures each year. A major problem in total joint reconstruction (TJR) is the occurrence of loosening of joint replacement devices. The vast majority of TJR implants are affixed to a skeletal number through the use of polymethylmethacrylate (PMMA) bone cement. This practice was pioneered by Sir

Reprinted from *SAMPE Journal*, May/June 1985, Courtesy of Society for Advancement of Material and Process Engineering of Covina, CA U.S.A.

John Charnley in the early 1960's. PMMA serves as a grouting agent. During the surgical procedure, it is introduced into the prepared bone cavity in the fluid state as a mixture of MMA powder and liquid monomer. As the mixture begins to polymerize, the implant is inserted and held in place until polymerization is complete. Hypotension and intraoperative deaths have been associated with the use of PMMA cement [1]. Other patients have been shown to be allergic to PMMA through patch test sensitivity testing [2]. But by far the greatest problems are associated with post operative implant loosening. Therefore, elimination of the bone cement is a worthy goal.

Unquestionably, bone cement is the weak link in TJR. It is a brittle material riddled with porosity, seams, internal and other defects. It can be contaminated by bone marrow and blood, all resulting in a degradation of mechanical performance. Additionally, there is overwhelming evidence documenting adverse tissue reactions and bone resorption around the bone cement sheath. The tissue reaction is thought to be incited by the existence of particulate PMMA debris within the joint tissues. The histological reaction to this debris is one of bone resorption or dissolving bone [3,4]. As such, it is the primary cause for implant loosening.

It is believed that a mechanical breakdown of the interface between implant and bone cement is the precursor to loosening by setting up a mechanism for the generation of PMMA wear debris. Cyclic loading of the implant causes relative movement between implant and cement sheath. Since the bond between cement and implant is weak, the interface fails. This is not surprising given the large modulus mismatch of PMMA and metal implant and the poor adhesive quality of bone cements.

Loosening becomes progressive. As the cement sheath continue to erode, debris is generated at a rate faster than surrounding tissues can accommodate it. Osteocytic cells differentiate into osteoclasts which attack and resorb bone cells and results in the formation of a fibrous tissue which cannot support the implant. Gross movement of the implant will cause pain as it is stressed. At this point it becomes necessary to remove the implant, clean the joint capsule, and recement another implant into the remaining bone. The loosening phenomenon depends on a combination of factors, including patient activity, patient weight, implant design, and the technical skill of the surgeon [5]. Upon revision of the primary implant system much less supportive bone is available so the chances of a second revision are likely. This phenomenon can continue until revision is no longer possible and the patient becomes incapable of ambulation.

APPROACH

The concept of cementless fixation is not new. In fact, prior to the introduction of bone cement in the mid 60's to early 70's, most prostheses were inserted cementless. They relied on a press fit and other geometric considerations for stability. While implants were used without cement, they were not without problems. Some designs were not mechanically stable; others resulted in debilitating thigh and acetabular pain. The concept of biological fixation took hold in the late 60's and early 70's. Recognizing the disadvantages of cement fixation, researchers in Europe and the U.S. began work on implant systems that would form a physical bond with bone tissues [6–9]. This was in recognition of the fact that bone was observed to grow into any cracks, holes, or other surface irregularities of the older press fit designs. The early designs of Lord Modreporic and Judet relied on gross surface texturing into which bone would grow and eventually stabilize the implant. As can be observed in Figure 1, the entire length was textured. Both implants are cobalt, chromium, molybdenum alloy investment castings. The texturing is produced by investment casting identically textured wax models. The Judet wax model appears to be repeatedly pierced with a hot blunt tool, the Lord wax model has a single layer of polymer beads attached to it. While these systems incorporated novel features, they suffered predominately from poor design.

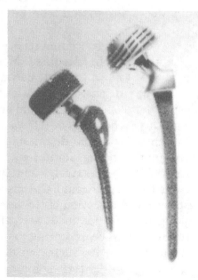

FIGURE 1. Judet femoral and acetabular prosthesis on left. Lord Madreporic implants on right.

Researchers in the U.S. have taken a different approach, that of microtexturing. The systems presently being investigated clinically are comprised of a variety of metallic, polymeric, and ceramic materials. The metal systems are of greatest interest due to their strength and long-term biocompatibility. They consist of either a sintered powder metal coating or sintered wire mesh coating. The use of powder metal techniques for the fabrication of porous metal structures for bone ingrowth attachment was first investigated by Hirschhorn and Reynolds [11] and Petersen et al [12]. Later Pilliar [13] developed the technology for applying a porous powder metal coating to a solid implant substrate. These coatings have been more thoroughly investigated in animals and subsequently in people than the others and have enjoyed the greatest commercial success. While following the pioneering work of Lord and Judet, the present day systems have been refined through improved implant geometry, optimization of the porous coatings, and improved instrumentation and insertion techniques.

In the early 70's Pilliar began his laboratory and animal investigations of the sintered metal powder coatings. From these studies, it was recognized that the long-term success of the arthroplasty depends in great measure on the optimization of the mechanics of the bone-implant interface [9]. Following these early studies, Pilliar in collaboration with Lunceford at the Moore Clinic in Columbia, South Carolina, developed the first endoprosthesis. It was based on the original press fit Austin Moore design and later became known as the Modified Moore implant. It was first implanted in 1976 and today remains the only FDA approved device commercially available for biological fixation (see Figure 2). The Modified Moore or Porocoat® AML® implant system, as it is known today, is based on the relatively successful experience of the uncoated cementless press-fit Moore device. The present design now consists of a round cross section in the distal region which progressively becomes oval towards the proximal or upper region of the implant. The round distal stem portion provides stability against rocking and bending motion within the medullary canal. The larger proximal portion effectively counters any rotary joint reaction forces imparted to the stem through the offset head. The collar rests on the medial aspect of the resection of the femoral head providing stability from sinking into the femur. Lastly, the proximal stem supports the porous sintered metal bead coating to provide for the progressive ingrowth of bone tissues. As such, the device provides the necessary attributes to satisfy the criteria for long-term stability; a mechanically stable anatomical design, biocompatibility of materials, and a sound mechanical interface with the host tissues.

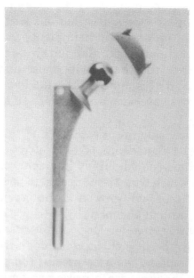

FIGURE 2. The Porocoat AML Total Hip System.

The stem is produced from a cobalt-chromium-molybdenum alloy meeting stringent chemical requirements of the ASTM F-75 specification. The powder metal coating is characterized as a random non-close packed array of 250 diameter spheres diffusion bonded together and to the implant substrate through a high temperature sintering operation as described by Pilliar [9]. The coating is 3/4 mm in thickness and has volume porosity of approximately 40%. The pore size ranges (a pore being defined as an interstice formed between three or more sinter bonded metal beads) from 100 to 400 with an average pore size of 250, well within the range considered to be optimal to support bone tissue ingrowth [10]. Interestingly, the volume porosity and average pore size increase with distance from the implant substrate. This reveals that the larger pores are located at the outer regions of the coating, adjacent to the prepared bone tissues. This density and pore size gradient is considered important in the efficient transfer of stress from the implant through the interface to the surrounding bone tissues. This efficient transfer of stress will also result in a reduction in implant stresses as they are shared with the bone [10,12]. Stress transfer to bone is important as weight bearing forces exerted through the implant can be several times the actual body weight.

An additional mechanical consideration is the maintenance of the anatomical stress distributions within the bone. Bone tissue reacts to stress and remodels to accommodate changes in stress. While it is a worthy goal to maintain stress distributions within the bone as anatomically as possible, most cemented implants constitute such a gross intrusion of the proximal femur that much bone remodelling must occur to accommodate the changes in stress distribution. With the AML® prostheses, radiographic analysis and in vitro photoelastic and strain gaging analysis have shown only minor adaptive bone modelling [14,15].

Figure 3 shows a low magnification SEM micrograph of the Porocoat® porous coating. The great depth of field of the SEM allows one to observe the three dimensional, highly interconnected structure porous of this coating into which bone tissue grows. In fact, it has been demonstrated that bone tissue will grow into the porous structure in very short times in both animal and man [16]. Because the secure fixation of the prosthesis requires time for bony ingrowth, are longer and more conservative than in the case of the cemented arthroplasty.

Insertion of the implant requires precise reaming of the proximal bone cavity as a tight press fit is necessary for initial stabilization. Initial stability will also allow for the time necessary for bone tissues to grow into the porous coating, further securing the implant. The broach used to prepare the femoral cavity has the same general shape as the implant but is slightly undersized. This creates an interference fit between the implant and femoral cavity. The straight stemmed implant must be driven into the cavity using a mallet. This procedure assures close bone tissue apposition to the porous coating to foster bone growth into it. Post operative patient weight bearing is initially more conservative than with the cemented systems. If a tight pressfit has not been achieved micromovement of the implant might require a longer time period for bone ingrowth fixation to occur. Postoperative pain may be greater than with the cemented system. This is thought by many to be beneficial as it is a reminder to the patient to exercise caution during the early weight bearing period and ambulation. On the other hand, postoperative stability of the cemented implant is at its best but degrades with time. The pain free mobility of these implants unfortunately gives the patient a false sense of security which could result in over stressing leading to mechanical instability. Biologically fixed implants usually get better with time.

CONCLUSIONS

To date, long-term results have been excellent. Of the 20,000 AML implantations, very few have required revision. This was usually in

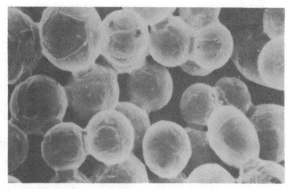

FIGURE 3. Scanning electron micrograph of the Porocoat® porous coating. Metal spheres are approximately 250 microns in diameter.

cases of infection which may necessitate implant removal. Upon revision though, virtually all the original bone stock is available for reimplantation of a new cementless device. For this reason, cementless THR is considered a conservative approach.

The fundamental problem of implant loosening in a cemented hip arthroplasty can be adequately addressed through the use of porous coated implants. Implants such as the Porocoat® AML1® offer new hope to those suffering from debilitating joint disease. Fixation of the uncemented prosthetic implant can occur through bone tissue ingrowth into a porous coating resulting in a mechanically sound long lasting bond. While there is still much room for improvement, this implant system meets the basic criteria of geometric design, biocompatability, and a means for bony attachment necessary for optimal performance of a joint replacement prosthesis.

REFERENCES

1. K. C. Kim and M. A. Ritter, *Chemical Orthopaedics, 88,* 154 (1972).
2. R. Ross, W. G. Thilly, and D. A. Kaden, *Journal of Bone and Joint Surgery, 61,* 1203 (1979).
3. M. D. Willert, Tissue Reactions around Joint Implants and Bone Cement, In *Symposium on Arthroplasty of the Hip, p. 11–21,* Edited by G. Chapcal, Stuttgart, Thieme (1973).
4. M. G. Willert, J. Ludwig, and M. Semlitsch, J. Bone and Joint Surgery, 56-A, 1368 (1974).
5. T. A. Gruen, G. M. McNeice, and M. C. Amstutz, *Clin. Orthorp., 141,* 17 (1979).

6. G. Lord and P. Bencel, *Clin. Orthop., 176,* 67 (1983).

7. R. Judet, *et al., Clin. Orthop., 137,* 76 (1978).

8. J. Galante, *et al., J. Bone and Joint Surg., 53A,* 101 (1971).

9. R. M. Pilliar, M. U. Cameron, and I. Macnab, *J. Biomed. Eng., 10,* 126 (1975).

10. J. D. Bobyn, R. M. Pilliar, and M. U. Cameron, *Clin. Orthop., 150,* 263 (1980).

11. J. S. Hirschhorn and J. T. Reynolds, "Powder Metallurgy Fabrication of Cobalt Alloy Surgical Implant Materials," In E. Korostoff, (ed.), *Research in Dental and Medical Materials,* New York, Plenum, p. 137 (1969).

12. C. D. Peterson, *et al.,* "Union between Bone and Implants of Open Pore Ceramic and Stainless Steel. A Histologic Study," *Trans of Orthopaedic Research Soc.,* New York (1969).

13. F. E. Kennedy, J. P. Collier, and L. A. Kormornik, "An Experimental Study of Stress Distribution in Bone Cement used to Grout Standard and Porous-Coated Prostheses. *Advances in Bioengineering,"Am. Soc. of Mechan. Eng.,* New York, p. 75 (1979).

14. C. A. Engh and J. D. Bobyn, "Biologic Fixation of Hip Prosthesis; Review of the Clinical Status and Current Concepts," *Advances in Orthop. Sur.,* p. 136 (1984).

15. J. P. Collier, *et al.,* "Stress Distribution in the Human Femur, the Role of Femoral Prosthesis Geometry and the Mechanics of Fixation," *Trans, 30th Annual O.R.S.,* Atlanta, Georgia (1984).

16. J. P. Collier and M. Mayor, "The Histology of Tissue Ingrowth into Porous-Metal-Coated Femoral Hip Prostheses in Five Humans," *Trans. Society of Biomaterials,* p. 79 (1983).

New Material Concepts in Orthopedics

J. C. BOKROS
CarboMedics, Inc.
Austin, Texas

INTRODUCTION

THE REPLACEMENT OF bone destroyed by disease or trauma is a multifaceted problem. The replacement material must be biologically benign in the broadest sense. It must not produce a chronic foreign-body inflammatory response which can increase the probability of infection and inhibit healing, and the properties that confer biocompatibility must not be changed in an adverse way by the in vivo environment.

Although bone can accept small deviations in stress from the normal and remodel to sustain such stresses, large deviations from normal physiologic limits can lead to degeneration and loss of bone. Accordingly, mechanical contrivances fashioned by man to replace natural joints, in order to succeed, must sustain the stresses that are applied in normal function and, at the same time, transmit the load to the supporting bone in such a way that the bone is subjected to the same sorts of stresses that were responsible for its evolution in the first place.

For proper long-term function, not only must the mechanical properties of materials used in construction of the prosthesis be appropriate, but it must also either have surface characteristics that allow bone to grow into the surface and become mechanically locked or have surface chemical properties that promote the chemical attachment of bone to it. An ideal surface might incorporate mechanical interlocks as well as chemical attachment. This paper deals with new concepts that address

Reprinted from *SAMPE Journal,* July/August 1984, Courtesy of Society for the Advancement of Material and Process Engineering, Covina, CA U.S.A.

the problems encountered in the engineering of bone replacement and summarizes some early clinical results.

PYROLYTIC CARBON

A variety of carbons including vitreous (glassy), pyrolytic, and vapor-deposited carbons and carbon fibers, have been used in the construction of artificial joints. Of the bulk forms of carbon, the dense, isotropic carbon deposited at low temperature along with silicon (LTI-Si carbon*) is the strongest. Comparisons of the properties of carbons and methods of fabrication have been published in two recent reviews [1,2].

Clinical use of LTI-Si carbon in the cardiovascular field has been extensive. Through 1983, more than 790,000 LTI-Si carbon parts have been supplied for use in 580,000 prosthetic heart valves. Since it was introduced in 1968, fewer than two dozen mechanical failures have been reported, so the failure rate during the 16 years of clinical use is substantially less than 1 in 10,000.

LTI-Si carbon has been evaluated extensively for use in implant dentistry. The application of LTI-Si carbon as a dental implant is relevant to orthopedic applications because dental implants are seated directly into bone without the use of cement. The implant protrudes through the gingiva and supports the forces of mastication which can be considerable. The good performance of the LTI-Si carbon dental implant is due mainly to the fact that the surface that interfaces with bone does not present itself as a foreign body, and its inherent surface roughness allows bone ingrowth and mechanical attachment (see for example Figures 2 and 3 in Reference 3). Further, since the modulus of elasticity of the LTI-Si carbon posts is near that of bone [4–6], the load transmission from the implant into bone is near physiologic so the loss of crestal bone common with stiffer and less compatible dental implants is minimal. This is evidenced by a sclerotic peri-implant line visible on radiographs that resembles a lamina dura (see Figure 10 in Reference 7).

Early experience with LTI-Si carbon dental implants have been reported in References 3 and 7. The design that finally evolved has a simple conical shape with grooves provided for ingrowth (Figure 1). Actuarial data for 89 patients (Figure 2) shows a cumulative success rate of 88% over a four year period [8].

Encouraged by the good performance of LTI-Si carbon as a dental

---

*Available commercially under the trade name Pyrolite® carbon, CarboMedics, Inc., Austin, Texas.

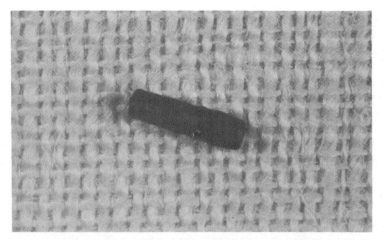

FIGURE 1. Post-type LTI-Si carbon dental implants.

implant material, work has been directed to the replacement of small joints in the hand and foot with LTI-Si carbon implants. Results from replacements of the metacarpophalangeal joint of baboons with uncemented LTI-Si carbon prostheses indicate that the implants were well tolerated for nine months, at which time, the implants were retrieved [9]. Histological examination showed attachement by direct

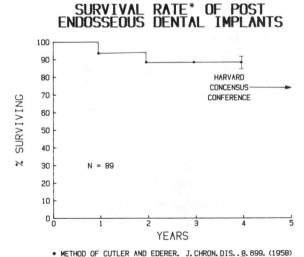

FIGURE 2. Actuarial data for LTI-Si carbon post-type dental implants.

apposition of both bone and fibrous tissue. There was no evidence of bone resorption around the implant stems and functional fixation was obtained with all the implants. No foreign body reaction or wear particles were observed in the adjacent soft tissue. In comparison, two cemented implants of the same configuration both showed evidence of bone resorption and/or gross implant loosening.

Preliminary experience with non-cemented LTI-Si carbon replacements of the metacarpophalangeal joint in humans is also reportedly good. Results from 39 patients (104 joints) with up to five years followup have demonstrated satisfactory clinical results and biologic acceptance of the implants [10].

Replacements for the thumb and great toe followed the development of prosthetic metacarpophalangeal joints (Figure 3). A number have been implanted in humans and are functioning well, but the terms for these implants are currently less than about a year [11].

In another effort aimed at the development of an improved hip-joint prosthesis, Cook and co-workers [12] compared the effect of both LTI-Si carbon and metal (Ti-4A1-6V) articulating surfaces on cartilage. They implanted prostheses of the sort shown in Figure 4 in the hips of adult mongrel dogs. After one year, the acetabular cartilage that interfaced with LTI-Si carbon was in good condition whereas the cartilage that interfaced with the titanium alloy showed considerable degeneration. Additional work, as yet unpublished, has confirmed the original results

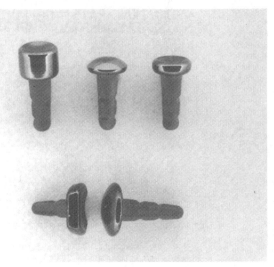

FIGURE 3. LTI-Si carbon replacements for the thumb and toe (upper thumb; lower toe).

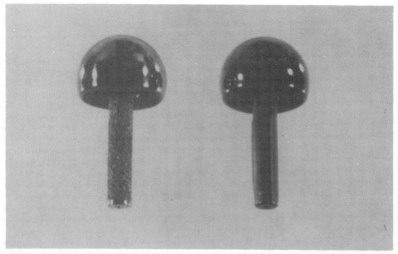

FIGURE 4. Prosthesis implanted as a hemi-arthroplasty in the hips of mongrel dogs.

and endoprostheses with LTI-Si carbon-surfaced head are under test for future use in human clinical trials (Figure 5).

CARBON COATED POROUS TITANIUM

Although LTI-Si carbon materials are satisfactory for use as small joint replacements, it is not possible to fabricate total joint replacements from LTI-Si carbon that are as large as is required for either the hip or the knee. For these applications, a solid titanium alloy (Ti-6A1-4V) has been selected because of its relatively low elastic modulus compared to cobalt or iron based alloys, to provide direct fixation of the prostheses to bone without cement, selected locations on the prosthesis are surfaced with porous titanium. The morphology used, shown in Figure 6, is quite different from that obtained by sintering together spherical particles (Figure 7). The channels that interconnect the pores shown in Figure 6, at the same density, are larger than can be attained with spherical particles. The microstructure sought (Figure 6) is not unlike the pore structure present in cancellous bone (Figure 8).

Although the structure of porous titanium has a morphology that allows bone ingrowth and attachment (see Figures 3, 9, 11, 12 and 13 in Reference 13), the large metallic surface area is of concern because of the potential for high levels of metal-ion release into the adjacent tissues and the uncertainty as to the long-term effort of such ions on

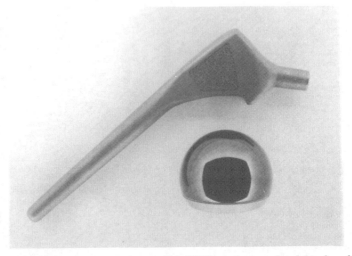

FIGURE 5. Titanium endo-prostheses with LTI-Si carbon surfaced head and incorporating porous regions for biological fixation.

the viability of the boney tissues growing in the pores. Griffin has studied the corrosion rate of both solid and porous titanium surfaces and found that, for the uncoated specimens, the porous titanium corroded several times faster than solid titanium with the same geometric area [14]. However, after coating with a special form of impermeable vapor-

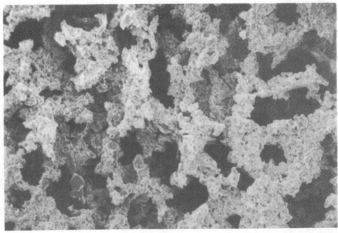

FIGURE 6. Porous titanium surface. The density is 50% and the average pore size is 200 microns.

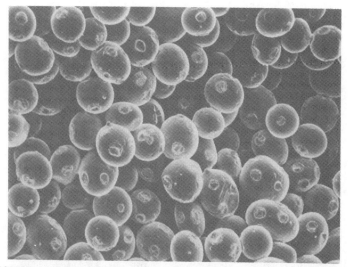

FIGURE 7. Morphology of surface obtained by sintering spherical particles.

deposited carbon**, both the solid and porous specimens corroded at about the same rate which was substantially less than the corrosion rate of the uncoated solid titanium specimens (Figure 9).

Although there is yet no long term evidence of adverse affects of titanium metal ion release on tissues, the data in Figure 9 suggests that, should such affects become evident, carbon coating is effective in reducing the release of metal ions from porous titanium surfaces. An example of the use of carbon-coated porous titanium as a biological fixation surface on a hip-joint prosthesis is depicted in Figure 5.

FIXATION WITH HYDROXYLAPATITE

The good compatibility of hydroxylapatite with bone [15–17] and its apparent ability to form strong bonds with bone has received considerable attention, especially since there appears to be an increase in the rate of bone ingrowth into porous hydroxylapatite surfaces [17,18]. Such observations could be of clinical importance because an increase in the rate of bone ingrowth could reduce the time before recipients of

---

**Biolite® carbon, CarboMedics, Inc., Austin, Texas.

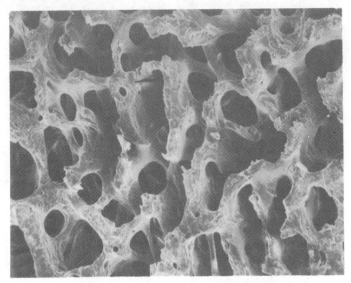

FIGURE 8. Structure of cancellous bone.

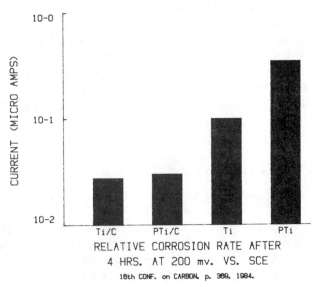

16th CONF. on CARBON, p. 369, 1984.

FIGURE 9. Corrosion rates of uncoated solid titanium (Ti) and porous titanium (PTi) compared with carbon coated solid (Ti/C) and carbon coated porous titanium (PTi/C) [14].

hip or knee prostheses could bear weight and thus reduce their recuperation period.

Heretofore, efforts to coat orthopedic prostheses with a variety of ceramic materials including hydroxylapatite has not led to any widely accepted concept. After trying a variety of coating methods including plasma flame spraying, Jarcho and Kay [19] developed a propietary sintering process in which special sintering agents (activators) are used to obtain tightly adherent, impermeable hydroxylapatite coatings which can be either pure hydroxylapatite or hydroxylapatite co-sintered with other constituents. In order to promote early bonding of tissue to titanium implants, the areas on the prosthesis selected to be ingrowth surfaces are first coated with porous titanium and then coated with a hydroxylapatite based material by sintering. The mor-

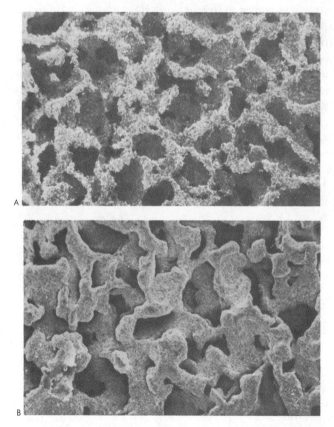

FIGURE 10. Porous titanium surface a) before and b) after coating with a hydroxyl-apatite based material (courtesy Jarcho and Kay, [19]).

phologies of porous titanium surfaces before and after such coating processes are shown in Figure 10. The concept is ready to advance to limited clinical evaluation as soon as results from animal tests (in progress) are fully evaluated.

CONCLUSION

Advances in the understanding of prosthesis/bone mechanics and the utilization of new material concepts are providing the basis for the development of improved orthopedic prosthetic devices. The biocompatibility of LTI-Si carbon together with the similarity of its mechanical response to that of bone explains, for the most part, the success of small LTI-Si carbon joints implanted without cement. Further, the compatibility of carbon surfaces with cartilage has the potential for expanding the usefulness of endo-prostheses by delaying the time before a full total hip replacement is required.

The development of specialized pore morphologies in titanium which are coated with a thin, impermeable carbon to reduce ion release is providing the kind of biofixation required in larger hip and knee prostheses. This concept alone is intriguing; the possibility that the rate of fixation may be enhanced through the use of special forms of calcium phosphate materials sintered into the pore structure adds to the exciting potential for such ideas.

The aforementioned concepts together with the development of biologically based bone cements and grouts could provide the impetus for a significant advance in orthopedic prosthetics before the end of this decade.

REFERENCES

1. A. D. Haubold, H. S. Shim, and J. C. Bokros, "Carbon in Medical Devices," in *Biocompatibility of Clinical Implant Materials*, D. F. Williams (Ed.), CRC Press, Inc., Boca Raton, Florida, Vol. II, pp. 3–42 (1981).
2. J. C. Bokros, "Carbon in Medical Devices," in *Materials Science Monograph; Ceramics in Surgery*, P. Vincenzini (Ed.), Elsevier, Amsterdam, Vol. 17, pp. 199–214 (1983).
3. J. C. Bokros, *Carbon, 15,* 353 (1977).
4. D. T. Reilly and A. H. Burstein, *J. Bone Joint Surg., 56-A,* 1001 (1974).
5. P. S. Walker, *Human Joints and Their Artificial Replacements,* Springfield, Charles C. Thomas (1977).
6. K. Piekarski, *J. Appl. Physics, 41,* 215 (1970).
7. J. N. Kent and J. C. Bokros, *Dental Clinics in North America, 24* (3), (1980).

8. R. M. Meffert, San Antonio, TX, Private Communication (1983).

9. S. D. Cook, et al., *Orthopedics, 6* (8), 952, (1983).

10. R. D. Beckenbaugh, *Orthopedics, 6* (8), 962, (1983). Also private communication (1984).

11. S. Kampner, et al., "Pyrolytic Carbon—An Alternative Implant Material in Orthopedic Surgery," presented at AAOS Meeting, Atlanta, GA (1983).

12. R. C. Anderson, et al., "An Evaluation of LTI Carbon and Porous Titanium Load Bearing Prostheses," *Transactions,* Joint 9th Annual Meeting of the Society for Biomaterials and 15th International Biomaterials Symposium, April 27–May 1, 1983, Birmingham, AL, Vol. VI, p. 80 (1983).

13. R. C. Anderson, et al., *Clin. Ortho. and Rel. Res.,* No. 182, Jan-Feb, pp. 242–257 (1984).

14. C. Griffin, Austin, TX (1984), to be published.

15. M. Jarcho, *Clin. Orthoped., 457,* 259 (1981).

16. H. W. Dennissen, et al., *J. Biomed. Mater. Res., 14,* 713–721 (1980).

17. P. Ducheyne, *J. Biomed. Mater. Res., 14,* 225 (1980).

18. R. L. Salsbury, et al., "A Comparison of the Rate of Bone Bonding and Durapatite Implants in Rats," *Transactions,* Joint 7th Annual Meeting of the Society for Biomaterals and the 13th International Biomaterials Symposium, p. 113 (1981).

19. M. Jarcho and J. F. Kay, private communication, Calcitek, Inc., San Diego, CA (1983).

Influence of Mixing Technique on Some Properties of PMMA Bone Cement—Clinical Practice, Producer's Advice, Material Investigations, Improvements

P. Eyerer
Institut für Kunstoff-Prüfung und Kunststoffkunde
Universität Stuttgart
Pfaffenwaldring 32
D-7000 Stuttgart 80, West Germany

R. Jin
Hefei Polytechnical University
Hefei, PR China

INTRODUCTION

THE MIXING TECHNIQUE of bone cement and its influence on the cement's properties has often been a subject of research: Charpley [1]; Lee et al. [2]; Debrunner [3]; Haas et al. [4]; Debrunner [5]; Lee et al. [6]; Henßge [7]; Lee [8]. In spite of many publications on this subject, important questions are unanswered:

- How do the mixing conditions of bone cements differ within the clinical practice?
- What are the derived property variations?
- How accurate is the advice of different producers?
- Is it possible to improve the mixing technique?
- Is there any correlation between the property variations and the loosening of endoprostheses?

Presented at ANTEC '85, The Society of Plastics Engineers, Inc. 43rd Technical Conference, April 29–May 2, Washington, D.C. USA

The following investigations should help to find some answers to these questions.

MATERIALS

Six different hospitals in Germany provide us with pieces of bone cement separated from the dough they mixed for joint operations. Palacos R, Refobacin, Sulfix 6, AKZ and CMW bone cement were used. We received round pieces 3–5 cm in diameter and about 5 mm thick. They were separated from handmixed dough for the hip joint cup. We also obtained residual parts of the injection processed dough.

METHODS

Density measurements were made following the ASTM 792-66 procedure. After conditioning, bone cement cubes of about 5 × 4 × 3 mm in size were cut off. The porosity was calculated from density. Hardness (DIN 53456) and ultimate flexural strength (DIN 53435) characterize the mechanical properties. The average molecular weight ($\bar{M}_w$) describes the polymerization process.

RESULTS

Density measurements of hand processed cement samples of the 6 hospitals show variations from 1,110 g/cm³ to 1,270 g/cm³, Figures 1 and 2; this refers to a porosity range of 1 to 15%. Further it is shown, that the variation of the injection processed samples is remarkably lower and the average density is higher. Ultimate flexural strength, Figure 3, and hardness indicate differences up to 100% concerning the extreme values of density. The $\bar{M}_w$ of samples from three hospitals varies little, the mean values are almost identical. This expresses a relatively comparable chemical reaction during polymerization. The main source of influence is the amount of air (porosity) mixed in during stirring. Because of these results we analyzed the mixing procedure and quantified the following parameters: sequence of the single components, mixing time, Figure 4, mixing velocity, Figure 5, kneading of dough by hand, quantity of dough, cement thickness, applied pressure. Although many of these parameters were investigated before some new points of interest arose. One example is the influence of mixing velocity on porosity. An optimized mixing technique, Table 1, resulted in obviously higher density values, Figure 6. The porosity could be reduced to 1 to 4.5% with low variation. Jasty et al. [9] and Burke et al. [10]

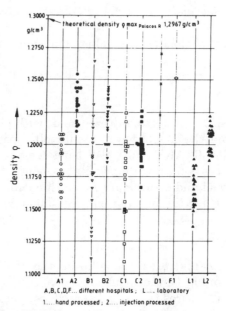

FIGURE 1. Density of refobacin-palacos R samples, mixed during hip total endoprostheses operations by theatre nurses *before* optimizing the mixing technique (each point is another sample).

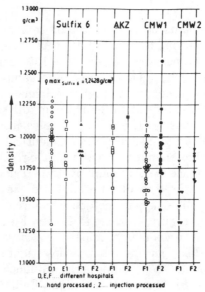

FIGURE 2. Density of different PMMA bone cement samples, mixed during hip total endoprostheses operations by theatre nurses *before* optimizing the mixing technique (each point is another sample).

92

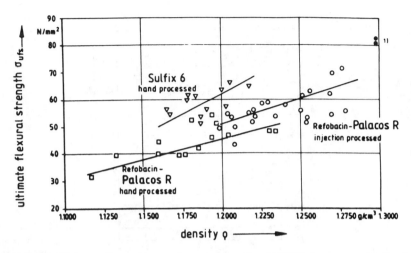

FIGURE 3. Ultimate flexural strength versus density of PMMA bone cements, 1) polymerized under pressure.

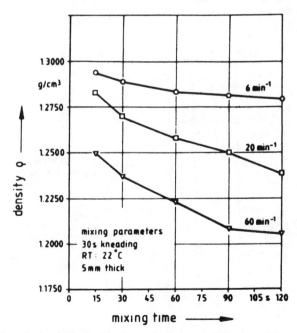

FIGURE 4. Correlation between density and mixing at different mixing velocities for palacos R. Mixing parameters: 30 s kneading; 5 mm thick; RT: 20°C.

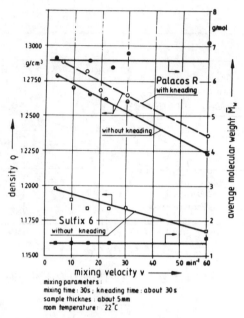

FIGURE 5. Influence of mixing velocity on density and average molecular weight of PMMA bone cement.

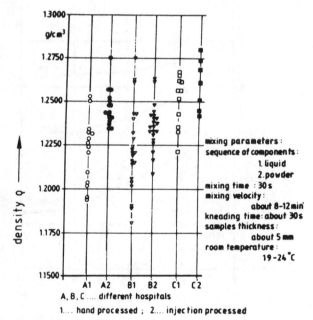

FIGURE 6. Density of refobacin-palacos R samples, mixed during hip total endoprostheses operations by theatre nurses *after* optimizing the mixing technique (each point is another sample).

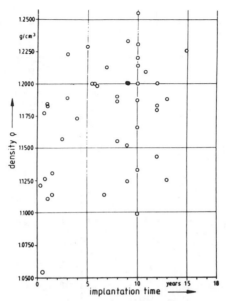

FIGURE 7. Density of palacos R bone cement of retrieved hip cups as a function of in vivo implantation time.

showed, that by centrifugating the mixed dough for 2 minutes at 4000 rpm, the porosity decreases depending on the viscosity of the dough. Due to its high viscosity Palacos did not exhibit any porosity reduction after the described procedure [9], Table 2. On the other hand our developed optimized mixing technique shows similar improvements without any new equipment and above all it is applicable to any type of bone cement without in principle depending on its viscosity. Of course it has to be adapted. An analysis of 43 in vivo implanted and loosened Palacos bone cements (implanted and loosened Palacos bone cements (implanted 6 month to 15 years) indicates no clear correlation between loosening and porosity, Figure 7. Further extensive investigations are essential.

CONCLUSIONS

- the mixing conditions of the participating hospitals differ remarkably, Figures 1 and 2,
- the resulting property variations expressed in ultimate flexural strength can rise to factor 2, Figure 3
- the advice given by the bone cement producers is inadequate partly, sometimes inaccurate and/or partly contradictory.

Table 1. Optimized mixing parameters for palacos R bone cement.

Mixing Parameters	Palacos R Optimized Values
Mixing cup	Porcelain; 6 cm diameter 6 cm high
Mixing tool	Chamfered sheet with handle
Dough quantity* (powder)	10 to 40 g
Sequence of components	1. Liquid vice versa 2. Powder is also possible
Mixing time	30 s
Mixing velocity	About 10 min^{-1}
Taking out the dough of the mixing cup within	About 10 s
Kneading time (rolling and pressing)	About 30 s
Thickness	About 5 mm
Pressure during polymerization	In work
Room temperature	22 °C

*Corresponding to producer's advice the quantity of MMA was 1:2 of the powder quantity.

- improvements within single parameters lead to an optimized mixing technique; the porosity of hand processed bone cements can be reduced from an average value of 8 ± 6% to 2.5 ± 1.5%, Table 1,
- a correlation between the measured property variation (especially high porosity) and the loosening of prostheses cannot be concluded definitely; further investigations are necessary, Figure 7.

Table 2. Influence of centrifugating PMMA bone cements at 4000 rpm after mixing the dough on resulting porosity [9].

	Porosity %		
Bone Cement Centrifugation Time	0	30 s	120 s
Simplex P	8.2−15	3.1−5.1	2.4−3.5
A K Z	10.2−12.2	7.8	6
Palacos R	10−12	10−12	10−12

ACKNOWLEDGEMENTS

For intensive cooperation and important discussions we thank Drs. R. Ascherl (München), K. -H. Dittel (Stuttgart), E. F. Gauer (Heidelberg), J. Haasters (Essen), U. Holz (Stuttgart), F. Lechner (Garmisch-Partenkirchen), U. Weber (Gießen). We also thank the company Kulzer (Wehrheim), Merck (Darmstadt) and Sulzer (Winterthur/CH) for providing us with bone cement for our laboratory tests. We are very grateful to Dr. Ege, Kulzer, as well as Dr. M. Semlitsch and R. Streicher, Sulzer, for many useful discussions.

REFERENCES

1. J. Charnley, *Acrylic Cement in Orthopaedic Surgery*, Edinburgh-London, E. S. Livingstone (1970).
2. A. J. C. Lee, R. S. M. Ling, and J. D. Wrighton, *Clin. Orthop.*, *95*, 281 (1973).
3. H. U. Debrunner, Interner Techn. Report 6/75, Bern (1975).
4. S. S. Haas, G. M. Brauer, and G. Dickson, *J. Bone Jt. Surg.*, *57-A*, 380 (1975).
5. H. U. Debrunner, *Arch. Orthop. Unfall Chir.*, *86*, 261 (1976).
6. A. J. C. Lee, R. S. M. Ling, S. S. Vangala, *Arch. Orthop. Traumat. Surg.*, *92*, 1 (1978).
7. E. J. Henßge, *Knochenzement Symp.*, 23.–25.4.84, Göttingen.
8. A. J. C. Lee, *Knochenzement Symp.*, 23.–25.4.84, Göttingen.
9. M. Jasty, N. F. Jensen, and W. H. Harris, *2nd World Congress on Biomaterials*, 27.4.-1.5.84, Washington.
10. D. W. Burke, E. I. Gates, and W. H. Harris, *J. Bone and Joint Surg.*, in print.

Advances in Biomedical Adhesives and Sealants

HENRY LEE
Lee Pharmaceuticals
South El Monte, California

ABSTRACT

The development of adhesive filling materials for dentistry over the past 25 years is reviewed. Epoxy resin based adhesive filling materials which bond to enamel, dentin, and cementum are described and their benefits to dentistry presented. Adhesives for keratinized surfaces such as fingernails and hooves are reviewed.

INTRODUCTION

BIOMEDICAL ADHESIVES AND sealants may be divided into three main categories: (1) adhesives and sealants which may be cured outside or away from the body, (2) adhesives and sealants which must be cured on various surfaces of the body, and (3) adhesives and sealants which must be cured within the body.

Adhesives and sealants which may be cured outside or away from the body presents a somewhat easier task as a wider range of raw materials may be considered and heat and pressure can be used to achieve a cure, and the cured product can be subjected to extraction processes to remove residual traces of catalysts or traces of unreacted monomers, etc.

Adhesive and sealants which must be cured on or in the body present the requirements that they must cure at body temperatures in useful periods of time, that they must cure with acceptable reaction exo-

Reprinted from *SAMPE Journal,* July/August 1984, courtesy of Society for Advancement of Material and Process Engineering, Covina, CA U.S.A.

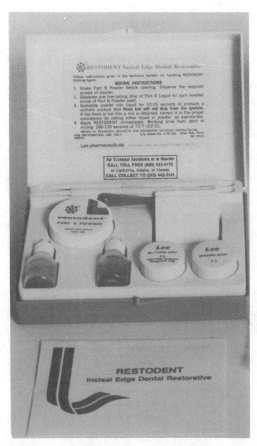

FIGURE 1. Kit of adhesive filling material for repairing biting edge of anterior teeth. Loss of the incisal edge of anterior teeth due to a blow in the mouth poses a severe aesthetic problem for youngsters as their teeth are not yet developed sufficiently to permit placement of a crown (cap). This dental restorative can build up the tooth and replace the missing tooth structure in a simple 20 minute procedure requiring no drilling or anesthesia. The adhesive filling material must bond to etched enamel in 0.5 grams masses at room temperature in 60 seconds.

therms, and must possess low orders of toxicity prior to cure, during cure, and after cure as well as have the set of physical and chemical properties dictated by the application.

Adhesives and sealants for use on or in the body may be further divided into the types of tissue or the type of implant which must be bonded. These applications may be divided into four categories: (1) adhesives and sealants for keratinized, exteriorized soft tissue (skin

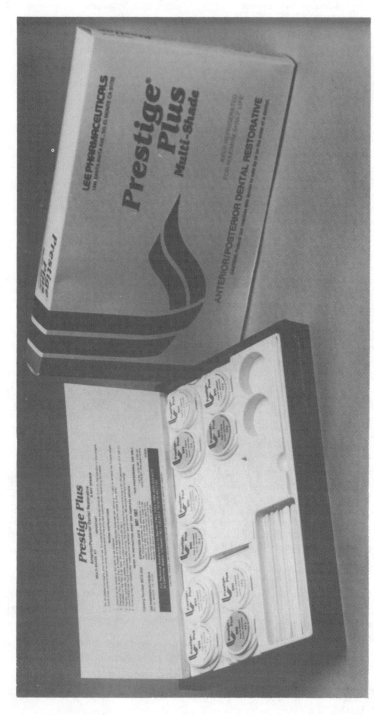

FIGURE 2. Epoxy resin based filling material supplied as two container adhesive kits. Six sets of containers provide for six shades of white to permit matching natural tooth structure. Close matching of index of refraction of cured resin and inorganic fillers leads to pearlescent, semi-translucent restoration which picks up the color of adjacent tooth structure so that the filling material blends into the tooth.

and fingernails and hooves), (2) mineralized and exteriorized tissue (teeth), (3) interior hard tissue (bones) and (4) interior soft tissue.

Further classifications may be made based on the type or rate of bleeding or strength or keratin-like nature of the soft tissue, etc.

The entire field of biomedical adhesives and sealants is in a state of ferment. We know that the use of plastics and polymers as implant materials is moving ahead steadily [5], but the use of adhesives and sealants has moved slower because of the special requirements posed above.

There is a definite need for numerous adhesives and sealants within the body. One need only spend an hour with a surgeon and he will start to outline products he would like to have for reinforcing tissue or for bonding tissue, etc. However, developments in this field run slow because of the many problems outlined above.

Workers in the area of biomedical adhesives and sealants are making progress in the area of adhesives and sealants applied to the exterior of the body, and in so doing are solving many of the problems that face the formulation of adhesives and sealants for use within the body.

For the purpose of this article I shall confine my remarks to the area of dental materials and fingernail repair and lengthening materials, as this is the area of much of my own personal present involvement [5–10] after numerous years in the industrial and aerospace adhesives and sealants arena [1–4]. It may seem mundane to work in these areas after working on encapsulants for naval motors intended to be flooded by battle damage, or on adhesives for ablative shield for missiles [2,3] but the technical problems in the dental and nail care field are just as intense and pose numerous added technical challanges as outlined above even if the end use does seem more mundane.

TWENTY YEAR PROGRAM

In the past twenty years or so, since 1961, the dental profession has had its own "moon shot" program underway. This program was the development of adhesives which could be used in the mouth to bond to enamel, dentin, and cementum.

The purpose of materials which would bond to enamel, dentin, and cementum are numerous. In the first place, conventional filling materials in use until a few years ago would leak at the margin of the restoration and permit secondary decay to start, so that the fillings often had to be replaced in five or seven years, depending on the patient's oral hygiene, etc. In addition, the filling materials required that the tooth be prepared with numerous undercuts to hold the filling material in the cavity since it was not adhesive. Also, because the filling could leak at the margins, it was often a practice to drill the cavity much larger than needed just to remove decay, but instead to extend the filling area into a region of the tooth where the action of the tongue and the sweep of food across the tooth was such that there was a tendency for the area to be swept clean, so that there was less chance of debris accumulating and less chance of food and bacterial getting into the margin of the cavity and causing decay. These practices were codified under the terms "extension for retention" and "extension for prevention."

Recognizing the short comings of time honored practices, the dental profession reasoned that if we had the technology to build airplanes and rockets using synthetic adhesives and sealants, and the engineering skills to put a man on the moon, then there had to be a way to develop dental adhesives which would permit the dentist to only

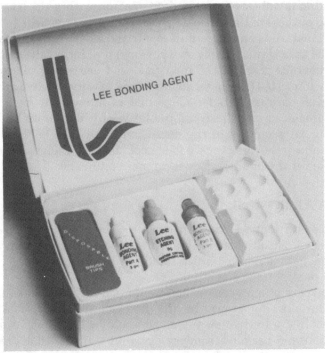

FIGURE 3. Epoxy resin based adhesive supplied in dropper bottles with mixing wells. This material may be used with adhesive filling materials to improve bond to enamel and to seal margins created by polymerization shrinkage.

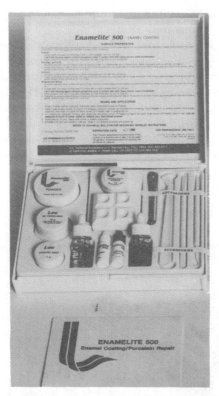

FIGURE 4. Epoxy resin based adhesive coating kit for enamel. This kit permits the restoration of cavities in the enamel of teeth created by various erosion forces. Usually these are referred to as cervical erosions as they occur near the cervix of the tooth where it emerges from the gum. Usually enough enamel has been eroded to expose the dentin. Drilling in this area is difficult as the pulp of the tooth is not as well protected as on the biting surface of the tooth. By use of adhesives, restorations can be made with no drilling in many cases. The adhesive also bonds to dental porcelain so that chips on porcelain crowns can be repaired without removing the crown, which is an expensive procedure.

remove the decay and apply an adhesive filling material. The profession hoped to be able to eliminate the sacrifice of sound tooth structure which the conventional material imposed on them. Two national symposia of dental and scientific disciplines were conducted to bring the problems into focus [11,12].

Since the time of these symposia the dental materials has been working steadily. The National Institute of Dental Research sponsored some early research grants and contracts for the study of certain fundamentals of adhesion, and the measurement of certain essential parameters such as surface tension data on numerous synthetic monomers, critical surface tension data on enamel and dentin and cementum under different oral conditions and after various forms of preparatory treatment such as drilling and etching with acids, etc. These grants and contracts were not negotiated with the dental schools but with industrial and aerospace companies so as to bring the latest ideas from outside the profession into the profession. By so doing, the government, under the guidance of the dental specialists at NIDR and under the guidance of certain devoted dental materials chemists at the National Bureau of Standards and at certain dental schools such as Indiana University and Marquette, as well as specialists in the Naval Research Laboratory,

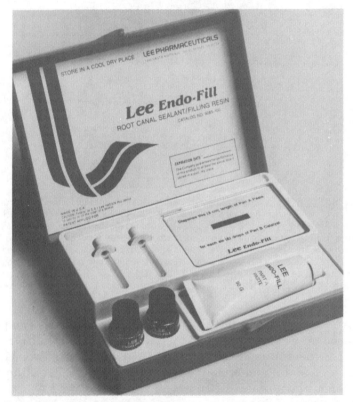

FIGURE 5. A root canal sealant which is used to fill and seal the root canals of teeth undergoing endodontic treatment. The silicone rubber formula can be applied conventionally on a gutta percha point, or can be injected with a special syringe. The material is opaque to X-rays, and low in toxicity. It prevents fluids and bacteria from entering the treated tooth at the apex. It can be removed as needed to bond in a post for building up a broken down tooth.

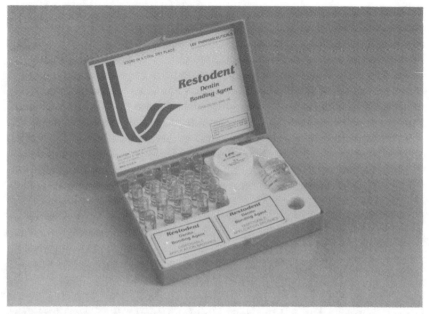

FIGURE 6. A kit of polyurethane adhesive for bonding filling materials to dentin and cementum.

served to attract numerous non-dental polymer chemists and adhesive specialists to the problem of the dental profession.

The program has been a success. The dental materials chemists now offer to the profession materials which will bond to etched enamel and to unetched dentin and cementum. Materials are also available which will bond to dental gold, dental stainless steel, and to dental porcelain. Filling materials which bond directly to tooth structure are available from numerous supplies. Other filling materials are offered in kits which permit dispensing small amounts as needed. The materials sets in 30 to 180 seconds, or in some cases up to 5 minutes, depending on the working time needed by the dentist. The filling materials are of either the two-component type, or of the ultraviolet or visible light cure type. The use of the light cured materials frees the dentist from time pressures imposed by the short set time of the two component materials. This permits the dentist to carve or shape the restoration to tooth contour before curing it, for example.

Modern dental filling materials of the synthetic resin type are a modern composite, usually based on an aromatic epoxy resin which has been modified to cure at room temperature in small masses (approx.

0.15 grams to 0.5 grams). By use of mineral or glass fillers which are opaque to X-rays and which have a refractive index close to that of the cured epoxy, the chemist can provide a semi-translucent, pearlescent filling material of great durability, opaque to X-rays, and adhesive to tooth structure. (If a synthetic resin based filling material is not opaque to X-rays, the filling will resemble "decay" on X-ray examination and it is difficult to differentiate secondary decay from the filling material.) Filler contents in excess of 80% by weight are achieved by means of selective grading of particle sizes and by treatment of the filler with organo-functional silanes. The silane also improves the integrity of the mechanical properties over a long service life in a moist environment. Compressive strengths of 30,000 to 60,000 psi are achieved despite cure in small masses at only 37°C.

Adhesion to dentin has been one of the hardest problems to solve, as dentin is only 65% by weight mineral, the rest is essentially "wet leather." However, clinically useful strengths are now being achieved by organic adhesives which either chelate with the calcium in the hydroxy apatite crystals in the dentin or by adhesives which react with active hydrogens on the protein. In this sense, these dentin adhesives are a breakthrough in the field of not only biomedical adhesives, but in the field of adhesives in general, since so many of our industrial and aerospace adhesives bond by means of Van der Waal's forces, rather than primary chemical bonds or ionic bonds.

FINGERNAILS

Another area of biomedical adhesive for exterior application is that for fingernails. Adhesives are now available which will bond to fingernails, that are low in toxicity, have good set times, have a modulus of elasticity similar to the natural nail, and are natural appearing in color. They come in kits with directions adequate for the typical consumer to comprehend. Adhesives are also available for bonding plastic nail tips for nail extension. These are easy to apply and also easy to remove. The application may seem mundane to most engineers, but most will admit they have heard the expression from a loved one "Oh darn, I broke a nail!" Well, now that problem has been solved too.

FUTURE

For those chemists who tend to laugh at such applications as fingernail lengthening and repair, let us pose the problem of developing an adhesive for horse shoes, which the farrier can apply with one hand

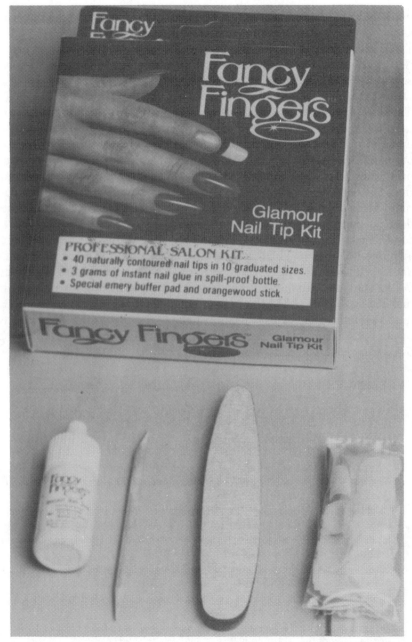

FIGURE 7. A kit of plastic nail tips and a special cyanoacrylate adhesive provide fast repairs of broken nails.

while holding up the leg and foot of a 2000 pound horse! And which can then take the pounding on concrete and stone.

For those chemists who are interested in biomedical adhesives for within the body, let us say that much work remains to be done. We have solved many of the toxicity problems and handling problems and formulation problems of materials intended for application on the body. The development of injectible silicone for filling root canals shows that adhesives and sealants can be cured within the body successfully. But applications such as this do pose problems which are a magnitude of order more difficult. The silicone root canal filling material required over 10 years of work compared to the two or three required on a filling material. Besides taking rather more work to develop they take much more time to prove out clinically. This means that the expense to develop them may well be beyond the ability of smaller companies to fund. Yet it is these smaller companies who have made most of the developments in biomedical adhesives and sealants to date. And once developed then the appropriate profession must be taught to use them. Often the new product cannot bear a price sufficient to permit its marketing. In this sense, the area of biomedical adhesives and sealants may resemble that of the "orphan drugs," materials that are vitally needed, yet their cost is too great for any organization to supply at a price the consumer can afford.

REFERENCES

1. Henry Lee and Kris Neville, *Epoxy Resins—Their Application and Technology*, McGraw-Hill Book Co., New York, 305 pp. (1957).
2. Henry Lee and Kris Neville, *Handbook of Epoxy Resins*, McGraw-Hill Book Co., New York (1967).
3. Henry Lee, Donald G. Stoffey, and Kris Neville, *New Linear Polymers-The Chemistry and Technology of Ten New Commercial Polymers*, McGraw-Hill Book Co., New York, 374 pp. (1967).
4. Charles Cagle; Henry Lee, and Kris Neville, Consulting Editors, *Handbook of Adhesive Bonding*, McGraw-Hill Book Co., New York (1973).
5. Henry Lee and Kris Neville, *Handbook of Biomedical Plastics*, Pasadena Technology Press, Pasadena, California (1971).
6. Henry Lee, et al., *Handbook of Dental Composite Restoratives*, Lee Pharmaceuticals, South El Monte, California (1973).
7. Henry Lee, *Adhesive Dental Composite Restoratives*, Pasadena Technology Press, Pasadena, California (1981).
8. Henry Lee, Editor, *Cyanoacrylate Monomers—The Instant Glues, A Monograph*, Pasadena Technology Press, California (1981).
9. Henry Lee, *The Bonded Orthodontic Appliance—A Monograph*, Pasadena Technology Press, Pasadena, California (1981).

10. Henry Lee, *Technique Manual: Modern Methods of Restorative Dentistry,* Quintessence Publishing Co., Berlin, West Germany (1982).

11. Ralph W. Phillips and Gunnar Ryge, Editors, *Adhesive Restorative Dental Materials,* Clearing House, US Dept. of Commerce, Springfield, VA (1961).

12. *Adhesive Restorative Dental Materials-II,* Public Health Service Publication No. 1494 (1966).

High Performance Tecoflex Polyurethanes in Biomedical Applications

MICHAEL SZYCHER AND VICTOR POIRIER
Thermedics, Inc.
Woburn, MA

ABSTRACT

Tecoflex polyurethanes are high-performance polymers that exhibit the elastic properties of crosslinked rubbers, yet are truly melt-processable thermoplastics. This family of biomedical-grade polymers can be molecularly varied to produce a range of products from soft and flexible to hard and rigid. Since all Tecoflex grades are thermoplastics, they can be extruded into tubing or film, injection or compression molded into fabricated items, or solution spun into elastic monofilaments. This unusual combination of properties makes them valuable in critical biomedical applications such as artificial hearts, cardiovascular catheters, pacemaker lead insulation, etc.

INTRODUCTION

POLYURETHANE MACROMOLECULES—PLASTICS and elastomers—are not only useful as consumer products, but also function as life-sustaining components and diagnostic devices. The artificial heart may be today's most dramatic example of polyurethanes in medical applications, but other segments of the medical industry are equally dependent on biomedical-grade polyurethanes, such as pacemaker lead insulation, diagnostic and therapeutic catheters, as well as an array of implantable devices.

But the body's acceptance of polymeric materials is highly complex:

Reprinted from *SAMPE Journal,* July/August 1984, courtesy of Society for the Advancement of Materials and Process Engineering, Covina, CA U.S.A.

it treats most materials like foreign invaders. Therefore, polymers must be "biocompatible," that is, implant biomaterials must have good tissue compatibility, adequate attachment to tissue where required, and have good thromboresistance (resistance to clotting).

One of the most crucial requirements in medical applications is the need to develop biomaterials which are compatible with blood. Fortunately, the unique molecular architecture of Tecoflex makes the surface of this material appear innocuous to living organisms, thus circumventing blood clotting, or adverse immunologic responses that may be inimical to life.

This paper reviews the history of the artificial heart, and the search for a biomaterial capable of reliably flexing over 400 million times, or the equivalent of ten year's pumping. In addition, this communication also focuses on the crucial role played by the polyurethanes, since these elastomers are among the few biomaterials capable of surpassing the dual requirements of blood compatibility and long-term flexure endurance, necessary for the successful clinical use of artificial hearts.

DEVELOPMENT OF THE ARTIFICIAL HEART

Heart and cardiovascular disease accounts for approximately 750,000 deaths in the United States annually, as well as the permanent disabling of millions of other individuals. Despite strong efforts aimed at the prevention of disease, many people continue to face certain death. Dramatic advances in drugs, surgery and mechanical intervention have helped alleviate some of the complications of cardiovascular disease; however, patients with end-stage disease are still subject to limited alternatives. One alternative is heart transplantation, which has limited application because of the immunological rejection phenomenon; should immunologic rejection be circumvented within the coming years, there would still remain a decided lack of healthy donor hearts, since most are available as a result of accidents. It is estimated that only 1500 to 2000 biologic hearts are available for transplant each year for 60,000 potential patients who need them. Obviously, the most viable alternative would be permanently-implantable artificial hearts, which are needed to fill the gap.

Recognizing the desirability of artificial hearts, the National Heart, Lung and Blood Institute (NHLBI), Department of Health, Education and Welfare, established a program for the development of an artificial heart in 1964. An organized effort was initiated to develop implantable artificial heart devices to meet discreet clinical needs in the treatment of heart disease. This planned development ranged from devices for temporary mechanical circulatory assistance to those for total permanent cardiac replacement.

Such expectation had a sound physiological basis; of all major organs of the body, the heart performs only one function—pumping of blood. All other major organs perform a variety of metabolic and endocrine activities. By contrast, the heart can be viewed as strictly a fluid-moving device. Conceptually, an impaired natural heart could be replaced by a totally artificial device, if some major problems could be overcome.

Among the problems to be resolved were the manufacture of devices small enough to fit the anatomical constraints of the human thorax, the development of control consoles capable of anticipating cardiac cycle, the manufacture of a prosthesis that is not only reliable and durable, but also capable of overcoming the body's immunologic response mechanism and tendency to clot blood at the mere surface contact with any substance deemed alien to itself.

Because death and disability from heart disease are most commonly due to the pumping inadequacy of an infarcted left ventricle, with the remainder of the heart providing adequate function, an effective tem-

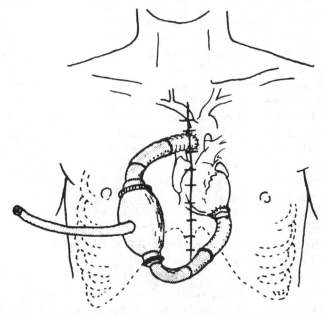

FIGURE 1. Thermedics' temporary Left Ventricular Device is implanted in parallel between the left ventricle and the ascending aorta. In this fashion, the artificial heart provides mechanical support to the failing left ventricle, allowing the natural heart to rest and regain strength.

porary left ventricular assist device was considered a major priority at Thermedics. The goal was to develop a single Left Ventricular Assist Device (LVAD) for short-term use. Eight years ago, development of this device was completed, and we began implanting LVADs in critically ill patients for whom all accepted medical procedures had been exhibited. The LVADs were implanted between the left ventricular apex, and the ascending aorta, as shown in Figure 1.

The LVADs were implanted to take over all left ventricular work, allowing the natural heart to rest and regain strength. Over the last series of patients—people who otherwise would have died—almost half regained pumping function and survived varying lengths of time. One man, now in his mid-sixties, is alive five years later because of this device.

The pump is connected between the apex of the left ventricle and the ascending aorta. This arrangement facilitates unloading of the left ventricle, making it a passive rather than active pumping chamber. Briefly, oxygenated blood from the lungs is collected in the left atrium and allowed to flow through the mitral valve into the left ventricle during diastole (the period when the heart is not ejecting). When the LVAD is connected, the left ventricle will not eject in the normal manner through the aortic valve into the arterial system, but will preferentially pass blood into the LVAD, which represents a relatively low resistance collecting chamber. The LVAD is then activated to eject the blood into the aorta. Thus, the left ventricle is relieved of most of the work of pumping and is able to "rest."

For the longer term, Thermedics is developing and testing in animals an implantable, electrically driven artificial heart system powered by an external battery belt, intended for long-term use in critically ill patients with irreversibly damaged natural hearts. For this next phase, a permanently implantable, fully ambulatory Ventricular Assist Device (VAD) is being developed. This new system, shown in Figure 2, will address a larger population of cardiac patients.

We are following a plan whose end goal is the development, and clinical application, of artificial heart devices that will not require large external support systems and, thus restore cardiac patients to a high quality of life. Over the past 17 years, our laboratories have progressed from pneumatically powered temporary assist devices to electrically driven heart pumps that can be powered by miniature portable battery packs and will not require a noisy, external support console.

The most important requirement for a long-term system is that the implant allow the patient a high quality of life. In order that the patient is able to move freely and lead as near normal life as possible,

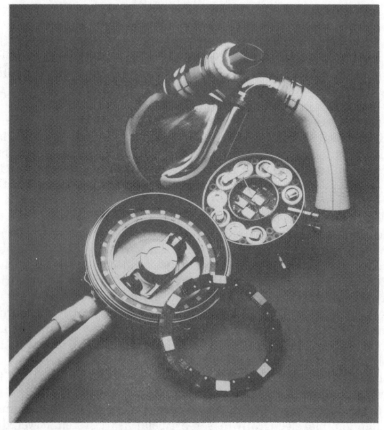

FIGURE 2. Components of Thermedics' artificial heart include: the pump housing, the internal battery pack, the low-speed torque motor, and the five-layer printed circuit board (containing the electronic modules) which controls the beat rate of the artificial heart.

the system must be self-contained and miniaturized. Microelectronics allow that to happen.

Thermedics does not plan to remove the natural heart, but rather to implant the artificial heart to work in synchrony with the natural heart. This is because the natural heart is part of a sophisticated feedback control system to regulate blood pressure. If, for example, a person runs up a flight of stairs, the heart increases the blood flow to support the increased effort. By attaching the artificial heart in parallel to the natural, we are able to take advantage of that feedback mechanism. The natural heart is also there as a back-up, so that the patient will not necessarily die in the event of failure of the artificial system. And there is a psychological advantage to the patient in retaining the natural heart because the patient perceives the artificial heart as merely assisting his own heart.

The development, and clinical testing of artificial hearts, we made possible by the use of a space-age polymer, the polyurethane elastomers. These versatile polymers have been fabricated into artificial heart bladders and continually flexed in our mock circulatory loops, with the oldest bladders now exceeding 500 million flexes, the equivalent of more than 12.5 years of continuous pumping. The story of these remarkable polymers is discussed in the next paragraph.

HIGH PERFORMANCE TECOFLEX POLYURETHANES

One of the most crucial requirements since the inception of the artificial heart program has been the need to develop biomaterials specific to chronic implantation. Major problems include the propensity for thrombus formation at the blood-materials interface, long-term flexing reliability, and the tendency of the body to reject foreign objects.

Fortunately, some synthetic polymers can be designed to appear innocuous to living organisms, thus circumventing any adverse immunologic response that may be inimical to life. Flexing surfaces necessary in most pump designs present special problems since the flexing characteristics of the polymer must be outstanding to survive 42 million flexes per year; this requirement, coupled to nonthrombogenicity, introduces a secondary level of complexity. Polymers intended for cardiac implantations lasting for ten years must reliably flex over 400 million times, a requirement that extends beyond the capability of most biomaterials.

In 1979, a second-generation biomedical-grade thermoplastic polyurethane elastomer was introduced by Szycher and collaborators. This polyurethane, trade named Tecoflex, is considered a second-generation elastomer, since it is an aliphatic polymer. Aliphatic polyurethanes represent a substantial advance over older, more conventional aromatic polyurethanes, since the aliphatic polyurethanes do not yellow upon exposure to ultraviolet (UV) light, and do not decompose to form carcinogenic byproducts, such as 4,4'-methylene dianiline (MDA).

Tecoflex polyurethane elastomers are rubbery reaction products of organic isocyanates, high molecular weight polyols, and low molecular weight chain extenders. The products are the condensation reaction between a reactive moiety, the isocyanate, and compounds containing active hydrogen sites, such as hydroxyl and amine groups. Typically, the reaction proceeds in two sequential steps. In step one, the iso-

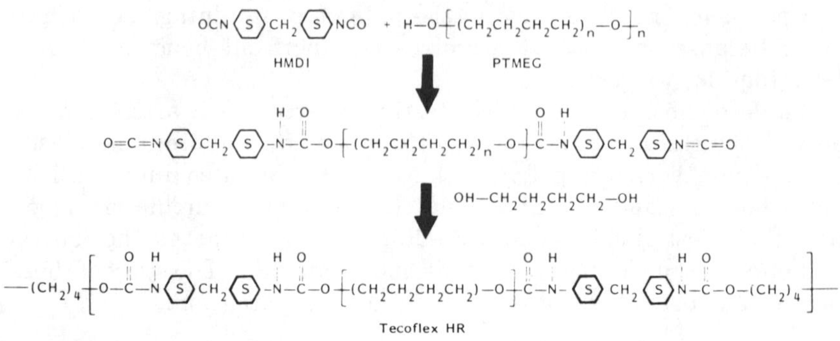

FIGURE 3. Macromolecular synthesis of Tecoflex. Ingredients are reacted in step-wise fashion to produce regularly repeating segments of soft and hard regions.

cyanate is prereacted with a high molecular weight polyol to form a "prepolymer." In step two, the chain extender, or curative, is added to the prepolymer, resulting in rubbery, thermoplastic polyurethane polymers exhibiting the elastic propeties of crosslinked rubbers. The reaction sequence is shown in Figure 3. Tecoflex thermoplastic polyurethane elastomers consist of essentially linear primary polymer chains. The structure of these primary chains comprise a preponderance of relatively long, flexible "soft" chain segments which have been joined end-to-end by rigid "hard" chain segments through covalent chemical bonds. The soft segments are diisocyanate-coupled, low-melting polyether chains. The soft segments include single diurethane bridges resulting when a diisocyanate molecule couples two polyether molecules, soft segments formed by the reaction of diisocyanate with the small glycol chain extended component.

The polar nature of the recurring rigid, hard, urethane chain segments results in their strong mutual attraction, aggregation, and ordering into crystalline and paracrystalline domains in the mobile polymer matrix. The abundance of urethane hydrogen atoms, as well as carbonyl and ether oxygen partners in polyurethane systems, permits extensive hydrogen bonding among the polymer chains. This hydrogen bonding apparently restricts the mobility of the polyurethane chain segments in the domains and thus their ability to organize extensively into crystalline lattices. As a consequence, semi-ordered regions result, which are described as "paracrystalline." Association of the electrons of the polymer structures represents another binding forces. The more weakly attractive van der Waals forces are also operative in all parts of the polymer chains. The polymer chains are long enough to get entangled in each other.

The lateral effect of all the foregoing states and forces, particularly paracrystallinity and hydrogen bonding, is to tie together or "virtually cross-link" the linear primary polyurethane chains. That is, the primary polyurethane chains are cross-linked in effect, but not in fact. Concurrently, of course, the virtual linkages also lengthen the primary polyurethane chains. The overall consequence is a labile infinite network of polymer chains which displays the superficial properties of a strong rubbery vulcanizate over a practical range of use temperatures.

Virtual cross-linking is a phenomenon that is reversible with heat and, depending upon polymer composition, with solvation, offering many attractive processing alternatives for thermoplastic polyurethanes. Thermal energy great enough to (reversibly) break virtual cross-links, but too low to appreciably disrupt the stronger covalent chemical bonds that link the atoms in the primary polymer chains, can be applied to extrude or mold the polymers, and a solvent which solvates the polymer chains, reversibly insulating the virtual cross-links, carries the primary polymer chains into solution separate and intact for such application as coating or scientific study.

CONCLUSIONS

Tecoflex biomedical-grade elastomers are currently being evaluated in many critical clinical applications such as diagnostic and therapeutic catheters, interventional radiology, cardiac pacemaker insulation leads, and intravenous catheters. Polyurethane elastomers are seen as the polymer candidate of choice in these clinical applications because of their hemocompatibility, flexure endurance, high strength, and processing versatility.

At Thermedics, we have been developing a family of novel, biomedical-grade, cycloaliphatic-based thermoplastic polyurethane elastomers. The cycloaphatic nature of these second-generation elastomers precludes the thermodydrolytic formation of MDA (a carcinogen) during steam sterilization. The processing versatility of this family of polymers makes them particularly suitable for a wide variety of existing or new medical products. The combination of purity, strength, and processability make these new thermoplastic elastomers particularly amenable to medical devices which must interact chronically in a highly corrosive environment such as the human body.

Tecoflex polyurethanes have been proven non toxic, and when in direct contact with circulating blood, its unique molecular structure enables it to preferentially adsorb albumin, a natural circulating serum protein. This feature results in passivation of the Tecoflex surface to prevent undesirable blood clotting. Commercial quantities of Tecoflex have been supplied to major device manufacturers to satisfy variety of special medical products requirements.

Artificial Skin: A Fifth Route to Organ Repair and Replacement

I. V. YANNAS
Professor of Polymer Science and Engineering
Massachusetts Institute of Technology
Cambridge, MA 02139

D. P. ORGILL
Massachusetts Institute of Technology

INTRODUCTION

THE DESIGN OF biomaterials has relied extensively, and with considerable success, on the concept of the inert and permanent prosthesis. Ideally, the latter is a device which replaces a diseased or damaged tissue or organ and restores physiological function over the lifetime of the patient without altering the structure and function of tissues adjacent to it and without itself undergoing changes in structure or function. This concept has motivated a great deal of interdisciplinary research, some of it ingenious, which has led to the design of several useful prostheses.

An alternative approach to the design of biomaterials, which is much less used, puts aside the twin requirements of biological inertness and engineering permanence. This approach focuses instead on the controlled interaction between the biomaterials device and host tissue. It aims toward regeneration of the damaged or diseased tissue and the simultaneous metabolic disposal of the device. We shall refer to such a device as a biodegradable regeneration template.

The current surgical treatment of the patient who has suffered deep and extensive burns is prompt closure of wounds, after thorough exci-

Presented at ANTEC '85, The Society of Plastics Engineers, Inc. 43rd Annual Technical Conference, April 29–May 2, Washington, D.C., U.S.A.

119

sion of necrotic tissue, in order to control two life-threatening processes, i.e. extensive fluid loss and massive bacterial infection. A further essential requirement, control of scar formation, is rarely life threatening in a direct way but it frequently leads to physchological devastation of the massively disfigured individual and limits dramatically the individual's ability to function in society.

Currently, large excised wounds are treated with the split-thickness autograft. Although other approaches have been used (see Discussion), the autograft usually performs in a very satisfactory way by adequately controlling fluid loss and infection.

The autograft is often unavailable for prompt use, however, as happens with patients who have suffered deep burns over a substantial fraction of the body surface area. In addition the process of harvesting it from a previously intact donor site leaves the latter scarred. Furthermore, the surgical operation involved in harvesting the autograft is a serious one, normally requiring support services such as a blood bank.

The biomaterials device described here competes well with the autograft. It is a bilayer polymeric membrane which promptly closes skin wounds in animals and humans and simultaneously serves as a template for the construction of a functional extension of the skin. The top layer of the membrane is a silicone elastomer while the bottom layer is a highly porous, covalently cross-linked network of bovine hide collagen and glycosaminoglycan (GAG) (Figure 1). We have achieved reproducible conditions under which autologous epidermal cells, seeded onto the membrane before grafting, synthesize mature neoepidermal tissue *in vivo* while mesenchymal cells from the wound bed synthesize a neodermal tissue that differs from conventional scar tissue. Whereas the silicone layer is eventually ejected spontaneously or removed nontraumatically and is recovered intact, the collagen-GAG layer is biodegraded within 4 weeks or less and is replaced by neoepidermal and neodermal tissue. These conditions are obtained by controlling several physicochemical and biological parameters of the bottom layer, including the average molecular weight between covalent crosslinks, the ratio of collagen to GAG, the pore structure, the intensity of banding of collagen fibers and the density of autologous epidermal cells seeded before grafting.

Our 11-year design effort has developed in two stages. Stage 1 is a non-cellular, aseptic polymeric membrane capable of being produced in large quantities and of being stored over indefinite periods of time. When grafted on deep wounds without any additional manipulation Stage 1 membranes have been shown to reliably protect animals and humans from fluid loss and infection. Stage 1 membranes do not pre-

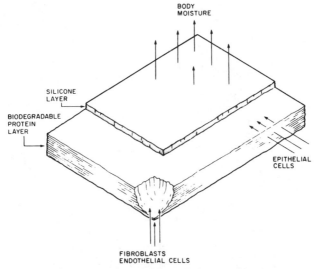

FIGURE 1. Structure of Bilayer Polymeric Membrane.

vent scar formation unless the silicone layer is eventually replaced with a thin autoepidermal graft. Stage 2 membranes, prepared by seeding Stage 1 membranes prior to grafting with a small number of autologous epidermal cells, promptly control fluid loss and infection equally well but, in addition, reduce contraction and scar formation without need for subsequent manipulations, such as harvesting auto-epidermal grafts.

In this paper we review briefly the biomaterials design principles which were relied upon in our effort. We then summarize in very condensed form selected experimental results of animal and human studies with Stage 1 and Stage 2 membranes. Emphasis is placed on presentation of recent results obtained wth Stage 2 membranes. A detailed presentation of our experimental procedures and results of our ongoing 11-year effort is currently being published in *Journal of Biomedical Materials Research* [4,6,7].

BRIEF SUMMARY OF DESIGN PRINCIPLES

A detailed discussion of the physicochemical aspects of wounds closure by appears elsewhere [1]. Briefly, it is essential to achieve intimate physicochemical contact between graft and wound bed in order to prevent proliferation of bacteria in microscopic air pockets at the graft-wound bed interface. Achievement of efficient wetting requires use of a

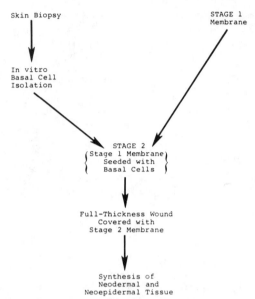

FIGURE 2. Iterative design of a non-cellular two layer polymeric membrane.

membrane with sufficiently low flexural rigidity and critical surface energy. Maintenance of the graft-wound bed bond is achieved by migration of mesenchymal cells from the wound bed into the graft and early synthesis of connective tissue, the latter acting as a "biological adhesive" at the graft-wound interface. Control of moisture flux through the graft is also an indispensable prerequisite for maintenance of a strong bond between graft and wound bed [1].

These essential requirements have been met by iterative design of a non-cellular two-layer polymeric membrane which is referred to here as Stage 1 (Figure 1). The top layer is a moisture-curing silicone elastomer while the bottom layer is a highly porous covalently crosslinked network of purified bovine hide collagen and chondroitin 6-sulfate [2,3] which may optionally be seeded with autologous epidermal cells (Figure 2). Functionally, the top layer imparts mechanical strength to the graft, prevents bacterial entry into the wound, and controls the moisture flux; it remains intact and is eventually ejected as a result of neoepidermal tissue synthesis or is peeled off nontraumatically by the surgeon at a time of election. The bottom layer is, however, enzymatically degradable and acts as a tissue support medium utilized by the wound bed to construct neodermal tissue (Stage 1) or neoepidermal as well as neodermal tissue (Stage 2). The rate of enzymatic degradation of the bottom layer must be controlled [4,5] to match approximately the rate of neodermal tissue synthesis [4]. The volume fraction of pores is controlled to exceed 96% while the mean pore size exceeds 50 μm. Failure to meet each of these requirements results in grafts which do not control infection adequately and do not lead to neodermal tissue synthesis.

The limiting dimensions of the graft need to be considered with respect to the migration rate of mesenchymal cells (originating in the wound bed) through the thickness direction and of epithelial cells (originating at the wound edge) along the plane of the membrane. For example, endothelial cells and fibroblasts migrate at rates of about 0.4 mm/day and 0.2 mm/day, respectively. We find that a 0.5-mm thick collagen-GAG layer is populated by these mesenchymal cells within 2 to 5 days following grafting.

At approximate observed speeds of 0.25 mm/day, epidermal cells, advancing from opposite wound edges in the plane of the membrane, between the collagen-GAG and silicone elastomer layers (Figure 1), typically close a 1.5-cm wound gap in guinea pigs within about 30 days, a period roughly equal to an optimal biodegradation time constant [4]. However, the very large wounds which are seen with patients who have suffered extensive burns often exceed 30 cm. Coverage of such large wounds by epidermal cell sheets advancing from the wound edges would require a period of time too long to be clinically acceptable.

We have approached the problem of epithelialization of large wounds in two ways. In one approach [6], which has been used with over 50 patients who had sustained massive third-degree burns, the burned area was originally excised down to viable tissue and grafted with Stage 1 membranes. At a time of election, up to 46 days, the silicone layer was peeled off nontraumatically, exposing a newly synthesized layer of neodermal tissue. The exposed neodermal tissue was then covered with a thin layer of autoepidermal tissue, harvested with a dermatome. The layer of autoepidermal tissue was sufficiently thin to prevent scar formation at the donor site (Figure 2).

Another approach, which has been used so far only in our work with animals (Stage 2), involves seeding of the porous collagen-GAG layer of the polymeric membrane prior to grafting with a small quantity of uncultured autologous epidermal (basal) cells. Following grafting of the wound with the seeded membrane, these cells have been shown to proliferate at the interface of the two layers of the membrane, forming sheets of mature keratinized neoepidermis within less than 14 days following grafting. Seeding of a properly constructed collagen/GAG layer appears to overcome the limitation of the size of wound which can effectively be treated. This design is a distinct improvement over Stage 1 since it overcomes the current need for eventual harvesting an auto-epidermal graft in the treatment of large wounds. Quite importantly, Stage 2 membranes reduce the wound closure time from greater than 20 days to less than 14 days.

ANIMAL SKIN GRAFTING WITH STAGE 1 MEMBRANES

Three major structural parameters of the collagen/GAG layer have been placed under control. The bound GAG content of the collagen/GAG network, determined by hexosamine assay [2], was controlled by adjustment of reaction conditions during the high temperature treat-ment step under vacuum (following freeze drying), and by adjustment of the conditions during treatment in a glutaraldehyde bath [2]. Cur-rently used Stage 1 membranes have a bound GAG content of 8.2 ± 0.8%-wt. The average molecular weight between crosslinks, $\bar{M}_c$, partly controls the biodegradation time constant; the latter can be deter-mined by use of a collagenase assy [7]. *In vitro* data have been empir-ically correlated with animal data [5], and a preliminary relation between $\bar{M}_c$ and fractional weight loss of subcutaneous implants has been obtained [5]. Currently, M_c of the collagen-GAG layer, calculated from the tensile modulus measured under conditions of ideal rubber elastic behavior [2], is 13,000 ± 3500. The pore volume fraction of the freeze dried membranes is higher than 0.96 and mean pore size is 150 ± 30 μm; both values have been determined by application of quantitative stereological procedures to scanning electron photomicro-graphs of the freeze-dried collagen-GAG layer [3]. The pore structure has been controlled by use of a freeze-drying process which was devel-oped following a detailed comparative study of other dehydration proce-dures [3]. Bilayer membranes currently in use have Young's moduli in the range 7–40 × 10^4 N/m^2 while moisture permeability ranges be-tween 1 and 10 mg/cm^2/hr (values obtained in the hydrated state) [8].

Although the above-mentioned physicochemical characteristics have been arrived at after considerable experimentation we wish to empha-size that additional studies, currently ongoing, may dictate modifica-tion in the level of these variables.

Full-thickness wounds closed with Stage 1 membranes remained free of infection and exudation. Histological studies showed extensive cel-lular migration inside the graft. No evidence of inflammation in the area of the wound was observed after about 4 days following excision and grafting. There was no gross indication of rejection, neither was any histological evidence of an immunogenic response detected over

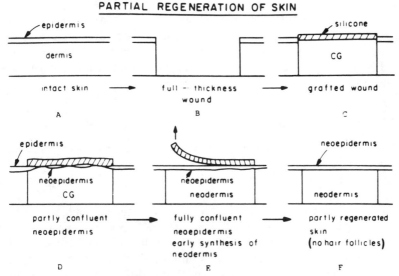

FIGURE 3. Partial regeneration of skin.

more than 30 days of observation following grafting. Lymphocytes were almost never observed. There was also no tissue necrosis nor was there thrombosis or alterations in vascular histological characteristics. By comparison, homografts were usually rejected by the animals between 9 and 14 days after grafting.

Wounds covered with Stage 1 membranes did not begin contracting until 10 ± 30 days in the animals with grafts. Autografts showed much less contraction (Figure 3).

Peeling of Stage 1 membranes at a 90° angle was resisted by forced as high as 4 N/m (4 g/cm) just 6 hrs after grafting with Stage 1 membranes, increasing to about 45 N/m (45 g/cm) favorably with the force that peels off conventional adhesive tape from itself. This was followed by a decay to zero peeling strength at the time of confluence by epidermal cell sheets (see below), which occurred between 30 and 40 days with these wounds. Low magnification study of the graft-wound interface following partial peeling showed copious tissue synthesis [8].

Extensive histologic observations show that the neodermis formed when either optimally designed Stage 1 or Stage 2 membranes are used is a well vascularized matrix comprising collagen fibers which appear to posses morphological characteristics similar to those of physiological dermis, rather than of scar tissue. The tissue interface between host and graft, is clearly elicited by use of polarized optical microscopy and by electron microscopic study of histological sections. When the design parameters are kept within certain limits the interface comprises loose strands of collagen fibers rather than a layer of well-packed fibers characteristic of fibrous scarring. Extensive control studies [5], suggest that at least 80% of the original collagen-GAG layer undergoes degradation within 3–4 weeks.

HUMAN SKIN GRAFTING WITH STAGE 1 MEMBRANES

Following primary excision of dead tissue, 49 burn victims received Stage 1 membranes as large as 15 × 25 cm [6]. Results with an initial group of ten patients are reported in detail in [6]. After being placed on the wound bed, the grafts were carefully sutured under a slight tension, avoiding wrinkling of the thin membrane. The subjects, 3 to 87 year-old males and females, with total third-degree burn size 50 to 90% body surface area, received Stage 1 grafts over 15 to 60% body surface area. No immunosuppression was employed. "Take" of Stage 1 membranes on the excised wound bed was 95 to 100%, providing continuous physiological closure without infection or rejection. Whenever the graft was next to intact epidermis the epidermal edge migrated between the two layers of the membrane over the distance of a few millimeters. Between 14 and 46 days later the silicone layer was removed from the vascularized neodermal tissue and the wound was closed with a thin autoepidermal graft (0.1 mm). "Take" of autoepidermis on the neodermis was 85 to 95%. Neither the donor site nor the grafted area showed significant contraction or scarring following such treatment. By comparison, following removal of split-thickness autografts (0.25–0.375 mm), which grafts include a fraction of the dermis in the conventional harvesting procedure, the donor sites are usually significantly scarred. The follow-up in this study ranged from 2 to over 16 months [6].

Histologic findings obtained by light and fluorescent microscopy showed a very favorable response of human host tissue to the collagen– GAG layer. Vascularized connective tissue tufts were shown to have grown into spaces of this layer and in 1–2 weeks the occupation of the lower layer of the graft by newly formed tissue appeared complete. Immunofluorescent microscopic findings confirmed the presence of basement membrane collagen in quantitative which were consistent with the presence of high levels of vasculature. The zone of transition from the normal host muscle or fat to the implanted collagen-GAG layer generally consisted only of several fibrous strands and was not characteristic of fibrous scarring. In a few cases thickened zones indicative of scarring were observed. The latter may be attributed to healing in the host bed of a wound partially damaged by burn, in which damaged tissue was incompletely excised [6].

STAGE 2 MEMBRANES: SKIN REGENERATION IN ANIMALS

After *in vivo* seeding with uncultured autologous basal cells, Stage 2 membranes were grafted onto full-thickness skin wounds. In the sterile environment of the wound closure, the basal cells reached confluence within 10–14 days and layers of keratinizing epidermal tissue became evident in the polarizing stage of the optical microscope at about the same time [8,9].

Repeated observations have left no doubt that the neoepidermal sheet nucleates and grows from the basal cells seeds rather than originating at the wound edge. Furthermore, there is no doubt that keratinization of such neoepidermal sheet over the entire wound area has progressed significantly before the 14th day.

Histologic studies of the interface between host tissue and Stage 2 grafts show a close similarity to the findings obtained with Stage 1 grafts. Well-vascularized connective tissue which resembles dermis eventually replaces the collagen-GAG layer in less than about 4 weeks. Collagen fiber bundles possess morphology which resembles that of physiological dermis and does not resemble scar [8,9].

The most striking long-term difference between the performance of Stage 1 and Stage 2 membranes is the gross appearance of the healed wound two months following grafting. The rectangular wound area grafted with a Stage 1 membrane was reduced to a linear scar as a result of strong contraction of wound edges. By contrast, grafting with Stage 2 membranes gave results which were quite similar, though not identical, to those obtained following grafting with unmeshed full-thickness autograft. Four months following grafting with Stage 2 membranes, the wound area was reduced to about 75% of the original excised area, compared to about 105% for the autograft (Figure 3). The perimeter of the wounds grafted with Stage 2 membranes consisted of scar tissue as did also the perimeter of wounds covered with autograft. The tissue inside the perimeter was clearly not scar and had almost identical appearance both with Stage 2 grafts and with autografts. Both were soft and extensible, were well vascularized and responded well to touch. Histologically, the tissue inside the wound perimeter was clearly not scar and appeared indistinguishable from intact guinea pig skin except for the absence of hair follicles. (The long-term area value reported for ungrafted wounds and for wounds grafted with Stage 1 membranes is about 25%) (Figure 2). This value corresponds to the area

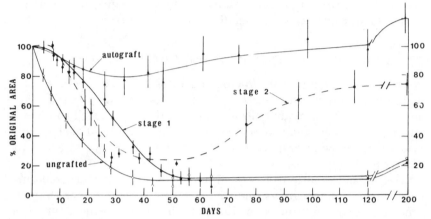

FIGURE 4. Kinetics of contraction of wounds grafted with stage 2 membranes.

occupied by scarred tissue between tattoo marks placed at the wound edge prior to inflicting the wounds.

There seems to be little doubt that two months after being grafted on full-thickness wounds, the collagen/GAG layer of Stage 2 membranes which has been seeded with basal cells has been replaced by new integument, comprising both a neoepidermal and a neodermal layer but lacking hair follicles.

The kinetics of contraction of wounds grafted with Stage 2 membranes have reproducibly (10 animals) followed a somewhat complex path (Figure 4). After a significant contraction of the wound area by day 30, the grafted wounds increased slowly but unmistakeably in size until, by day 120, the wound area approached 75% of the original (Figure 4).

Preliminary studies of the effect of viable epidermal cell density (seed cells) on the healing parameters showed that approximately 3×10^6 viable cells could be readily isolated from each cm^2 of skin biopsy. The viable cell density was adjusted so that 5×10^4 to 5×10^5 cells per cm^2 were seeded into the graft by the centrifugation method which we developed [9]. An area expansion factor of $6\times$ was thereby obtained when cells were seeded at $5 \times 10^5/cm^2$ and an expansion factor of $60\times$ was obtained at a seed density of $5 \times 10^4/cm^2$. We find, however, that whereas increasing the cell density about $5 \times 10^5/cm^2$ does not significantly affect the time, 10–14 days, normally required for wound closure by formation of a confluent neoepidermis, reduction of cell density to $5 \times 10^4/cm^2$ increases the closure time to approximately 21 days.

A preliminary comparison of properties of newly synthesized (regenerated) skin and intact (normal) skin shows several close similarities. However, differences are also apparent, striking among them being the absence of skin accessory organs, including hair (the guinea pigs have no sweat glands) (Figures 5, 6A, 6B).

DISCUSSION

Current treatment of patients who have suffered extensive skin loss emphasis fluid resuscitation and prompt closure of wounds with autografts, cadaver skin, or pig skin following the excision of dead tissue [10]. Failure to achieve closure of massive burn wounds within 3 to 7 days after injury significantly increases the probability that the patient will die [10].

Autografts provide prompt wound closure and leave minimal scarring. However, the patient's intact skin is often in short supply, and the operation to obtain it is undesirable. Homografts, obtained from cadavers and used immediately or after preservation in a skin bank [11] are also in short supply and, unless immunosuppressive agents are used, commonly are rejected early. However, the use of immunosup-

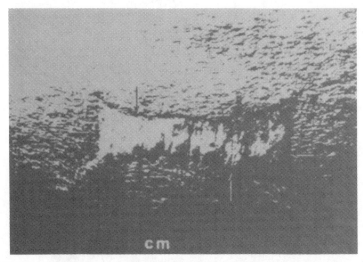

FIGURE 5. A rectangular segment of regenerated guinea pig skin (perimeter marked by arrows) surrounded by intact, partly shaven skin. Original size of excised, full-thickness wound, 3 × 1.5 cm.

pressive agents increases the risk of infection. Heterografts, obtained
from animals, especially pigs, are available commercially and are
widely used to achieve short-term wound closure. Normally they are
removed between the third and ninth day following application. A
number of natural and synthetic polymer membranes have been
employed in the treatment of burns but their use has not reliably
prevented infection [1]. A temporary skin dressing based on synthetic
polymers and peptides derived from collagen has been compared

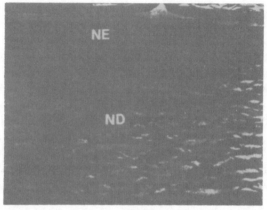

FIGURE 6A. Histological section of new skin. NE, Neoepidermis; ND, Neodermis, Mag.
275×.

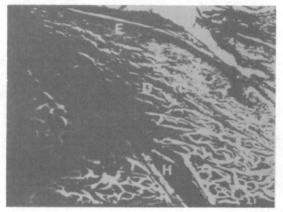

FIGURE 6B. Histological section of intact dermis. E, epidermis; D, dermis; H, hair fol-
licle. Mag. 275×.

favorably with human homograft and porcine heterograft, especially in covering graft donor sites; however, it requires removal about 7–10 days after application [12]. Recently, a culture of autologous epidermal cells was grafted into full thickness skin wounds in humans 5 weeks after harvesting [13]. A reconstituted collagen lattice populated by cultured autologous fibroblasts and epidermal cells has been grafted on rats at least 2 weeks after harvesting [14]. The latter two procedures require lengthy in vitro culturing of tissue prior to grafting.

By contrast with temporary dressings, where the obligatory removal exposes the wound bed once more to the risk of infection, Stage 1 membranes provide closure of full-thickness wounds in animals and humans without requiring eventual removal. This is achieved by synthesis of a stable well-vascularized neodermis in the aseptic environment provided by the silicone layer. Although the latter is eventually ejected spontaneously (small counts) or removed at a time of election (large wounds), the neodermis is not removed, but covered with thin autoepidermal grafts providing continuous physiological wound closure.

Efforts to prepare a long-term wound closure by culturing skin grafts *in vitro* [13,14], have shown great promise but they require use of dressings that must be eventually removed to be replaced by the cultured tissue. By contrast, Stage 2 membranes are designed to act as templates for synthesis of skin in vivo, making prompt and deliberate use of the host's wound tissue as an organ culture medium [9].

Human studies conducted over the past 2 years confirm and extend results from animal studies. They show conclusively that Stage 1 membranes are superior to cadaver and porcine skin grafts. When Stage 1 membranes are eventually covered with thin (0.1 mm) autoepidermal grafts, these membranes equal the split-thickness (0.25−0.4 mm) autograft in clinical performance at the graft size without generating a scarred donor site, as normally occurs after harvesting a split-thickness autograft [6].

Although not yet studied with human subjects, Stage 2 membranes provide a means for closing the largest full-thickness wounds without requiring use of autologous epidermal grafts, as is currently practiced when human subjects are grafted with Stage 1 membranes. This significant simplication in clinical procedure is achieved by seeding the membrane with a small number of cells from a skin biopsy before grafting. A neoepidermis is thereby generated in vivo inside the sterile environment of the bilayer membrane. In addition, autoepithelial wound closure is reduced from about 20 days, attainable with Stage 1 membranes, to less than 14 days.

Table 1. Comparison of new skin to intact skin in the guinea pig.

Property	Intact Skin	New Skin
Moisture permeability, in vivo, gm/cm/h[a]	4.5 ± 0.8	4.7 ± 1.0
Mechanical properties, In vitro tensile strength, Pa	31×10^6	14×10^6
Second derivative of stress-strain curve	+	+
Histological studies[b]		
Multilayered keratinizing epidermis	+	+
Intact dermal-epidermal junction	+	+
Skin accessory organs (eg., hair)	+	−
Dermal vascularization	+	+
Collagen morphology	wavy	less wavy
Epidermal thickness, μm	20–40	30–40
Dermal thickness, mm	0.8–1.3	0.9–1.4
Neurological test (pin prick)[c]	+	+
Vascularization test (blanching)[d]	+	+
Color[e]	white	white

[a] Measured value remained invariant, within experimental error, between 1 and 10 months following grafting.
[b] Performed 10 months following grafting.
[c] Positive results obtained by day 21.
[d] Positive results obtained by day 14.
[e] Color changes in the graft were as follows: red up to about 2 months; pink to off-white about 2–5 months; white, after about 5 months.

An important and reproducible result of the cell-seeding modification which defines Stage 2 membranes is attainment of substantial control of wound contraction (Figure 3). Scar synthesis appears also to be reduced, in the sense that conventional scarring eventually forms only at the perimeter of the wound. Scarring appear to be reduced within the wound perimeter. It appears that Stage 2 membranes induce synthesis of new, nearly physiologic integument within the wound bed.

Preliminary characterization shows that newly synthesized skin is strikingly similar, though not identical, to intact skin (Table 1) (Figures 5, 6A, 6B). Ongoing studies are directed towards biochemical characterization of macromolecular components in new skin, detail morphological analysis and elucidation of the kinetics of synthesis of the new organ mass.

REFERENCES

1. I. V. Yannas and J. F. Burke, *J. Biomed. Mat. Res.*, *14*, 65 (1980)
2. I. V. Yannas, J. F. Burke, P. L. Gordon, C. Huang, and R. W. Rubenstein, *J. Biomed. Mat. Res.*, *14*, 107 (1980).
3. N. Dagalakis, J. Flink, P. Stasikelis, J. F. Burke, and I. V. Yannas, *J. Biomed. Mat. Res.*, *14*, 511 (1980).
4. I. V. Yannas, J. F. Burke, C. Huang, and P. L. Gordon, *Fed. Proc. Fed. Amer. Soc. Exp. Biol.*, *38*, 988 (1979)
5. I. V. Yannas, J. F. Burke, C. Huang, and P. L. Gordon, *J. Biomed. Mat. Res.*, *9*, 623 (1975).
6. J. F. Burke, I. V. Yannas, W. C. Quinby, Jr., C. C. Bondoc, and W. K. Jung, *Ann. Surg.*, *194*, 413 (1981).
7. C. Huang and I. V. Yannas, *J. Biomed. Mat. Res.*, *Symp.*, No. 8, 137 (1977).
8. I. V. Yannas, J. F. Burke, M. Warpehoski, P. Stasikelis, E. M. Skrabut, D. Orgill, and D. J. Giard, *Trans. Am. Soc. Artif. Intern. Organs*, *27*, 19 (1981).
8. I. V. Yannas, J. F. Burke, M. Warpehoski, P. Stasikelis, E. M. Skrabut, D. Orgill, and G. J. Giard, *Trans. Am. Soc. Artif. Intern. Organs*, *27*, 19 (1981).
9. I. V. Yannas, J. F. Burke, D. F. Orgill, and E. M. Skrabut, *Science*, *215*, 174 (1982).
10. G. T. Shires and E. A. Black, eds., "Consensus Development Conference," *J. Trauma*, *19*, 855 (1979).
11. C. C. Bondoc and J. F. Burke, *Ann. Surg.*, *158*, 371 (1971).
12. E. A. Woodroof, M. J. Travis, A. R. Grossman, and R. H. Bartlett, *Advances in Biomaterials*, *3*, Winter, G. D., Gibbons, D. F., and Plenk, H., eds., Wiley, UK, in press.
13. N. E. O'Connor, J. B. Mulliken, S. Banks-Schlegel, O. Dehinds, and H. Green, *Lancet*, *1981-I*, 75 (1981).
14. E. Bell, H. P. Ehrlich, E. J. Buttle, and T. Makatsuji, *Science*, *211*, 1052 (1981).

Synthesis and Properties of Biomedical Graft Copolymers

J. L. WILLIAMS

Becton Dickinson Research Center
P.O. Box 12016
Research Triangle Park, NC 27709

1. INTRODUCTION

BIOMEDICAL APPLICATIONS OF polymers generally require that the polymer possess both biocompatible properties as well as engineering properties [1–5]. The requirement of biocompatible properties of the material often negates the use of a plastic that otherwise has excellent physical and processing properties. Graft copolymerization is one method of polymer modification that can build additional properties into the polymer without totally eliminating the desirable properties of the parent polymer. Since graft copolymerization takes place through covalent bonds, the modification is permanent and a variety of properties can be influenced through the proper selection of monomers for graft copolymerization.

2. EXPERIMENTAL

Monomer purification was carried out by either vacuum distillation or by pouring the monomer through a column containing amberlite which specifically absorbs any inhibitors present in the monomer.

Mutual irradiation grafting experiments were carried out in glass ampules which had been fitted with O-ring glass joints through which the grafting solution could be introduced. After introduction of the monomer solution, the ampoule was thoroughly degassed using the

Presented at ANTEC '85, The Society of Plastics Engineers Inc. 43rd Annual Technical Conference, April 29–May 2, Washington, DC U.S.A.

"freeze–thaw" method. After degassing, the sample was sealed under vacuum and irradiated.

In the case of pre-irradiation grafting, a double-tube arrangement was used with the two tubes being separated by a glass breakseal. The sample was contained in one tube which could be separately degassed and irradiated. Following irradiation, the monomer was placed in the second tube and degassed as above and finally sealed. At this point, the internal breakseal was broken and the grafting solution was poured over onto the sample. The tube assembly was then placed in a thermostatted bath and the grafting reaction allowed to proceed.

Following grafting, the ampules were cracked open and the films were thoroughly washed in solvent and finally in water. The percent graft was taken as the weight increase following grafting expressed as a percentage.

The samples were placed beneath a slow running stream of water to determine their visual wettability.

A laboratory extruder (Mechanical Engineering Department, Duke University) which had been fitted with a crosshead die was used in experimental tube preparation. Briefly, the device was a three-quarter inch screw extruder employing a hollow mandril through which air could be introduced to prevent tube collapse.

The substrates used in this investigation have been polyethylene (PE), polypropylene (PP), microporous polypropylene (MPP), and microporous polyethylene (MPE).

3. RESULTS AND DISCUSSION

A. Mutual Irradiation Grafting

Successful mutual grafting experiments have been carried out with a number of monomers (vinyl derivatives) which yield hydrophilic polymers or, in this case, grafts. Some typical grafting time curves for dimethylaminoethylmethacrylate (DAM) are shown in Figure 1. Over the dose range studied, the grafting level increases almost linearly with irradiation dose. The differences in the grafting rates observed are mainly due to diffusional effects in that the microporous films are more accessible than the corresponding dense monofilament Vexar material. In this case, Vexar which has a very large filament diameter limits the grafting rate due to slow diffusion of monomer into the fiber. This does not mean, however, that suitable surface grafting has not taken place at the surface.

The three main substrates (MPP, MPE, and PE) used in this study

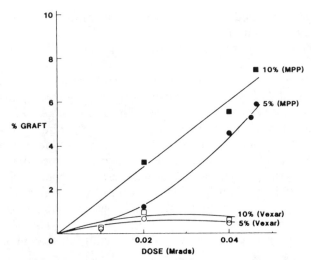

FIGURE 1. Concentration dependence of mutual irradiation grafting to Vexar and MPP in 5% and 10% DAM/10^{-2} MCuCl$_2$.

give similar overall grafting rates. In all mutual grafting cases with DAM, considerable solution gelation takes place beyond 0.05 Mrads. The use of copper chloride inhibits the polymerization in solution to a great extent but does not totally eliminate it at the higher irradiation doses.

The influence of monomer concentration on the grafting behavior for aqueous solutions of DAM is summarized in Figure 2. Clearly the grafting level continues to increase with higher monomer concentrations. Examination of the solutions for gel formation indicates that monomer concentrations below 30 percent are preferred to prevent excessive gel formation.

Several grafting experiments were carried out using comonomers of crotonic acid and vinyl acetate, and the results are presented in Figure 3. It is evident that the vinyl acetate grafts very rapidly in this system with a marked decrease in the grafting rate with increasing crotonic acid content. Samples grafted using 10 percent crotonic acid as the comonomer appear to have the best overall properties in terms of wettability and appearance.

B. Pre-irradiation Grafting

Considerable attention has been given to the possibilities of pre-irradiation grafting in the recent part of this study. This method offers at least two attractive advantages over the mutual technique. First,

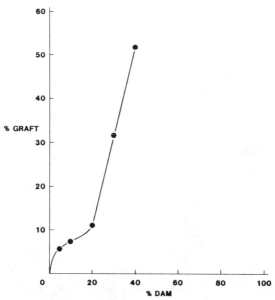

FIGURE 2. Effect of concentration on mutual irradiation grafted samples of MPP in DAM/10^{-2} MCuCl$_2$ at 0.01 Mrads/hr for 0.046 Mrads.

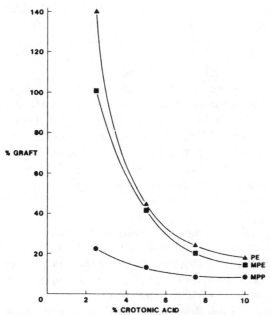

FIGURE 3. Effect of concentration of crotonic acid/vinyl acetate at 0.05 Mrads/hr for 1.04 Mrads.

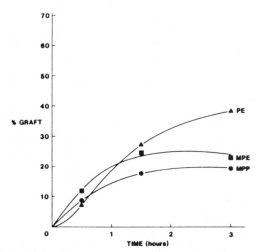

FIGURE 4. Pre-irradiation grafting in 50% DAM/50% MEOH at 40°C.

homopolymerization is minimized, thus, reducing not only monomer consumption but eliminating the need for exhaustive extraction of homopolymer. Secondly, the very nature of the method offers the possibility of having more growing chains at the substrate surface since there is no need for the inclusion of homopolymerization inhibitor in the grafting solution as required by the mutual technique for these highly radiation sensitive monomers.

Fortunately, the pre-irradiation technique appears to work quite well using aqueous solutions of DAM as shown in Figure 4. In fact, much higher grafting levels can be obtained using this system than found with the mutual method. This is not surprising in view of solution gelation which occurs using the mutual technique. As a general rule, however, the pre-irradiation method yields far lower grafting levels as compared to the mutual technique since radicals are not being continually generated during reaction which is true in the mutual method.

When methanol was used as a swelling agent instead of under otherwise identical conditions there was about a threefold overall decrease in grafting level. Examination of the grafting solutions following reaction reveals that they are very fluid therefore requiring only a moderate rinsing to remove residual monomer.

The influence of total dose on the grafting behavior for 100 percent DAM is depicted in Figures 5 and 6, for total doses of 2.5 and 6.8 Mrads,

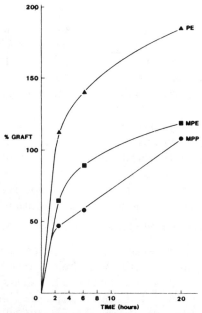

FIGURE 5. Pre-irradiation grafting in 100% DAM at 0.1 Mrads/hr for 2.5 Mrads at 40°C.

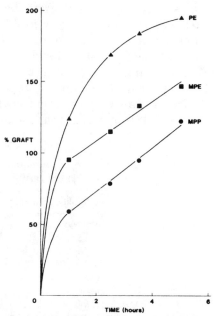

FIGURE 6. Pre-irradiation grafting in 100% DAM at 0.1 Mrads/hr for 6.8 Mrads at 40°C.

respectively. It is evident that there is a considerable increase in the rate of grafting between 2.5 and 6.8 Mrads. However, irradiation to 8.8 Mrads does not increase the grafting yields. This leveling tendency of grafting rate with dose is reasonable since it is known from separate studies that a steady-state radical concentration is generally reached at circa. 6.0 Mrads.

The pre-irradiation method offers a practical advantage in that the substrate can be passed through a conventional high-energy electron accelerator for irradiation and eventually brought into contact with the grafting solution in a continuous fashion. Unlike the mutual method this technique would not require special arrangements for simultaneous irradiation of substrate and solution.

C. Physical Properties and Characterization

A visual test has been devised for quick determination of the properties of the grafted samples in terms of their wettability following grafting. If a running stream of water beads on the surface, it is *not wettable;* is the sample surface wets but remains opaque, then it is *surface wettable;* and, finally, if the sample becomes totally translucent, it is termed *totally wettable.* The results of such tests on the DAM are summarized in Table 1. Clearly, the MPP starts out nonwettable (0 percent graft) and becomes surface wettable after a few percent graft. Total wet out takes place at about 30 percent graft. Beyond this grafting level, the substrates become completely wettable. Such materials might be useful in dialysis applications. For oxygenator requirements, however, the surface wettable films should suffice.

A sample of MPP containing 40 percent graft was used for a more extensive study of the true molecular water absorption behavior of the modified substrate. The actual water sorption isotherm is shown in Figure 7 obtained at 25 °C. It is apparent that the modified sample ab-

Table 1. The influence of grafting (DAM) on the wettability of MPP.

% Graft	Wettability Comment
0	Not Wettable
5	Surface Wettable
10	Surface Wettable
15	Surface Wettable
20	Total Wetting
25	Total Wetting
30	Total Wetting

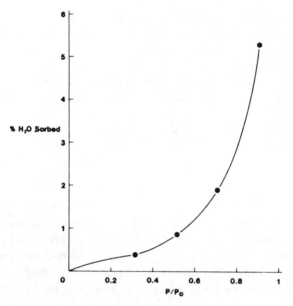

FIGURE 7. Water-sorption isotherm of pre-irradiation grafted MPP (47%) with DAM.

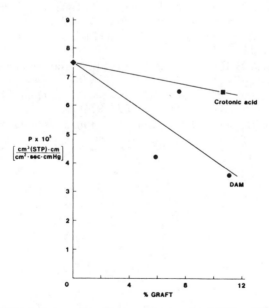

FIGURE 8. The influence of grafting on the air permeability of MPP at 25°C.

sorbs a considerable (>5 percent) amount of water even below unit activity. The MPP before modification would absorb less than 0.01 percent water almost 1000-fold less than following modification.

The air permeability was measured following graft modification to determine what effect the grafting might have on the transport properties. These results are presented in Figure 8 for both DAM and crotonic acid grafted on MPP. It is evident that only minor changes are brought about in the air permeability by the graft modification, thus, preserving the inherently high transport properties of these substrates.

4. CONCLUSIONS

In this investigation, emphasis has been given to developing grafting systems suitable for the grafting of hydrophilic type monomers to preformed substrates which have high oxygen and carbon dioxide transport. Irradiation initiation has been employed with special favor given to a pre-irradiation technique in the more recent part of this study.

5. REFERENCES

1. A. S. Hoffman, D. Cohn, S. R. Hanson, L. A. Harker, T. A. Horbett, B. D. Ratner, and L. O. Reynolds, *Radiat. Phys., 22,* 267 (1983).
2. B. D. Ratner, A. S. Hoffman, and J. D. Whiffen, *Biomatls., Med. Dev. and Artif. Org., 3,* 115 (1975).
3. B. D. Ratner, A. S. Hoffman, S. R. Hanson, L. A. Harker, and J. D. Whiffen, *J. Polymer Sci., 66,* 363 (1979).
4. A. S. Chawla and T. M. Chang, *ACS Polymer Preprints, 14,* 379 (1973); also in *Biomatls. Med. Dev. Art. Org., 2,* 157 (1974).
5. R. T. Greer, B. H. Vale, and R. L. Knoll, *Scanning Electron Microscopy, 1,* 633 (1978).

High Performance Medical Grade Silicone Elastomer

ELDON E. FRISCH
Dow Corning Corporation
Midland, Michigan

ABSTRACT

High performance medical grade silicone elastomer has been developed for use as a material of construction in dynamic medical implant devices. It has high strength and elongation, is very resistant to flaws and crack propagation and has excellent fatigue flex-life. These characteristics are particularly important to the durability of implants that flex or are subjected to motion such as in the flexible hinge finger, wrist, and toe joint implants designed by Alfred B. Swanson, M.D., and in the outer covering of breast implants.

Flexural durability and resistance to flaw propagation are attributable to excellent physical properties, including exceptionally high tear propagation strength (ASTM D624, Die B), and high resistance to crack propagation (ASTM D813). Laboratory flex-life evaluations of flawed and unflawed flexible hinge finger joint implants fabricated from this new elastomer and other candidate materials (including polyurethane, polyolefin, and silicone) confirmed that this new elastomer was substantially more durable. Biocompatibility evaluations to qualify this new material for clinical use included acute and chronic biocompatibility and biodurability studies. Rats were used as the experimental animal in the chronic biocompatibility study. Dogs were the experimental animal in the biodurability studies. Physical properties assessed in implanted and control specimens included tensile strength, ultimate elongation, tear strength (Die B), and flaw propagation characteristics.

High performance medical grade silicone elastomer was found to have excellent biocompatibility and biodurability. In biocompatibility studies, the health of test animals did not differ from that of control animals. In durability studies, the performance of characteristics evaluated in test and control speci-

Reprinted from *SAMPE Journal*, May/June 1985, Courtesy of Society for the Advancement of Material and Process Engineering, Covina, CA U.S.A.

143

mens were stable over the two year implant time. Lipid absorption stabilized at approximately 1.5%, a level reached relatively early after implantation and remaining constant thereafter. Lipid absorption did not reduce performance expectations. No evidence of biodegradation was detected. High performance medical grade of construction in all Silastic® brand bone and joint implants and in the cover of some designs of breast implants. Clinical data indicate the fatigue failures rarely occur.

INTRODUCTION

SILICONES ARE A generic class of polymeric materials containing alternating silicone and oxygen atoms in the backbone of the polymer chains. All silicon atoms typically have two organic ligands (polydiogranosiloxane). Generic silicones include substances that may vary widely in molecular structure and composition and formulated products that contain mixtures of silicones and non-silicone ingredients such as fillers and other additives. Generic silicones include fluids, antifoams, adhesives, elastomers, resins, and a wide variety of formulated compounds and greases.

The properties of most silicones remain essentially unchanged over a wide range of high and low temperatures. They remain flexible or fluid at low temperatures and retain their properties at high temperature. They are also resistant to moisture, oxidation, many chemicals, sunlight, and radiation. They have excellent electrical insulation properties. Because of their unique properties, silicones have become widely used in many of the demanding materials applications of our modern society.

Initial toxicological and biocompatibility studies conducted in the 1940's indicated that certain polydimethylsiloxanes and mixed poly-(dimethyl and phenylmethyl)siloxanes as a class were very low in toxicity and had a high degree of biocompatibility. When published [1], these data generated an unexpected interest in using silicones in many different health care applications, including the use of silicone elastomer as a material of construction for medical implant devices and artificial internal organs.

Silicone elastomers typically contain high molecular weight polydimethylsiloxane (molecular weight greater than 300,000) compounded with high surface area fumed silica (pure SiO_2, approximately 400 m^2/g), the only material known that adequately reinforces silicone elastomer to provide strong, highly elastic materials. During high energy mixing processes, the silica filler becomes coated and impregnated with silicone polymer.

Fabrication generally includes hot vulcanization which cross-links polydimethylsiloxane chains into an elastic, matrix network. Silicone elastomers that vulcanize by addition of hydrogen-to-vinyl to form cross-links contain a blend of two slightly different silicone polymers and a catalyst. When heated, silicone-hydrogen ligands, contained as small amounts of methylhydrogensiloxy copolymer in one polymer, react with silicone-vinyl ligands, present as methylvinylsiloxy copolymer in small amounts in a second polymer. Typical catalysts include trace quantities of rare metals, such as platinum. The cross-links are dimethylene radicals covalently bonded between silicon atoms of separate polymer chains. Organic peroxides may also be used as vulcanization catalysts.

Holter's [2] successful development of a silicone elastomer hydrocephalus shunt in 1955 heralded the current era of implant reconstructive surgery. A wide variety of silicone elastomer implants have subsequently been developed to facilitate or improve reconstructive surgery. By the mid 1960's implants made from medical grade versions of silicone elastomer as then available were used in most surgical specialties including plastic [3–6], orthopaedic [7–11], gynecologic [12], ophthalmic [13–15], and others.

Of the many implants developed, the silicone elastomer finger joint implant designed by Swanson [7–11] represented a particularly important advancement in the hand surgeon's armamentarium. This implant has two intramedullary stems joined by a flexible hinge-spacer. The availability of this implant has revolutionized the techniques for reconstruction of rheumatoid hands and has substantially improved the results. Swanson has also designed similar double-stemmed, flexible hinged implants for reconstruction of wrist and toe joints, and a wide variety of single-stemmed joint spacer implants for reconstruction of the trapeziometacarpal joint, the proximal head of the radius, the base of phalanx in the great toe, and a variety of other small joints in both upper and lower extremities.

All flexible bone and joint implants were initially made from medium hardness medical grade silicone elastomer, a material developed in the late 1950's. Its safety as an implant material had become well established by biocompatibility and biodurability [16] studies done in test animals and by a history of extensive clinical use.

Swanson [17] evaluated the durability of this early silicone elastomer in finger joint implants retrieved from clinical cases after various periods of time, and found no evidence of biodegradation and no correlation between implant performance and lipid content.

Weightman [18] constructed a hypothetical model to suggest that lipid absorption could weaken and possibly degrade silicone elastomer, but neither the findings from his laboratory studies, nor the studies of others supported his hypothesis.

HIGH PERFORMANCE SILICONE ELASTOMER

In the early 1970's technology was developed in Dow Corning's silicone elastomer research laboratories that permitted development of a silicone elastomer with strength and toughness previously unattainable. With this new technology an elastomer was developed with a combination of low modulus and excellent physical properties, particularly high tear propagation strength (ASTM D624, Die B) and very low flexural fatigue crack growth rates (ASTM D 813). These characteristics were deemed highly useful to extend the durability of dynamic, implantable medical devices such as the flexible hinge implants used in bone and joint reconstruction. The mode of fracture failure in flexible hinge implants in clinical use had been identified as propagation of surface flaws believed to result from articulation of implant against bone. Thus, an elastomer with low modulus, high tear propagation strength, high resistance to flexural fatigue crack growth, and an excellent profile of physical properties would logically improve flexural durability of flexible hinge implants in clinical use.

To satisfy the need for a more durable material, a new medical grade "high performance" silicone elastomer was developed from this technology. The safety requirements for a material of construction for implants were considered in the selection of all ingredients. The new elastomer contained no types of chemical bonds not also found in the earlier medical grade silicone elastomer used initially.

The physical propeties of high performance medical grade silicone elastomer and conventional medium hardness medical grade elastomer are compared in Table 1.

The new elastomer has a four-fold increase in tear propagation strength (ASTM D624, Die B) 1.339 kg/m vs 5.357 kg/m (75 ppi vs. 300 ppi) and an increase in crack growth resistance (ASTM D813) by a factor of approximately 600. Growth of the initial 2.0 mm (0.080 in.) long cut (ASTM D813) in specimens prepared from earlier elastomer, typically exceeded 12.7 mm (0.5 in.) after only 7,333 cycles and had an extrapolated average crack growth rate equal to approximately 1.46 m (57.3 in.)/10^6 cycles. By comparison, when tested in an identical manner, in specimens prepared from medical grade high performance silicone elastomer the length of the prescribed 2.0 mm (0.080 in.) cut consistently remained less than 12.7 mm (0.5 in.) after 10^6 cycles, in all specimens. With "H.P." elastomer the average length of the initial

Table 1. Typical properties of medical grade high performance and medium hardness silicone elastomer.

Property	Method	High Performance	Medium Hardness
Tensile strength	ASTM D412	1.0343×10^7 Pa	8.274×10^7 Pa
Ultimate elongation	ASTM D412	700%	450%
Modulus at 100% elongation	ASTM D412	2.0685×10^6 Pa	1.3790×10^6 Pa
Tear initiation strength, Die C	ASTM D624	5.3569×10^3 kg/m	Varies widely
Tear propagation strength, Die B	ASTM D624	5.3569×10^3 kg/m	1.3392×10^3 kg/m
Crack growth, 10^6 cycles	ASTM D813	2.7 mm (1.80 in.)	1459 mm (57.3 in.) Extrapolated
Durometer, Shore A	ASTM D2240	52	50
Specific gravity	ASTM D924	1.15	1.14

2.0 mm (0.080 in.) cut was 4.7 mm (0.188 in.) at 10^6 cycles, an average growth of 2.7 mm (0.1 in.)/10^6 cycles. Testing by ASTM D813 was made part of batch-to-batch quality assurance for medical grade high performance silicone elastomer with a pass or failure requirement that the initial 2.0 mm (0.080 in.) cut must remain less than 12.7 mm (0.5 in.) after 10^6 cycles in all 12 specimens tested simultaneously. Non-silicone elastomer candidates were also considered. A polyurethane thermoplastic elastomer (Tecoflex® brand) and a polyolefin elastomer (Hexsyn®, Goodyear Rubber) were also tested in keeping with ASTM D813. The polyurethane failed in less than 2000 cycles and the polyolefin in less than 100.

The flex life of Swanson-designed finger joints prepared from the earlier medical grade silicone elastomer and medical grade high performance silicone elastomer were compared. Flexural durability testing was done in a machine which flexed the implants through a 90° arc (0° to 90° and back to 0°) at a rate of 16.67/s (1000/min.). When unflawed implants were tested the number of flexes required to initiate a flaw in both materials was essentially equal, exceeding 150,000,000 cycles. However, with implants flawed prior to testing by a 1.57 mm (0.062 in.) long through-and-through cut made in the center of the hinge perpendicular to the long axis, medical grade high performance silicone elastomer flexed more than 100 times longer prior to failure than conventional medical grade medium hardness silicone elastomer. Flawed implants made from the conventional material typically had separated completely at 90,000 cycles, while the cut in the implants made from high performance elastomer demonstrated some cut growths at 9,000,000 cycles, but the implants had not separated. Finger joints molded from both polyurethane (Tecoflex® brand) and polyolefin (Hexsyn®) failed early in flex-testing.

Biocompatibility Evaluations

To qualify high performance elastomer for use in implants, biocompatibility evaluations were conducted. Studies included acute and subacute tissue reaction in rabbits and mice as described in USP XIX for Class VI plastics. Subchronic tests were also done by placing samples intramuscularly and subcutaneously in rabbits for 7, 30, and 90 days. Histopathological evaluations of pertinent tissue specimens found no adverse reactions in any of the tests.

The material was also evaluated by direct contact cell culture testing done with WI-38 human embryonic lung cells [19,20]. The new elastomer elicited no cytopathic reactions.

Chronic biocompatibility was evaluated in a 2-year or life time study in albino rats. Four groups of 100 animals each (50 males and 50 females) were used. One group each received identically shaped implant specimens of medical grade medium hardness silicone elastomer, and USP polyethylene respectively, implanted intramuscularly, subcutaneously, interperitoneally, and in bone marrow. The fourth received sham surgery only, at the same sites. All animals that died before 2 years were appropriately assessed. At the end of 2 years all surviving animals were sacrificed. All tumors were evaluated and classified. No detectable differences in the biocompatibility of the three implant substances were detected in this study and the reactions in all of the implant groups were essentially the same as in the sham surgery group.

Biodurability Evaluation

Biodurability of medical grade high performance silicone elastomer was evaluated by subcutaneous implantation of test specimens in dogs for periods of up to 104 months.

MATERIALS AND METHODS

The study started with 20 sets of test specimens, all prepared from the same lot of elastomer, each set consisting of 5 tensile strength specimens, 5 Die B tear strength specimens, and 10 flaw propagation specimens.

All specimens were sterilized with ethylene oxide at the start of the study. Sterilized control specimens were tested to obtain base line values for all of the tests. Control specimens were stored dry at 37°C, and were tested identically to test specimens. Test specimens were retrieved and tested at 2, 4, 8, 16, 32, and 104 weeks. Control specimens were evaluated at 32 and 104 weeks.

A predetermined number of control and implanted specimen sets were solvent extracted initially and terminally to facilitate quantitative and qualitative observations of extractable materials and weight changes. The preimplant extractions were done for 16 hours with a refluxing 2:1 mixture of chloroform and methanol in a Soxhlet extractor. This solvent mix was selected to facilitate extraction of both polar materials of biological origin, and non-polar materials (lipid or silicone) not chemically bound into the cross-linked, polymeric matrix. Weight loss from pre-implant extractions was monitored. Post-implant extractions were done by immersion for 48 hours in 25 ml of the same solvent mix at room temperature rather than at reflux to avoid degrad-

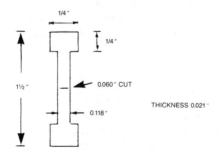

START AT 40% ELONGATION (10 INCHES
PER MINUTE) REPEAT THROUGH 20
CYCLES—INCREASE ELONGATION 5%—
REPEAT SEQUENCE UNTIL FAILURE OCCURS

TEST END-POINT IS NUMBER OF CYCLES
TO FAILURE

FIGURE 1. Flaw propagation test.

ing any biological materials which may have been absorbed. Weight changes were again monitored, and silicon content in the decanted solvent was determined by atomic absorption spectroscopy. Biological materials were assessed by thin layer chromatography. Precision, accuracy, and reproducibility of the extraction and analytical techniques were not evaluated and determined, thus only qualitative findings are considered pertinent. All physical property testing was done by ASTM methods except for the fatigue flaw propagation test. Because of its relatively large size it was deemed impractical to implant the test specimens prescribed in ASTM D813. A flaw propagation test with a smaller specimen was specifically designed for this experiment and was not a standard test method. In flaw propagation testing, specimens were uniformly tested for fatigue flaw propagation characteristic by cyclic and progressive elongation of a small specimen with a central cut (Figure 1).

The end-point of the test was measured as a number of cycles at which separation of the specimen occurred at the location of the central cut.

Implantation and Removal—The specimens were implanted in subcutaneous tissue in dogs along the lower back and flank areas on both sides of the spinal column. At predetermined times specimens were removed from each dog, weighed and physical properties measured within 7 hours.

Physical Property Measurements—Physical properties of nonextracted, implanted and control specimens measured at various time intervals are shown in Figures 2–6. Measurements from implanted specimens were compared to evaluate the effect of increasing implant time. These values were also compared to the test results from control specimens.

Findings

All physical property test values varied randomly and inconsistently during the study. Variations were attributed to experimental error of the study design. None of the physical properties of high performance elastomer evaluated in this study appeared to change as a result of subcutaneous implantation in the dog.

Tensile Strength—Tensile strength data (ASTM D412) for test and control specimens are shown in Figure 2.

Values varied from a low of 1.0356×10^7 Pa (1502 psi) for 32 week implanted specimens to a high of 1.1900×10^7 Pa (1726 psi) for 104 week control specimens. Base line tensile strength was 1.1528×10^7 Pa (1672 psi) compared to 1.1542×10^7 Pa (1674 psi) for 104 week im-

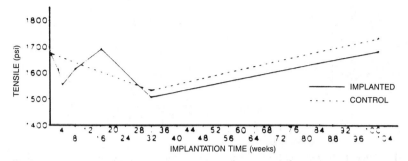

FIGURE 2. Tensile strength of high performance silicone elastomer after implantation.

planted specimens. Non-implanted specimens (base line and two control) averaged 1.1425×10^7 Pa (1657 psi) compared to 1.1129 Pa (1614 psi) for all implanted specimens.

Elongation—Average elongation data (ASTM D412) for implanted and control specimens are shown in Figure 3.

Values varied from a low of 576% for 32 week implanted specimens to a high of 812% for two week implants. Base line specimens averaged 683% compared to 716% for 104 week implants. Non-implanted specimens (one base line and two control) averaged 676% compared to 700% for all implanted specimens.

Tensile Stress—Average tensile stress data (ASTM D412) at 200% elongation for test and control specimens are shown in Figure 4.

Values varied from a low of 4.9437×10^6 Pa (717 psi) for two week implanted specimens to a high of 6.6608×10^6 Pa (821 psi) for 32 week control specimens. The value for base line specimens was 5.2609×10^6 Pa (763 psi) compared to 4.9989×10^6 Pa (725 psi) for the specimens implanted 104 weeks. The average value for all implanted specimens

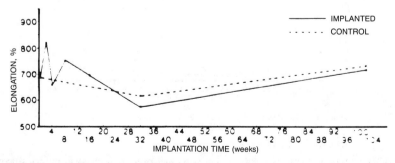

FIGURE 3. Elongation of high performance silicone elastomer after implantation.

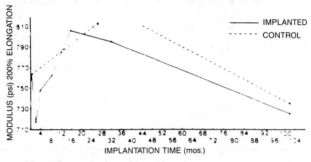

*32 week control modulus value was 821

FIGURE 4. Modulus of high performance silicone elastomer after implantation.

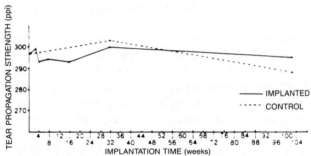

FIGURE 5. Tear propagation strength in high performance silicone elastomer after implantation.

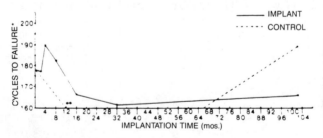

*Starting at 40% elongation, 20 cycles, and increasing elongation 5% with each additional 20 cycles

**32 week control value was 33 cycles

FIGURE 6. Accelerated fatigue flaw propagation resistance in high performance silicone elastomer after implantation.

was 5.2333 × 10^6 Pa (759 psi) compared to 5.3229 × 10^6 (772 psi) for non-implanted specimens.

Tear Propagation Strength—Average tear propagation strength data (ASTM D624, Die B) for test and control specimen are shown in Figure 5.

The highest value was 5.410 × 10$_3$ kg/m (303 ppi) in 32 week control specimens. The lowest was 5.1605 kg/m (289 ppi) in two year control specimens. The values for base line and 104 week implanted specimens were essentially identical, 5.2855 × 10$_3$ kg/m (296 ppi). The averages for all implanted specimens for all non-implanted specimens were also the same, 5.2855 × 10$_3$ kg/m (296 ppi).

Flaw Propagation Resistance—Average flaw propagation resistance data for test and control specimens are shown in Figure 6.

The lowest value was 133 cycles in 32 week control specimens. The highest value was 190 cycles in four week implanted specimens. The value for base line specimens was 178 cycles compared to 166 cycles for specimens implanted 104 weeks. The value for all implanted specimens was 174 cycles compared to 166 cycles for non-implanted specimens.

EXTRACTION STUDIES

Soxhlet and Immersion Extraction—Average weight loss from Soxhlet extraction of 80 base line specimens was 2.13%. Extraction typically removes all polydimethylsiloxane not chemically bound into the cross-linked elastomer network matrix. The average weight loss from immersion extraction of 80 control specimens stored dry, 40 for 32 weeks and 40 for 104 weeks, was 1.73%. Since these specimens logically contained the same quantity of extractable extraction with static solvent was less effective than Soxhlet extraction and left an average of 0.4% by weight residual extractable silicone. The relatively high variation seen in weight loss from static solvent extractions also indicates the ineffectiveness of this method. Static solvent extraction did not appear to provide the accuracy and precision required for quantitative materials balance studies.

The silicon content in solvent extracts from the 80 control specimens, measured by atomic absorption, indicated that the average weight loss of silicone was 1.73%. While this average should and did match well with the measured weight loss, large variations were found between measured weight loss and atomic absorption determinations in three of the four specimen sets indicating that the techniques used did not provide the accuracy required for precise quantitative evaluation.

In the 80 specimens that had been Soxhlet extracted prior to implantation the average weight gains were 1.12% after 32 weeks and 1.98% after 104 weeks with considerable specimen-to-specimen variation. Weight losses from terminal 48-hour, room temperature, solvent immersion extraction averaged 1.21% and 1.71% respectively. These data would indicate that lipid absorption in extracted, implanted specimens is approximately 1.16% at 32 weeks implantation and 1.85% after 104 weeks.

In the 80 specimens implanted without previous extraction, average weight gains were 1.06% at 32 weeks and 1.31% after 104 weeks. Weight loss from the terminal solvent immersion extraction averaged 2.85% and 2.95% respectively and included both extracted silicone and lipid. The average weight loss of silicone as determined by atomic absorption techniques in these specimens was 1.83% vs. 173% found by immersion extraction of control specimens. High variation from specimen-to-specimen were again found. These data indicate that lipid absorption in implanted, unextracted specimens after 32 weeks was approximately 1.04%, and after 104 weeks 1.22%. Further, the residual silicone content in specimens implanted for either 32 or 104 weeks is essentially the same as the residual silicone in control specimens.

Thin layer chromatographic analysis of the absorbed lipids indicated they consisted of 80% to 90% triglycerides and 10% cholesterol. Smaller amounts of partial glycerides and free-fatty acids were also found. No phospholipids were found. No significant differences in lipid composition were found between specimens which had been implanted with and without prior solvent extraction.

CONCLUSIONS

High performance medical grade silicone elastomer was found to have excellent biocompatibility and biodurability. The findings from subacute, acute, subchronic, and chronic biocompatibility assessments indicated that the material has characteristics suitable for its use as a material of construction for permanent implants.

In biodurability assessment, none of the physical properties monitored (tensile strength, ultimate elongation, tensile stress at 200% elongation, tear propagation strength, Die B, and flaw propagation resistance) changed in a consistent or progressive manner as a consequence of subcutaneous implantation in dogs for up to 2 years duration.

The differences in physical properties between implanted specimens and control specimens stored dry at 37°C when tested at 32 and 104 weeks were small, generally less than the differences found between test values from testing done at various time intervals. The findings from this study indicate that changes in physical properties of medical grade high performance silicone elastomer from 2 years subcutaneous implantation in the dog either do not occur or are very small and are thus not a factor in performance of implants fabricated from this material.

Extraction studies demonstrated that medical grade high performance silicone elastomer contains approximately 2% by weight of polydimethylsiloxane which is not chemically bound into the cross-linked polymeric matrix, and may thus be extracted with an appropriate solvent by Soxhlet extraction techniques. The technique of room temperature static solvent extraction as used for extraction after explanation was less efficient and less predictable than the preimplant extractions done with refluxing solvent in a Soxhlet extractor. When these differences are taken into consideration there is no apparent difference between the content of free silicones in these specimens after 104 months implantation and the content at the time if implantation. Thus, there did not appear to be a significant loss of silicone to tissues or systemic circulation, nor generation of free silicone during the implant period.

Lipid absorption after 32 weeks implantation was approximately 1.1% and after 104 weeks implantation approximately 1.5%, based on averages of specimen weight gains while implanted and that portion of weight loss upon terminal extraction attributable to nonsilicone material. This finding was consistent in specimens which had been implanted both with and without prior solvent extraction.

Lipid absorption appeared to occur relatively early after implantation and probably became constant when the silicone elastomer became saturated with lipids in the specific implant environment. The absorbed lipids consisted of 80% to 90% triglycerides and 10% cholesterol. Smaller amounts of partial glycerides and free fatty acids were also found. No phospholipids were found. No significant differences in lipid composition were found between specimens which had been implanted with and without solvent extraction.

This study indicated that medical grade high performance silicone elastomer had excellent biodurability during two years subcutaneous implantation in the dog.

These laboratory findings have been confirmed by clinical experience. High performance medical grade silicone elastomer has been used as a material of construction for Silastic® brand flexible implants used in bone and joint reconstruction since 1975 and in the outer cover of some breast implants for several years. Biocompatibility and fatigue failure complications have been minimal.

REFERENCES

1. V. K. Rowe, H. C. Spencer, and S. L. Bass, *J. Indust. Hyg. & Tox.*, *30*, 6:332 (1948).
2. H. LaFay, *Readers Digest, 57,* 29 (1957).
3. J. Safian, *Plast. and Recon. Surg., 37,* 446 (1966).
4. T. D. Cronin and F. J. Gerow, "Augmentation Mammaplasty: A New 'Natural Feel' Prosthesis," *Excerpta Media International Congress Series No. 66, Proceedings of the Third International Congress of Plastic Surgery,* Washington, D.C., pp. 41–49 (1963)
5. T. D. Cronin, *Plast. and Recon. Surg., 37* (5), 399 (1966).
6. G. B. Snyder, E. H. Courtiss, B. M. Kaye, and G. P. Gradinger, *Plast. and Recon. Surg., 61,* 854 (1978).
7. A. B. Swanson, *Inter-clin, Inform. Bull., 6,* 16 (1966).
8. A. B. Swanson, U.S. Patent No. 3,452,765.
9. A. B. Swanson, U.S. Patent No. 3,875,594.
10. A. B. Swanson, *Flexible Implant Resection Arthroplasty in the Hand and Extremities,* St. Louis, The C.V. Mosby Co., 1973.
11. A. B. Swanson, *J. Bone Joint Surg., 54A,* 435 (1972).
12. W. J. Mulligan, *Int. J. Fertil., 11,* 424 (1966).
13. H. A. Lincoff, I. Baras, and J. McLean, *Arch. Ophthal., 73,* 160 (1965).
14. H. A. Lincoff, *et al., Mod. Prob. Ophthal., 15,* 188 (1975).
15. H. A. Lincoff and J. McLean, *Am. J. Ophthal., 64,* 877 (1967).
16. J. W. Swanson and J. F. LeBeau, *J. Biomed. Mater. Res., 8,* 357 (1974).
17. A. B. Swanson, *et al., Orthopedic Clinics of North America, 4* (4), 1097 (1973).
18. B. Weightman, *et al., J. Biomed. Mater. Res. Symposium,* No. 3, pp. 15–24, John Wiley & Sons, Inc. (1972).
19. R. E. Wilsnack, *Biomater. Med. Devices Artif. Orangs, 4* (3 & 4), 235 (1976).
20. R. E. Wilsnack, F. S. Meyer, and J. G. Smith, *Biomater. Med. Devices Artif. Organs, 1* (3), 543 (1973).

Materials for Ligament Replacement

JAMES M. MORAN
Cleveland Research Institute at
St. Vincent Charity Hospital and Health Center
Cleveland, Ohio

ABSTRACT

Damaged ligaments and tendons present a difficult restorative procedure to the orthopaedic surgeon. Current techniques involving repositioning of the patient's viable soft tissues to assist or replace damaged structures have not met with overwhelming success. As a result, the utility of foreign substances in these procedures is being investigated. The materials may be permanent or degradable and may be used as actual ligament replacements or to augment the patient's own tissues. Despite promising early clinical results such devices must still be considered experimental.

INTRODUCTION

OVER THE PAST decade replacement of damaged ligaments and tendons have been the focus of increased research activity. This work may have been stimulated by the success of other biomaterial applications or our growing national interest and participation in athletic activities. But perhaps the most compelling reason may be our enhanced appreciation of the degenerative changes resulting from long-term joint instability.

Until the 1950s treatment of ligamentous injuries consisted primarily of immobilization for up to a year followed by a return to limited motion using a protective restraining device. More recently aggressive surgical intervention has been employed for certain chronic and acute injuries in the hope that complete recovery can be achieved. Reinforce-

Reprinted from *SAMPE Journal*, May/June 1985, courtesy of Society for the Advancement of Material Process Engineering, Covina, CA, U.S.A.

ment and reconstruction have been performed in the knee, ankle, elbow, and hand and shoulder. Autografts (tissues transplanted from one site to another in the same person) are the prime material source. However, autografts are not always available, may not be large enough, may be weaker than the original structure, or may stretch, resulting in instability or inadequate muscle strength [1].

These problems have spurred the development of ligament replacement materials which potentially strength durability, possibly resulting in decreased postoperative immobilization and speedier recovery [2]. Distinctly different design philosophies are apparent. Some prostheses are meant to be biologically or mechanically degradable and serve as a temporary framework upon which the body can deposit connective tissue (induction prostheses), while others are intended to be permanent replacements or supplements to other tissues.

CHARACTERIZATION OF NATURAL LIGAMENTS

Regardless of the material type or intended role in load transmission, the overall goal remains to be replacement of a well "designed" and durable natural material. Most ligaments are composed of parallel fibers of collagen, a fibrous protein. The fiber bundles are wavy in the unloaded state but straighten out under tension.

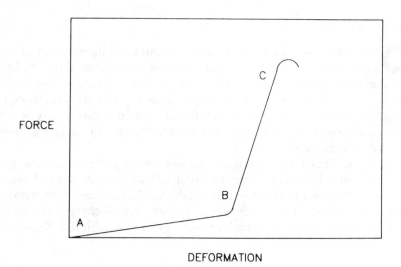

FIGURE 1. Ligament force–deformation curve.

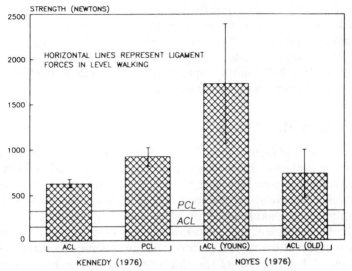

FIGURE 2. Cruciate ligament strength.

The typical shape of a force-deformation curve is shown in Figure 1. The toe of the curve (A-B) reflects straightening of the bundles and is thought to be the range of normal physiologic loading [3], the linear portion (B-C) is used to specify elastic stiffness or, alternately, elastic modulus using a stress-strain curve. The force-deformation response can be altered by numerous factors including age of the tissue donor, strain rate, and the particular anatomic structure being tested.

Mechanical tests of ligaments may be broken down into three broad categories. First, the most complex studies involve the use of intact cadaver joints and mechanical simulation of normal joint kinetics to study ligament loads. Second, for tests of individual structures, all of the ligaments and joint capsule are severed with the exception of the ligament of interest. A tensile test is then usually performed. In the final test type the ligament is isolated from its bony attachments and the specimen is mounted in standard tensile testing machine.

Figure 2 presents ultimate force data for the human anterior cruciate ligament (ACL) and posterior cruciate ligament (PCL) as determined by a test of the second type [4,5]. The horizontal lines represent the forces calculated to occur in the ligaments in the knee of a 700N individual who is walking on level ground [6]. Failure strains are in the 25–40% range [7].

Recent guidelines proposed for the strength of autograft reconstruction of human anteriocruciate ligaments might reasonably be applied to ligament replacement materials as well. It has been suggested that 445N is a reasonable upper bound on force transmission in normal activities, while 1000N is an upper bound for strenuous activities [1]. Above 1000N damage would be expected to occur.

LIGAMENT REPLACEMENTS

A wide range of factors must be studied before human implantation of ligament replacement devices is permitted by the Food and Drug Administration. *In vitro* laboratory tests generally focus on mechanical properties, effects of sterilization, tissue culture studies, and fixation of the implant to the skeleton. Animal studies may then be conducted to investigate tissue toxicity, systemic effects, mechanical degradation, strength of attachment, and performance in specific reconstructive applications. A brief survey of the characteristics of materials currently under investigation for ligament replacement applications follows.

Carbon Fibers

Carbon fibers have been found to perform well as a degradable scaffold upon which ligaments may be regenerated. Biocompatibility is excellent and no allergic, carcinogenic or biologic problems have been reported. Flexion causes the ligament to fragment over time while collagen continues to be deposited by the host. In early experiments in sheep, carbon fragments were found to collect in regional lymph nodes [8], but this may have been a species-related phenomenon, as this finding has not as yet been documented in other animals or humans.

The ligaments consist of 10,000–96,000 seven micron diameter carbon filaments. The strength of the ligament is roughly 6 KN for the average sizes. In animal studies the strength of the carbon ligament-new host tissue composite has been found to be 33–160% of that of the replaced natural structure [9,10]. Wide variation results from differences in species, surgical technique, duration of implantation, and method of ligament attachment. Of particular importance is the application. In animal studies the ligament has not fared well in anterior cruciate ligament substitutions, but the opposite is true for tendon replacements.

Coated Carbon Fibers

In order to overcome potential problems associated with carbon fragment migration, a coated ligament has been developed. The coating of polylactic acid (PLA) is gradually replaced by collagen over a period of about two weeks. Although fibers may break, their movement is confined by the PLA until the collagen sheath is formed, and by the sheath thereafter.

An implant currently undergoing clinical trials in the United States consists of 10,000 seven micron diameter filaments sprayed with a diluted PLA solution [11]. It has a tensile strength of 450 N. Needles are attached to both ends of the strand to aid implantation. Reported applications are repair of the Achilles tendon, knee extensor mechanism, medial collateral ligament, and anterior cruciate ligament [2].

Polyethylene

In 1974 ultra high molecular weight polyethylene (UHMWPE) was used for the first anterior cruciate ligament commercially marketed. It consisted of a 178 mm long rod of UHMWPE, 6.4 mm in diameter, threaded on both ends. The portion of the rod in the joint space was tapered to 4.8 mm. Also included were stainless steel grommets to protect the rod from abrasion where it emerged from the bone and stainless steel sleeves used to line the bone drill holes. It was held in place by fixation nuts which threaded onto the rod and butted against the sleeves.

It did not prove to be very successful, as many patients complained of pain and reoperation was required in a high percentage of cases [13,14]. Although some continue to provide excellent results seven years after implantation, clinical use has been stopped [15]. In a retrospective comparison of the clinical results to a design analysis it was determined that the yield point, creep behavior and fatigue strength of UHMWPE were inappropriate for this application [14].

Polyethyleneterephthalate (Dacron)

Dacron, in the form of velour, mesh and woven tape has been widely investigated for use in ligament replacement applications. In canine ACL replacement studies, fraying and breakage have occurred, with failure rates ranging from 33–66% depending on time of implantation and weave type [2,16]. Bone grows around fibers inside the anchorage holes but fraying occurs where the ligament emerges from the hole. Rupture occurs before host tissue has sufficiently strengthened the prosthesis. In direct comparison animal studies, carbon fibers have been found to out-perform dacron [10,17]. Nevertheless, a short term clinical study has shown dacron tape to perform as well as autologous tissues in the correction of chronic human knee instability [18].

Dacron has also been used to augment patellar tendon grafts in canine knee ACL reconstruction in the hope that it might protect the graft from stretching and failure in the initial phases of healing [19]. In fact, the augmented grafts did not perform as well as the plain grafts. It was thought that the Dacron shielded the graft from load and therefore the graft resorbed. Long term results showed the dacron could not carry the load alone and eventually failed.

Xenografts

Xenografts are tissues transplanted between members of different species. In current ligament replacement applications bovine tendons and ligaments are transplanted to humans. The xenografts are treated with glutaraldehyde before implantation. Glutaraldehyde cross-links the collagen proteins and blocks sites of enzyme degradation and immune response. The xenograft eventually evolves into a composite of xenograft collagen which only functions mechanically and host collagen which functions mechanically and biologically.

The strengths of the bovine grafts are very similar to those of the tissues they intended to replace, but they do have a higher modulus of elasticity [20]. This is probably a result of the glutaraldehyde induced cross-linking. Early data from clinical trials in the United States is available. One of the nineteen centers involved in the evaluation of this device reported fourteen failures out of eighteen implantations [21]. While this trend did not follow through in the remaining centers it does highlight the potential for poor results due to the technically demanding surgical procedure.

Xenografts have also been used on conjunction with dacron sleeves, which cover the graft ends inside the bone tunnels. In a study of rabbit ACL reconstructions one rupture occurred in sixteen animals [22]. At one year the implants remained firmly anchored in bone and new collagen had grown into the implant in the joint space.

Others

Many other materials and combinations of materials have been reported for use in ligament repair and reconstruction. The following briefly summarizes some of this data.

A 6 mm diamond braid polypropylene tape has been used as a ligament augmentation device (LAD) [15]. It has a tensile strength of 1370N and a 7% deformation after one million applications of a 500N load. It has been used to augment the middle third of the patellar tendon in ACL reconstructions.

In goats the failure load of the reconstructed ligament has increased

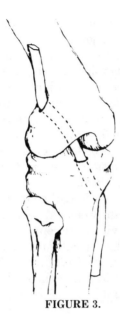

FIGURE 3.

from 360N immediately after surgery to 1100N at twelve months.

Dexon (polyglycolic acid) resorbable suture has been braided to form a temporary ligament [23]. It serves to protect the repaired ligament during healing. Thirty size 00 strands have a strength of 825N. In a study of canine ACL repair, the repaired ligaments had a strength of 530N four months after surgery compared to a normal canine ACL strength of 1360N.

A composite leader has been used to lengthen patellar tendon grafts for ease of transfer [24]. It consists of a core of aramid fibers (Nomex) embedded in Teflon and surrounded with Proplast, a porous Teflon-carbon fiber composite.

IMPLANTATION

An overall impression of the manner in which devices for ACL repair are implanted can be gained from Figure 3.

It is important that the bone tunnels be approximately colinear so that the ligament does not bear against the bone edge where it emerges from the tunnels. The hole is also usually chamfered to remove sharp edges which may excessively abrade the implant. If a collateral ligament on the side of the knee is also involved, a single loop of material might be used for both repairs. Similar procedures are used for the reconstruction of other joints.

Many different techniques are employed to initially fix the implant to the bone. Bone screws and staples are frequently used to hold the end tabs of the ligament in place. The implant may also be sutured to surrounding soft tissue or folded over and sutured together to prevent being pulled into the tunnel. In some instances an interference fit between the implant and tunnel, reinforced with cyanoacrylate, is used. An expanding carbon rivet has been developed for use with carbon fiber implants [25]. Long term fixation is generally intended to be provided by bone growth into the prosthesis.

Postoperative care varies and is still evolving, but currently entails immobilization for up to eight weeks. A rehabilitation program is implemented and athletic activity is discouraged for at least six months.

Regardless of the steps taken to carefully design and test a ligament replacement or augmentation device, success ultimately hinges on the skillful technique employed by the orthopaedic surgeon and cooperation on the part of the patient.

CONCLUSIONS

It has been estimated that it could take seven to eight years at a cost of $4–5 million to bring a ligament replacement from the initial concept to the market [26]. The ideal device will combine a balance of strength and stiffness with abrasion resistance, biocompatibility, and susceptibility to bone and soft tissue ingrowth.

Most designs are still undergoing the clinical trials required by the Food and Drug Administration, so it is not clear whether or not a solution to the problem of ligament reconstruction is at hand. However, in light of the limitations found to date in laboratory and animal tests it is apparent that both patients and surgeons will need to develop reasonable performance expectations. While a relatively high degree of normal function may be recovered, it is doubtful that patients will return to their pre-injury status.

REFERENCES

1. F. R. Noyes, D. L. Butler, E. S. Grood, R. F. Zernicke, and M. S. Hefzy, *J. Bone and Joint Surg., 66-A*, 344 (1984).
2. R. M. Rubin, J. L. Marshall, and J. Wang, *Clin. Orthop. and Rel. Res., 113*, 212 (1975).
3. Y. C. Fung, *Biomechanics: Mechanical Properties of Living Tissues*, Springer-Verlag, New York, p. 210 (1981).

4. J. C. Kennedy, R. J. Hawkins, R. B. Willis, and K. D. Danylchuk, *J. Bone and Joint Surg., 58-A*, 350 (1976).

5. F. R. Noyes and E. S. Grood, *J. bone and Joint Surg., 58-A*, 1074 (1976).

6. J. B. Morrison, *J. Biomech., 3*, 51 (1970).

7. L. Claes, Aktuel, *Probl. Chir. Orthop., 26*, 10 (1983).

8. D. H. R. Jenkins, *J. Bone Joint Surg., 60-B*, 520 (1978).

9. E. M. Keating, S. Saha, S. Pal, and J. A. Albright, Transactions of the 29th Orthopaedic Research Society, 95 (1983).

10. L. Claes, C. Burri, R. Neugebauer, J. Piehler, and W. Mohr, Aktuel., *Probl. Chir. Orthop., 26*, 101 (1983).

11. J. Aragona, J. R. Parsons, H. Alexander, and A. B. Weiss, *Am. J. Sports Med., 11* (1983).

12. A. B. Weiss, M. Hatam, and H. Alexander, *Contemporary Orthop., 7*, 39 (1983).

13. M. Scharling, *Acta Orthop. Scand., 52*, 575 (1981).

14. E. H. Chen and J. Black, *J. Biomed. Mat. Res., 14*, 567 (1980).

15. J. C. Kennedy, *Clin. Orthop. and Rel. Res., 172*, 125 (1983).

16. J. F. Meyers, W. A. Grana, and P. A. Lesker, *Am. J. Sports Med., 7*, 85 (1979).

17. J. R. Parsons, H. Alexander, J. S. Ende, and A. B. Weiss, Transactions of the 29th Orthopaedic Research Society, *96* (1983).

18. J. Mockwitz and H. Contzen, *Aktuel. Probl. Chir. Orthop., 26*, 110 (1983).

19. J. T. Andrish and L. T. Woods, *Clin. Orthop. and Rel. Res., 183*, 298 (1984).

20. W. S. Berg, T. M. Stahurski, J. M. Moran, and A. S. Greenwald, *Orthop. Trans., 7*, 279 (1983).

21. W. C. McMaster, *Am. Acad. Orthop. Surg.*, Cassette 84AA0S-7 (1984).

22. R. Gambardella, J. Jurgutis, and M. Nimni, G. J. Marshall, E. Gendler, A. Sarmiento, and J. Sweeny, Transactions of the 30th Orthopaedic Research Society, *110* (1984).

23. H. E. Cabaud, J. A. Feagin, and W. G. Rodkey, *Am. J. Sports Med., 10*, 259 (1982).

24. G. W. Woods, C. A. Homsy, J. M. Prewitt, and H. S. Tullos, *Am. J. Sports Med., 7*, 314 (1979).

25. A. E. Strover, Aktuel., *Probl. Chir. Orthop., 26*, 127 (1983).

26. A. B. Weiss, H. Alexander, M. Blazina, R. Larson, E. M. Lunceford, and W. C. McMaster, *Contemporary Orthop., 7*, 99 (1983).

Machining Bioglass® Implants

JUNE WILSON, G. E. MERWIN, AND L. L. HENCH
University of Florida
Gainsville, Florida

ABSTRACT

A range of surface active materials which bond to living tissues have been studied since their original invention by L. L. Hench in 1969. Clinical trials are now in progress at the University of Florida and devices made from Bioglass® materials will become widely available. Machining of this glassy material by surgeons is unprecedented but essential in the operating room. Experiments which demonstrate that this can be easily and satisfactorily done under operating room conditions are described.

INTRODUCTION

A T A RECENT conference held in Holland, a mixed group of participants discussed at length the use of different materials to provide treatment for disease and alleviation of symptoms in a very specific organ—the ear. Their contributions and discussions have now been published [1]. The conference was notable for its specificity and for the variety of disciplines which were represented. For what seemed like the first time clinicians and materials scientists were able to concentrate on the same problem, identify areas of concern and raise their mutual awareness of the other's difficulties.

The ear consists of three main parts; outer, middle and inner ear (Figure 1). The outer ear is the visible part, the pinna which collects sound from the outside world and relays it to the eardrum as vibrations. The eardrum, which separates the outer from middle ear, transmits the vibrations to a series of small bones or ossicles, three in

Reprinted from *SAMPE Journal*, May/June 1985, courtesy of Society for the Advancement of Material and Process Engineering, Covina, CA U.S.A.

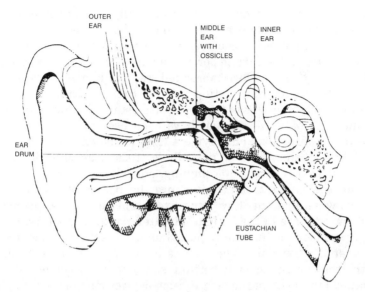

FIGURE 1. The ear showing division into three parts.

number, which cross the space which is the middle ear. Since the eardrum will vibrate properly only if the atmospheric pressure on each side is equal, there is a connection from the middle ear to the outside via the eustachian tube. The third hearing bone connects with the inner ear, passes the vibrations to the inner ear fluids which results in stimulation of the nerve endings and the perception of sound.

The eustachian tube makes its presence known in conditions such as swimming and flying, where atmospheric pressure varies and unless the pressure on both sides of the eardrum is continuously equalized, the well-known consequences, pain and discomfort occur. However, the presence of a channel between mouth, upper airway and middle ear can also permit the passage of bacteria into the middle ear cavity especially during periods of respiratory infection which are frequent in children.

The condition, known as otitis media, or middle ear infection can, if it is recurrent or chronic, have a serious effect on the small, sound transmitting bones of the middle ear, causing adhesion of scar tissues to the wall and bones and eventual destruction of the bones themselves. Since the function of these bones is exclusively mechanical, it seemed likely that, in patients whose ossicles have been destroyed, a manmade material could be fabricated to replace them. Since the late fifties, many materials have been tried, with varying degrees of success. Many types of materials have and are being used, noble metals, stainless steel, polymers, composites based on polymers, porous polymers, ceramics both solid and porous and, most recently, glass ceramics and bioactive glasses. Once fabricated, the implant must be fixed in place in the middle ear, resting against the ear drum on one side attaching to the remains of the ossicle (the staples) which connects to the inner ear. Many techniques have been used to achieve this. The whole range of metals and polymers used in the ear consists of inert materials and, since they do not adhere of themselves to tissue, they have been fixed in place by crimping, adhesives, by scar tissue surrounding the implant or growing into the porous structure. Unfortunately, when implants have been fixed in place by these means, the long-term response in the patient has often not been good. Scar tissue as it grows holds the implant in place but absorbs the movement which it is meant to transmit. Where pores in the implant allow tissue ingrowth, they must be of a certain size and thus compromise the mechanical integrity of the device. Such devices may break into pieces as tissue invades and without effective adhesion to the ear drum, they can eventually penetrate and extrude into the outer ear, leaving a severely damaged eardrum. The implant ceases to function and must be replaced if the patient is to hear again. The most recent advances with ceramics, glass ceramics and bioactive glasses have crossed the boundary which separates inert from active materials and have given the surgeon materials which of themselves adhere to tissue, do not provoke a scar tissue and do not need adhesive nor ingrowth to keep them in place. These materials are a major advance in biomaterials science but present a new problem in the operating room.

Patients, and their middle ear cavities come in all shapes and sizes and no manufacturer of implants can hope to do more than approximate the range of shapes and sizes needed. All implants must be amenable to contouring in the operating room by the surgeon when he directly examines the middle ear of the anesthesized patient. Implants made from polymer and composites provide no problem and can be shaved and shaped with scalpels and surgical instruments. However ceramic and glass materials are not so easily contoured. They require special instruments, such as a diamond bit or burr and the burr may need cooling whilst in operation. Ceramic implants have been successfully shaped by the surgeon, usually these are of alumina, using the drill system which is used for drilling bone. Ceravital® implants, which are a glass-ceramic and Bioglass® implants, which are a glass, are now available and appear to present to the surgeon a more diffcult shaping problem. It is especially notable in the case of Bioglass® implants that there is some apprehension in approaching a clear glass material with a water cooled diamond blurr. Such apprehension on the part of the surgeon translates into cost to the patient since the longer it takes to shape and contour the implant, the longer the time the patient is in the operating room under anesthesia and the higher the cost on his hospital bills, to say nothing of damaged, shattered or otherwise lost implants which will already have cost more than $100.

It was with this situation in mind that we have investigated the machinability of Bioglass® implants under operating room conditions. We have looked at the ease of machining, speed of machining and the final finish. It is essential that our implant of bioactive material have a final finished surface which is smooth and without flakes or fragments which would cause unwanted tissue reactions. We have compared these measurements with those taken for Ceravital® under identical conditions since the materials are very similar, the major and most obvious difference being that Ceravital® is a poly crystalline glass-ceramic material and Bioglass® is a transparent glass.

MATERIALS

Bioglass® implants are now in clinical testing at the University of Florida and this material was used for the machining tests described. Bioglass® implant compositions have been specially designed to elicit a bond of living tissue to the surface of the implant [2]. The interfacial bond that forms is stronger than the cohesive attachment of the fibers of the tissue itself. Consequently, implants made from Bioglass® do not loosen with time as do biologically inactive implants.

The implants are made by melting a mixture of 45% (weight percent) SiO_2, in the form of high purity glass sand, 24.5% CaO, in the form of $CaCO_3$, 24.5% Na_2O, in the form of Na_2CO_3 and 6% P_2O_5 in the form of phosphoric acid at 1350°C in covered Pt crucibles, homogenizing for 24 hours, and pressure casting in machined graphite molds. This established the implant's primary shape which is a disc attached to a strut of variable length but usually between 1 and 2 mm in diameter. (See cover.) Bioglass® and Ceravital® implants were used for the machining study. The drill system used was the Shea Microdrill system which has a fast/slow speed control and which may be irrigated during drilling. The diamond burr used was 2.84 mm.

METHODS

The most usual requirement in the operating room is that the strut be made shorter. It may also be necessary to reshape the sides of the disc to fit the cavity. In these experiments the implants were hand held by the surgeon who was wearing surgical goves, mimicking conditions in the operating room. Measurements were made with a micrometer before and after drilling. Drilling was at slow and fast speeds with and without irrigation. A further experiment allowed the surgeon to use whichever technique he felt was appropriate to achieve a good finish. This last experiment, while not amenable to quantitation, does of course most closely simulate the conditions in the operating room.

To allow for slight differences in the strut diameters measurements were calculated as total volume of material removed per second of drilling. Usual time was 10 sec in each experiment. The number of experiments possible with Ceravital® was limited since few devices were available because of cost. They are included because they are already available and provide a basis for comparison.

Ceravital® glass-ceramic drilled at slow speed with a 2.84 mm diamond burr, without irrigation.

1. 0.068 mm^3 removed per second
2. 0.076 mm^3 removed per second
3. 0.071 mm^3 removed per second

Ceravital® glass-ceramic drilled at fast speed with 2.84 mm diamond burr, without irrigation.

1. 0.131 mm^3 removed per second

Ceravital® glass-ceramic drilled at slow speed with 2.84 mm diamond burr, with continuous irrigation (as suggested by the manufacturer).

1. 0.062 mm^3 removed per second
2. 0.119 mm^3 removed per second

Bioglass® glass drilled at slow speed with 2.84 mm diamond burr, without irrigation.

1. 0.165 mm^3 removed per second
2. 0.149 mm^3 removed per second
3. 0.116 mm^3 removed per second
4. 0.126 mm^3 removed per second
5. 0.136 mm^3 removed per second

Bioglass® drilled at fast speed with 2.84 mm diamond burr without irrigation.

1. 0.393 mm^3 removed per second
2. 0.383 mm^3 removed per second

Bioglass® glass drilled at slow speed with 2.84 mm diamond burr with continuous irrigation.

1. 0.070 mm³ removed per second
2. 0.134 mm³ removed per second
3. 0.186 mm³ removed per second

These results are shown in Figure 2.

As far as the *speed* of removal is concerned there appeared to be no difference in the rate at which a strut could be shortened whether irrigation was used or not. Irrigation while drilling did not make the implant harder to handle and more difficult to see and is probably a factor in the spread of results in the experiments with irrigation. The gradual increase in rate of removal of both materials probably represents increasing confidence on the part of the surgeon. However there seemed to be less flaking at the edge of the Bioglass® implant with irrigation. However flaking was not particularly notable in any experiment.

It is clear from the results that more Bioglass® material is removed per unit time consistently and with a fast drilling speed a strut can be shortened very quickly. No significant flaking or chipping was seen with either material.

When the surgeon was able to concentrate on achieving a good finish it was clear that it was possible to produce a smooth, non-chipped sur-

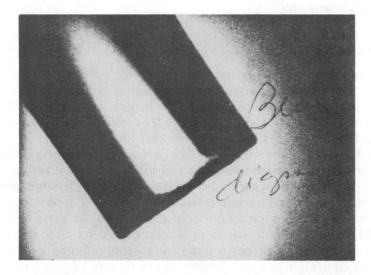

FIGURE 2. Rate of removal of Bioglass® and Ceravital® materials.

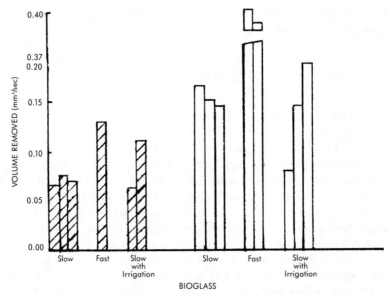

FIGURE 3. Bioglass® rod after shaping under operating room conditions.

face on the glass, providing the optimum materials conditions for the required tissue response in the patient (Figure 3). The glass-ceramic, being polycrystalline, presented a less smooth surface but again did not chip, crack or flake.

CONCLUSION

In spite of the popular conception that glassy materials are difficult to machine, we have shown that under operating room conditions a surgeon can shorten and shape small devices made from Bioglass® without problems and without risk to the device. The smooth final finish essential to the implant can be produced quickly and easily.

Similar experiments on Ceravital®, which is already in use, show that any surgeon familiar with that material will find the Bioglass® may be even easier to handle, a particular advantage being the transparency of the material, allowing precise placing and modelling in the ear.

Although our experiments have concentrated on the shaping of the middle ear prosthetic device, many other applications of the Bioglass® material are envisaged, particularly in orthopedic, dental and maxillofacial applications and our findings here will have relevance in those areas too.

REFERENCES

1. "Biomaterials in Otology: Proceedings of the First International Symposium," Leiden, the Netherlands, (April 1983).
2. L. L. Hench and E. C. Ethridge, *Biomaterials: An Interfacial Approach,* Academic Press, New York, NY (1983).

Advanced UV-Curable Polyurethanes for Wound Dressings

M. SZYCHER AND JONATHAN L. ROLFE
Thermedics Inc.,
Woburn, MA

G. C. BATTISTON AND J. VINCENT
United States Army Institute for Dental Research
Walter Reed Army Medical Center
Washington, DC

1. INTRODUCTION

FUTURE CONFLICTS MAY have to be fought without the advantage of overwhelming American Air supremacy. In the absence of air supremacy, it may not be possible to evacuate wounded American soldiers for proper medical treatment for at least several days. This situation implies that a wounded soldier would need to be treated in the field; the initial treatment would have to be performed by himself, by a buddy, or by an aid man.

Based on this scenario, we decided to develop a new field wound dressing. The new field wound dressing would need to be applied without the benefit of prior medical training, during combat, and under all imaginable climatic conditions. Furthermore, the new wound dressing needs to incorporate coagulants and extended-action therapeutic agent(s) to provide immediate and long-term stabilization of the wound. Presently available wound dressings do not meet these requirements. Under a research contract from the US Army Institute for Dental Research, Thermedics is developing a new field wound dressing based on an ultrafast curing polyurethane oligomer. When exposed to UV radiation

Reprinted from Vol. 30 SAMPE Proceedings, courtesy of Society for the Advancement of Material and Process Engineering, Covina, CA U.S.A.

during manufacture, it produces elastomeric films possessing oxygen and moisture vapor transmission characteristics resembling those of intact skin. Prior to cure, the urethane oligomer is precompounded with coagulants and extended-action therapeutic agents. This new family of biomedical-grade oligomers, when properly developed and tested, may become an ideal military field wound dressing for following reasons:

- Oligomer is synthesized from Nonexotic, off-the-shelf chemicals; thus the dressing will be inexpensive.
- All necessary manufacturing technology is present at Thermedics. Therefore, production lead time will be minimal.
- The ready-to-use field wound dressing will be dispensed from water-proof kits, carried in a standard-issue backpack.
- Field wound dressing may be applied under any conceivable climatic condition by non-medical personnel.
- Dressing is highly compliant for physical comfort and is highly abrasion resistant, even when wet.
- Dressing is moisture permeable but does not permit penetration of water or bacteria.

This unique combination of properties makes our new field wound dressing an innovative solution to the changing military medical priorities. At Thermedics, the research and biomedical staff are working closely with scientists at the US Army Institute for Dental Research in Washington D.C. to bring this exciting concept to clinical fruition.

2. RESEARCH OBJECTIVES

Contingency plans for future conflicts place unique demands on the military which are not experienced in the civilian community. Contrary to the treatment rendered to most casualties, it is most probable that soldiers wounded in future combat environments will face an entirely different situation. It will be common for evacuation of these patients to be delayed for 72 hours and possibly longer. During this critical post-wounding period, qualified medical personnel will not be immediately available to initiate therapy. It is during this time that care will be self administered or at best be provided by minimally trained personnel. It thus becomes critical that means are available to initiate therapeutic measures under these unusual circumstances. Less than half the number of soldiers killed in battle die outright as a result of explosions or high velocity missiles. The high morbidity and mortality associated with combat injuries is primarily attributable to post-wound medical complications, such as overwhelming infections and uncontrolled bleeding. Traditionally wounds have been treated with dressings. Wound dressings are usually composed of sterile, absorbent cloth pressure bandages, or a flat strip of elasticized, adhesive film, designed to cover and protect wounds.

The vast majority of maxillofacial wounds inflicted in combat are infected or become infected early on in their course of treatment. Presently available wound dressings are primarily limited to gauze pressure bandages. These materials provide minimally beneficial characteristics. They function as simple coverings that are not impervious to microorganisms, thus providing little protection from infection. By being absorbent, they may tend to desiccate the wound thus delaying healing. The material absorbed into the dressing may provide an excellent substrate supporting microbial growth. These materials may provide a mild measure of hemorrhage control by the application of pressure. However pressure must be maintained for long periods, thereby restricting movement so important in combat. For the situation described, our research objectives for the development of an ideal field wound dressing include:

1. Dressing which is soft and elastic, closely mimicking the mechanical properties of natural, intact skin.
2. Dressing should display adequate adhesion to intact skin, but be minimally adhering to clot, so it may be removed at will.
3. Dressing should control water vapor and oxygen exchange, resembling intact skin.
4. Dressing should gradually deliver broad spectrum antimicrobial agents that are non-toxic to the injured tissue.
5. Dressing should deliver a bolus of coagulant, to stop and control bleeding for prolonged periods.

These research objectives are based on the hypothesis that a field wound dressing, containing extended-action pharmacological agent(s), will provide immediate wound stabilization. This wound stabilization will be accomplished through: (a) hemostasis, (b) controlling infection, and (c) promotion of normal wound healing mechanisms.

We hypothesize that hemostasis will be rapidly reached through the incorporation of a coagulant such as Thrombostat (lyophilized thrombin). Infection control (from pathogenic bacteria, opportunistic invaders), will be accomplished by incorporation of pharmacological agent(s), such as gentamycin, or ampicillin anhydrate. Finally, promotion of normal wound healing mechanisms will be accomplished by the use of an abrasion-resistant, field-curable polymeric membrane, which is: (a) noninflammatory and nonantigenic to the wound, (b) compliant as skin, (c) similar to skin in oxygen permeability, and (d) similar to skin in water vapor transmission characteristics.

Incorporation of pharmacoactive agents is a key feature of the new wound dressing. The microencapsulation of drugs into a polymeric matrix was made possible by the development of a room temperature, ultrafast UV-curable polyurethane oligomer. This is a crucial consideration since most drugs are rapidly inactivated by mild heat. To insure full pharmacological activity, the drugs should not be subjected to heat. This requirement was met by incorporating the drugs into the liquid matrix of the uncured oligomer, followed by room temperature, UV-cure of the dressing.

Once cured, the wound dressing, containing drugs, becomes a sustained-release formulation. The dressing, once in contact with bodily fluids, provides immediate, direct and controlled doses of drugs, targeted to wound site, and thus minimizing problems inherent in systemic drug delivery. The technology involved in the selection and development of a sustained-release formulation will be discussed in the next few paragraphs.

3. SUSTAINED-RELEASE TECHNOLOGY

The need for devices that can deliver specific therapeutic agents to selected body sites at precisely controlled rates is best described by referring to Figure 1 which shows plasma drug concentration following the absorption of a therapeutic agent. Also shown are drug concentration levels above which a specific drug is toxic and below which it is not therapeutically effective. The difference between the two levels is known as the therapeutic index.

Plasma concentration of a drug after a single dose administration rapidly increases, then exponentially decays as the drug is excreted and/or metabolized. The drug is therapeutically effective only while the plasma concentration is above the minimum effective level, at which point another dose must be administered. The only way to increase length of therapeutic effectiveness is to increase initial loading. However, plasma drug concentration then exceeds the toxic level, and side effects become evident.

When a person swallows a pill, much of the drug may be distributed throughout the body; often only a small amount reaches the intended organ. To compensate for this inefficiency, doctors often administer large doses. That procedure is akin to flooding a skyscraper with water

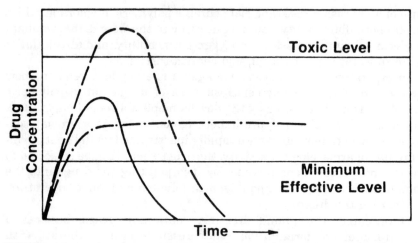

FIGURE 1. Drug concentration following absorption of therapeutic agent as a function of time. — safe dose; – – unsafe dose; · – · controlled release.

to extinguish a fire in a wastepaper basket on the twenty-fifth floor. Taking drugs orally or by injection has other disadvantages. When a drug is injected, much of its punch may be released in a single burst, flooding the blood stream; the level of drug then drops, requiring another shot and causing another burst; the result is a roller coaster pattern that can cause severe side effects.

A methodology that allows the plasma drug concentration to be maintained at any desired level for long periods of time, while never approaching the toxic level, clearly represents a significant advance in drug therapy. The new sustained-release systems are designed to overcome the above drawbacks; some can deliver the therapeutic level of conventional drugs with a tenfold, or even a hundredfold reduction in dose.

Current technology for the sustained release of pharmacoactive agents can be divided into three methodologies. These are diffusional, osmotic, and erosional. In diffusional devices a therapeutic agent is either dispersed in a polymer matrix or is placed in a core that is surrounded by a polymer membrane and release occurs by diffusion through the matrix or the polymer membrane. In osmotic devices a therapeutic agent is contained in a rigid housing and is pumped through a small orifice in the housing as a consequence of water penetration into the device through a semipermeable membrane driven by an osmotically active agent. In erosional devices the active agent can be chemically attached to a polymer backbone and released as its attachment to the polymer backbone cleaves by a hydrolysis reaction. The active agent can also be placed in a core and released by diffusion through a bioerodible polymer membrane or dispersed in a bioerodible matrix and released by diffusion from the matrix.

One type of diffusional device is the so called monolithic device. In a monolithic device the therapeutic agent is intimately dispersed (microencapsulated) in the rate-controlling polymer. Migration to the surface occurs by diffusion through pores within the matrix structure when exposed to an aqueous medium, such as bodily fluids. Our new wound dressing, which incorporates a coagulant and an antibiotic, can be properly classified as a monolithic sustained release device.

The recognition that drugs can be released from polymeric devices has resulted in a proliferation of research in the area of controlled delivery of bioactive agents. The ability of polymer matrices to meter drugs at controlled and reproducible rates for extended time periods provides significant benefits over conventional methods of drug delivery. Ideal drug administration requires that a constant level of the medicament be maintained throughout the course of therapy. This is rarely achieved in practice due to peak and valley blood concentrations which result from multiple dosing regimens. A schematic comparison of the two types of drug delivery is illustrated in Figure 2.

Referring to Figure 2, "Sustained" or "Controlled" drug delivery refers specifically to the precise control of the rate by which a particular drug dosage is released from a delivery system (ideally in a constant or neat-constant manner over a prolonged period of time) without the need for frequent, repeated administration, either orally or

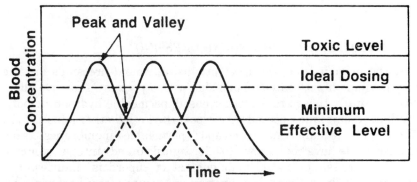

FIGURE 2. Hypothetical blood level pattern from a conventional multiple dosing schedule, and the idealized pattern from a controlled release system.

parenterally. Drug release rate that is constant over some fixed prolonged period of time follows zero-order kinetics in which the rate is
unaffected by the concentration. With orally ingested tablets and most
parenteral preparations (other than continuous i.v. infusions), there is
an initial rapid rate of release. This is followed by a steady decrease,
more or less in a first order manner, in which the rate is directly propor-
tional to the concentration until another dose must be administered to
maintain appropriate therapeutically effective drug concentration
levels in the blood. The steady decline in the rate of drug delivery until
another dose must be administered yields no therapeutic benefits.
Rather, it signifies a lack of control of the drug release by conventional
systems, including "sustained"–release preparations. In the latter
case, drug doses are released in "bursts" with consideration fluctua-
tions that give rise to "peaks" and "troughs" in the release profiles, and
consequently fail to provide constant drug concentration levels in the
blood. Furthermore, in many cases, orally ingested drugs (in contrast to
sublingual administration) are degraded rapidly and completely by the
liver prior to reaching the systemic circulation, thus diminishing the
therapeutic effectiveness over long periods of time. The advantages of
controlled-release devices are (1) reduced side effects due to the optimization of the blood concentration-time profile, (2) greater patient
compliance due to the elimination of multiple dosing schedules, (3)
reversibility of drug delivery which would allow for removal of the drug
source if needed, and (4) self-administration. In the case of our wound
dressing, only a small amount of coagulant is necessary to stop
bleeding since the pharmacological agent is directed at the precise
location. In addition, only a small amount of antibiotic is necessary to
prevent bacterial infection since the antibiotic is targeted directly at
the wound site.

4. DEVELOPMENT OF THE WOUND DRESSING

At the present time, the most promising wound dressings are the
polyurethane films, coated on one side with a pressure sensitive adhesive; generally these are polyether-based, permeable hydrophilic polyurethane membranes, coated with a polyvinyl ethyl ether adhesive [1].
These polyurethane moisture-vapor permeable membranes trade
named op-site have been shown to offer significant advantages over conventional dressings in the management of superficial injuries. The
hydrophilic polyurethane dressing protects wounds from bacterial contamination, while providing a suitable environment for rapid wound

healing [2]; patients seem more comfortable with the polyurethane dressing than with standard dressings [3], and rapid healing is produced by enhancement of re-epithelialization through increased mitotic division and migration of epidermal cells [4].

In spite of these impressive credentials, as a field wound dressing for high-velocity missiles, membrane-type wound dressings are impractical for two important reasons. First, application of these dressings often require two trained people and sometimes three [5]; a successful military field wound dressing should have the capability of being applied by only one person (the wounded soldier), or by a buddy. Second, membrane-type wound dressings act as occlusive dressings, devoid of pharmacological agents, such as coagulants. The management of bleeding, high-velocity missile wounds, often requires the presence of a coagulant to arrest bleeding, achieve hemostasis and, thus, stabilize the wound until more definitive medical treatment becomes available.

To prevent infection, systemic antibiotics must be administered within four hours after wounding when circulation is optimal [6]. If treatment is delayed, a milieu for bacterial growth develops resulting in complications associated with established infections [7]. Once infections are established it becomes difficult to systematically administer certain antibiotics for extended periods at levels that are safe, yet effective, at the wound site. Unless active locally, drugs are distributed throughout the body and the amount of drug hitting its target is only a small part of the total dose. This ineffective use of the drug is compounded in the trauma patient by hypovolemic shock, which results in a decreased vascular flow to tissues [8].

We are developing a field wound dressing reinforced with a nylon fabric which imparts to the dressing stretch properties (anisotropy) virtually identical to human skin. Our new wound dressing will be capable of being applied by one person, since it will be provided as a thin, pliable fabric-reinforced film, capable of being easily draped over complicated body contour. In addition, our new dressing will incorporate a coagulant, and a wide spectrum antibiotic.

Our wound dressing is based on an acrylic-terminated polyurethane oligomer, with a molecular weight between 2500 and 5000 Daltons. A high efficiency biocompatible photoinitiator is added at levels of less than one percent by weight, to provide a source of free radicals following UV bombardment. We have taken extraordinary measures to insure that all chemicals used in the composition are biocompatible, and in addition, that following UV cure there are few unreacted materials.

A common concern in the clinical use of unreacted materials is that there are repeated reports of toxicity, arising from the use of bone cements, such as polymethylmethacrylate, and also from the use of UV/ visible light-curable dental materials. Our review of the literature leads us to the conclusion that toxicity is traceable to the presence of leachable, unreacted monomers following apparent "cure" of the materials. Unreacted monomers, in contrast to the polymer, are low molecular weight cytotoxic fluids, capable of migration and leaching into surrounding tissue.

UV/visible light-curable dental materials depend on photochemical dissociation of a photoinitiator to produce free radicals. Either UV or visible light may be used to cleave the photoinitiator and thus initiate the polymerization reaction. Ultraviolet radiation is defined as that portion of the electromagnetic spectrum between 200 and 400 nm, and visible light is defined as that portion of the electromagnetic spectrum between 400 and 780 nm.

In the clinical use of radiation-curable composite restorative materials, two related factors are of concern: (1) rate and extent of the polymerization reaction, and (2) subacute toxicity to surrounding tissues. Radiation-curable composite restorative materials were initially screened for overt toxic effects; subcutaneous, intramuscular and intraosseous tests showed that implanted materials do not trigger inflammatory or allergic responses. Despite these favorable results in animal tests, the gradual exfoliation of clinical implants after five or more years suggest the possibility of subacute toxicity which manifests itself after prolonged times in situ. A recent study by Garcia, tested the biocompatibility of implanted polymethylmethacrylate (PMMA) in an animal model in which bone formation and resorption were independent of each other. Bone resorption was unaffected, but bone formation was seriously inhibited by the PMMA. Further, when three PMMA preparations varying in monomer content were tested, the data exhibited a dose-response relation, suggesting that inhibition of bone formation was due to the presence of leachable residual monomer.

Based on these findings, our UV-curable field wound dressing will be composed *only* of prereacted oligomers; prereacted oligomers, having molecular weights in the order of 2500 to 5000 Daltons, do not leach into surrounding tissues. Only low molecular weight monomers, such as methylmethacrylate (MMA), or hydroxyethylmethacrylate (HEMA), are sufficiently mobile to be leached by body fluids. To insure biocompatibility of both cured and uncured oligomers, we have undertaken a major test program designed to screen and identify any potential toxicity. Our initial tests were done in the laboratory (in vitro), and the specialized techniques employed, as well as the highly encouraging results, are discussed in the next section.

In Vitro Testing for Biocompatibility

A. GROWTH INHIBITION

African green monkey kidney cells (Vero) were grown in Dulbecco's modified eagles medium supplemented with 10% fetal bovine serum, 100 mm L-glutamine, 1% NCTC 109, 1% sodium pyruvate and penn-strep fungizone (DMEM) (M. A. Bioproducts, Walherville, MD). Cells were harvested by trypsin versine treatment, washed 3 times with Hank's balanced salt solution (HBSS) and viability count determined by trypan blue exclusion.

The vero cells were next suspended in DMEM at a concentration of 1×10^6 viable cells per ml. At this time 300 ml of the cell suspension was placed in each well of 24 well tissue culture plates and the plates were next incubated for 3 hr at 37°C in 10% CO_2 and 100% humidity to allow cell adhesion.

The media and non-adherent cells were then removed by aspiration and 300 ml of fresh DMEM was added to each well.

Samples of wound dressing were cut into 4 mm squares and placed in direct contact with the bottom of each well. The following samples were evaluated in triplicate: pre-cured wound dressings containing either 2, 4 or 6% photoinitiator; uncured wound dressings which were then cured *in situ* by exposure to UV light. All samples were evaluated visually at 24, 48, 72 and 96 hours for estimation of cell growth in approximation to the wound dressing by phase contrast microscopy. In addition, 100 ml of the media was removed from each well at each time frame, 100 ml of fresh media added as a replacement, and the media mixed with trypan blue. All samples were placed in a hemocytometer and the number of non-viable cells/100 ml was determined and compared to control wells which had been treated in an identical manner with the exception that no wound dressings had been placed in the wells.

At all observation periods, all formulations of the wound dressings appeared similar (Figures 3 and 4). It was observed that cell density increased as incubation time was extended. By 96 hours, all samples displayed cell monolayers which appeared to be in intimate contact with the wound dressing margins. The number of non-viable cells observed in media samples which had been exposed to the wound dressings was similar to the control wells (Table 1). As wound be expected, the number of non-viable cells/100 ml of media increased in both experimental and control wells as the incubation time was extended. These data suggest that the wound dressings tested had minimal to no adverse effect of tissue culture cells.

Table 1. Non-viable cells/100 ml of media removed from tissue culture wells.

	Incubation time			
	24 hr	48 hr	72 hr	96 hr
Control wells N = 12	0.16*	0.47	0.93	1.82
Experimental wells N = 24	0.21	0.46	1.01	1.79

*Mean non-viable cells per 100 ml.

B. CYTOTOXICITY (CHROMIUM RELEASE METHOD)

Vero cells were cultured and harvested as before, suspended in DMEM and total viable count was determined by trypan blue exclusion. All samples used in this procedure displaned > 98% viability. Following centrifugation, the cells were suspended at a concentration of 1×10^6 cells/ml and were labelled with medium chromate (^{51}Cr) with approximately 1.5u C per 10^6 cells. The sample was incubated for 90 minutes at 37°C in 10% CO_2, washed 2 times in HBSS and resuspended in DMEM. Following a 1 hour incubation, cells were again washed 2 times in HBSS and alliquated in DMEM at either 60,000 30,000 or 15,000 cells/200 ml. Samples (200 ml) of each cell concentration were plated in each well of 96-well tissue culture plates and exposed to either 1% SDS to determine total ^{51}Cr release, no exposure to determine spontaneous release and to 2 mm sg segments of selected wound dressings as the experimental group. Following a 24 hour incubation, the culture supernatant was removed using the Titerteh Supernatant Collection System and ^{51}Cr release was determined for all samples using a Model 1185 Gamma Comm (Tracor Analytic, Elhr Grove Village, IL).

The data obtained (Table 2) for all samples was similar, as the cell

Table 2. CR^{51} release expressed as mean CPM following 24 hour incubation.

Cell Concentration	Total Release	Spontaneous Release	Experimental Release
60,000/well	56783*	10179*	9569*
30,000/well	29172	5247	4598
15,000/well	16427	2506	2470

*Mean CPM. N = 3 for each group tested.

concentration decreased, the counts per minute (CPM) decreased proportionally. When the CPM of the experimental group was compared to the CPM in the spontaneous release group, the data were indistinguishable. Both groups displayed approximately 20% of the CP, obtained in the total release groups.

Within the limits of these studies it would appear that the previously mentioned wound dressing are noncytotoxic to tissue culture cells *in vitro* thus suggesting that one would expect no cytotoxicity *in vivo*. It would appear that these wound dressings would be biocompatable in an *in vivo* model system.

CONCLUSIONS

Sustained-release wound dressing are being developed by microencapsulating a variety of drugs into a UV-curable urethane oligomer. The uncured drug/oligomer system is a low viscosity thixotropic mixture, which may be closely applied to any contour of the human body following a ten second UV cure during manufacture. The ready-to-use wound dressing releases the drugs continuously and predictably when exposed to bodily fluids. This sustained-release wound dressing may be used to provide long/lasting therapeutic action capable of delivering pharmacoative agents such as coagulants and antibiotics. Most of these drugs are highly toxic, but in this case, since the drug is delivered only at the needed site in small concentrations, undesirable side effects are minimized.

REFERENCES

1. T. E. Lobe, *et al.*, *J. Ped. Surg.*, *15*, 6 (1980).
2. G. D. Winter, "Epidermal Regeneration Studies in the Domestic Pig," *Epidermal Wound Healing*, edited by Marbach and Rovee, Year Book Medical Publishers, Inc. (1972).
3. Y. Cavlak, *Aktuelle Traumatologie*, *10* (1980).
4. D. J. McCarthy, *J. Am. Pod. Assoc.*, *73*, 1 (1983).
5. W. Conkle, "Op-Site Dressing: New Approach to Burn Care," *J. Emerg. Nursing* (1981).
6. J. F. Burke, *Surgery*, *50*, 161 (1961).
7. G. Rodeheaver, M. T. Edgerton, M. B. Elliott, L. D. Kurtz, and R. E. Edlich, *Am. J. Surg.*, *127*, 564 (1974).
8. L. E. Gelin and J. R. Border, *J. Trauma*, *10*, 1078 (1970).

High Molecular Weight Citric Acid Esters as Effective Plasticizers for Medical-Grade PVC*

E. H. HULL
Special Chemicals Department
Pfizer, Inc.
2110 High Point Road
Greensboro, NC 27403

K. K. MATHUR
Materials Science Division
Pfizer, Inc.
P.O. Box 548
Easton, PA 18042

INTRODUCTION

RECENT STUDIES REPORTED by the National Toxicological Program have indicated two chemicals, di-2-ethylhexyl phthalate (DEHP or DOP) and di-2-ethylhexyl adipate (DEHA or DOA), to be hepatocarcinogens in rodents. Both of these compounds are used to plasticize PVC for a wide variety of applications in the food-contact and medical-device areas. DEHP, in particular, is used as the plasticizer for PVC in devices such as blood bags and medical tubing. It is known that DEHP is extracted into the fluids in contact with the plasticized PVC and that small quantities of the plasticizer or its degradation fragments are being introduced, in some cases, into the blood stream of the patient.

In early studies of the toxic effects of DEHP it was common to

Presented at ANTEC '84, The Society of Plastics Engineers, Inc. 42nd Technical Conference, April 30–May 3, New Orleans, LA U.S.A.
*Reprinted with permission from *Modern Plastics,* May, 1984. Copyright 1984, McGraw-Hill, Inc.

use massive or "kill" dosage levels of the plasticizer. The conclusion reached may well be objected to on the scientific grounds that (1) the dosage levels were far above those encountered in the real world and that (2) the animals employed may not necessarily show the same toxicological effect as would a human. Both of these objections appear to have been overcome in a series of studies conducted by Kevy and Jacobson. Rhesus monkeys were used in the later studies and it was reported that "abnormalities in hepatic scan and BSP (bromosulfophthalein) persisted for up to 26 months after transfusion as did histologic abnormalities. Patients undergoing maintenance hemodialysis receive a yearly dose of DEHP which is 10–20 times that which produced hepatotoxicity in the transfused rhesus [1]."

The focus of our program is to develop replacements for the phthalate esters which (1) show a low order of toxicity and (2) impart to PVC the proper balance of properties needed in the aforementioned applications. Citric acid, which occurs naturally in citrus fruits, appears to be an ideal precursor for this purpose. It is the only commercially available acid which affords four sites for esterification. This feature, in turn, provides an unusual degree of freedom in building the optimum molecular weight/polarity relationship needed to achieve the proper balance of properties in the plasticized PVC.

For some 25 years our company has been manufacturing and marketing four citric acid esters, primarily for use in food-contact films. Below is shown the general formula for citrate esters, together with trade names, generic names and some of the commercial uses of these four esters.

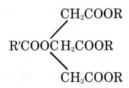

$$CH_2COOR$$
$$R'COOCH_2COOR$$
$$CH_2COOR$$

Citroflex	Generic Name	M.W.	Plasticizer for
C-2	Triethyl Citrate	276	Cellulosics
A-2	Acetyltriethyl Citrate	318	Cellulosics
C-4	Tri-n-butyl Citrate	360	Cellulosics
A-4	Acetyltri-n-butyl Citrate	402	PVC, PVDC

Citroflex A-4, in particular, is an excellent plasticizer for food films and is FDA approved for this purpose. It is, however, too extractable, particularly by soapy water, to be useful in many of the applications in the medical area.

It was obvious that esters of higher molecular weight than A-4 were needed; therefore a number of esters were prepared and screened for compatibility with PVC. Selection of the other precursors used in the ester synthesis was balanced on the following criteria:

1. Aliphatic
2. Straight carbon chain
3. Even-numbered carbon chain

These materials, in general, show lower orders of toxicity than their aromatic, branched-chain or odd-numbered carbon chain counterparts. Finally, but most importantly, the alcohols selected are commercially available.

Using these criteria, the homologous series of citrate esters, with alkyl units ranging from C_6 to C_{18} and alkoxy units ranging from C_2 to C_6 were synthesized. The series included mixtures of alkyl units, which are sometimes more effective than their pure counterparts. Esters with alkyl carbon chains ≥ 10 were found to be incompatible with the medium molecular weight PVC resin (inherent viscosity 0.96) used in our tests. However, mixed esters in which significant amounts of C_{10} alkyl chains are incorporated along with the C_6 and C_8 chains are compatible with PVC. We should note parenthetically that there are some targeted market areas for the esters with alkyl carbon chains ≥ 10, e.g. emollients, lubricants, etc., but that these areas are outside the scope of the present study.

In reference to the chain length of the alkoxy unit, esters with the C_6 alkoxy unit were eliminated owing to both the cost of the precursor(s) involved and to excessive processing costs of the ester. At this point, the majority of the candidates synthesized and tested were screened out, leaving four candidates for more rigorous testing as plasticizers for medical-grade PVC:

A-6	Acetyltri-n-hexyl Citrate	486
B-6	n-Butyryltri-n-hexyl Citrate	514
A-610	Acetyltri-n-(hexyl/octyl/decyl) Citrate	576
A-810	Acetyltri-n-(octyl/decyl) Citrate	612

PREPARATION AND TESTING OF PVC PLAQUES

Formulation	Parts by Weight
Resin (Medium Molecular Weight PVC)	100
Plasticizer	50
Stabilizer (Calcium/Zinc)	2.5
Lubricant (Stearic Acid)	0.25

The plastic stock was blended and two-roll milled for 5–10 minutes at 325° to 340°F. The milled stock was compression molded (3 min. at 340°–360°F and 32,000 psi) into 40- and 70-mil sheets, and conditioned for 48 hours at 75°F for evaluation. All tests were made with samples cut from 70-mil compression molded stock except for extraction tests which were conducted on 70-mil samples.

The performance data were obtained by accepted ASTM methods—any modifications are detailed below.

Tensile Strength Ultimate Elongation Modulus (100% elongation (ASTM D638)	Determined with Instron TT, 1100 series (2 in./min.) using a dumbbell-shaped specimen. Test carried out at 70° ± 5°F.
Hardness (ASTM D676)	Determined with Shore Durometer A (10 sec.) at 75° ± 5°F.
Torsional Flex (T_4 and T_f) (ASTM D1043)	Determined with Torsion Flex Tester of Clash and Berg design. T_4 is the temperature at which the Modulus of Rigidity is 10,000 psi; T_f is the temperature at which the Modulus of Rigidity is 100,000 psi.
Brittle Point (ASTM D746)	Determined by impact method using Scott Tester, Model E.
Volatile Loss (A/C) (ASTM D1203)	Determined on specimens 2 inches in diameter heated in activated carbon at 70°C for 24 hours. Results are expressed as percent of plasticizer lost.
Water Extraction (Tap)	Determined on specimens 2 inches in diameter suspended in appropriate liquid at 60°C for 24 hours. Results are expressed as percent of plasticizer lost.

Soapy Water Extraction (1% Ivory Flakes) Oil Extraction (ASTM No. 3)	Determined on specimens 2 inches in diameter suspended in appropriate liquid at 60°C for 24 hours. Results are expressed as percent of plasticizer lost.
Migration Loss (Silica)	Determined on specimens 2 inches in diameter heated in silica (100 mesh), at 70°C for 24 hours. Results are expressed as percent of plasticizer lost.
Volatile Loss (Air)	Determined by Oven Method (24 hr. at 100°C) on specimens 2 inches in diameter. Results are expressed as percent of plasticizer lost.

PVC PLASTISOLS

Formulation	PHR
PVC (Geon 121 or 178)	100
Plasticizer	As specified
Epoxidized Soybean Oil	3
Stabilizer (Calcium/Zinc)	1.5
Chelator	0.5
USP Grade $CaCO_3$	Where specified

Mixing Procedure: The primary and secondary plasticizers were charged to the Hobart Mixer and mixed for 30 seconds. While mixing at slow speed, PVC resin was added as quickly as possible. After 10 minutes of mixing, the stabilizer package was added and the mixing was continued for a total time of 20 minutes. The plastisol was deaerated on a Whip-Mix Model B high speed mixer for 5 minutes under vacuum.

Viscosity Measurements: The initial and time dependent viscosities were made on both Brookfield and Burrell viscometers. A Brookfield RVF-100 viscometer fitted with Spindle #5 was used at 20 rpm throughout the study.

The Brookfield stability was measured after 1

hour, 1 day, and 1, 2, 3, and 4 weeks of storage at room temperature (75 ± 5°F).

The Severs efflux rates were measured with a Burrell-Severs Model A-1200 rheometer equipped with a 0.166 cm diameter extrusion head.

The mass (grams) of plastisol extruded over a period of 100 seconds was determined at 30–90 psig.

RESULTS AND DISCUSSION

The four citrate esters selected were first characterized for typical properties as shown in Table 1. The four esters ranged in molecular weight from 486 to 612. The parameters of purity, color, odor, and neutralization number are basically dependent on processing capabilities. The values shown in this table are well within the usual specifications for high quality plasticizers. Properties such as specific gravity, refractive index, viscosity, pour point, flash point and solubility are inherent to the particular chemical compound, although impurities can change them significantly.

Table 2 shows the effect at 50 PHR of these citrate plasticizers on key ambient and low temperature properties of plasticized PVC in compari-

Table 1. Typical properties of citric acid esters.

Properties	A-6	B-6	A-610	A-810
Molecular Weight	486	514	576	612
Purity Weight-%	>99.0	>99.0	>99.0	>99.0
Color (APHA)	35	35	70	70
Neutralization Number	0.2	0.2	0.2	0.2
Moisture Weight-% (K.F.)	0.25	0.25	0.25	0.25
Specific Gravity @25/25°C	1.0046	0.9910	0.9742	0.9666
Refractive Index-25°C	1.447	1.445	1.450	1.450
Viscosity @25°C (cps)	36	28	47	50
Pour Point—°C	−57	−55	−51	−51
Flash Point-°F (C.O.C.)	465	400	460	485
Solubilities @25°C (g/100 ml)				
H₂O	<0.1	<0.1	<0.1	<0.1
Toluene	∂	∂	∂	∂
Heptane	∂	∂	∂	∂
Odor	Mild	Mild	Mild	Mild

Table 2. Performance properties of citrate esters, DEHP and DEHA.

Plasticizer	A-6	B-6	A-610	A-810	DEHP	DEHA
Hardness, Durometer, A (10 sec)	81	81	87	87	79	78
Tensile-psi	2978	2924	2743	2789	2748	1797
Ultimate Elongation-%	390	427	364	374	395	414
100% Modulus-psi	1574	1362	1656	1704	1368	1092
T_4 (10,000 psi)-°C	−9.1	−11.9	−6.9	−4.0	−8.4	−30.8
T_f (100,000 psi)-°C	−41.6	−48.7	−53.1	−59.7	−38.8	−66.5
Brittle Point-°C	−26.0	−33.5	−36.8	−37.8	−24.5	−56.5

son with DEHP and DEHA. The citrate esters imparted slightly higher hardness to PVC as compared with either DEHP or DEHA.

The ultimate tensile strength imparted by the citrates is significantly higher than that imparted by DEHA. The lower molecular weight citrate esters (A-6 and B-6) imparted higher tensile strengths than DEHP, while the results with higher molecular weight citrate esters (A-610 and A-810) were comparable to DEHP.

The ultimate elongation of PVC plasticized with A-6 was comparable to DEHP, while the B-6 and DEHA imparted a slightly higher value. The other two citrate esters (A-610 and A-810) imparted a slightly lower ultimate elongation.

On the low temperature torsional test, DEHA clearly imparted the best properties while the citrates were as good as or superior to DEHP.

The results of the brittle point test show DEHA to be superior to the citrates while they, in turn, are superior to DEHP.

In all of the transport properties (volatility, extraction and migration tests) DEHA is far inferior to DEHP. This set of properties would preclude the use of DEHA in the devices under consideration (Table 3).

In the volatility and migration tests the values for the first three citrates are lower than those for DEHP while the extraction test results are fairly comparable to DEHP. Of particular significance here is the soapy water extraction test which is reportedly the principal standard test which provides results that correlate best with those obtained with the various media encountered in medical applications.

In Tables 4 and 5 the results of some tests with citrate ester/epoxized soybean oil (ESO) blends are shown. ESO is commonly used in conjunction with DEHP at levels in the range of 1–5% (based on DEHP) as an aid in stabilization. We selected a ratio of 2.5/97.5 ESO/citrate as a base point in our studies. Test results on this combination are shown in Column 1. A significant improvement in properties, the soapy water extraction, is noted.

Table 3. Performance properties of citrate esters, DEHP and DEHA.

	A-6	B-6	A-610	A-810	DEHP	DEHA
Volatile Loss (Air)-%	2.6	1.7	0.3	0.1	4.8	7.1
Volatile Loss (A/C)-%	1.7	1.4	2.8	4.5	3.4	7.6
Water Extraction-%	1.9	1.7	1.5	3.3	0.7	1.5
Soapy Water Extraction-%	5.4	2.2	3.4	2.4	2.7	11.0
Oil Extraction-%	13.8	15.7	15.2	19.3	11.4	34.7
Silica Gel Migration-%	4.4	3.6	4.8	7.4	12.2	23.0

Table 4. Comparative performance properties of citrate esters/ESO blends.

Plasticizer	2.5 ESO 97.5 A-6	20 ESO 80 A-6	40 ESO 60 A-6	40 ESO 60 B-6	40 ESO 60 A-810
Hardness, Durometer A, (10 sec)	81	80	80	81	85
Tensile-psi	2907	3010	3079	3165	3097
Ultimate Elongation-%	422	424	420	428	395
100% Modulus-psi	1415	1429	1491	1514	1779
T_4 (10,000 psi)-°C	−9.5	−7.8	−7.7	−8.2	−5.4
T_f (100,000 psi)-°C	−41.8	−41.3	−39.3	−41.8	−50.3
Brittle Point-°C	−26.5	−25.5	−20.5	−24.5	−26.5

Table 5. Comparative performance properties of citrate esters/ESO blends.

Plasticizer	2.5 ESO 97.5 A-6	20 ESO 80 A-6	40 ESO 60 A-6	40 ESO 60 B-6	40 ESO 60 A-810
Volatile Loss (Air)-%	2.4	2.1	1.5	0.8	0.5
Volatile Loss (A/C)-%	1.3	1.6	1.4	0.9	1.1
Water Extraction-%	1.3	0.9	0.6	0.8	1.0
Soapy Water Extraction-%	2.9	2.9	6.4	4.8	3.8
Oil Extraction-%	13.0	11.6	10.1	10.0	12.9
Silica Gel Migration-%	5.7	5.3	4.7	4.0	2.5

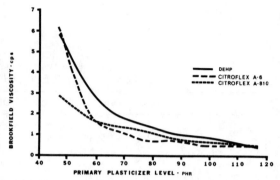

FIGURE 1. Brookfield viscosities at varying plasticizer levels in GEON 178 system.

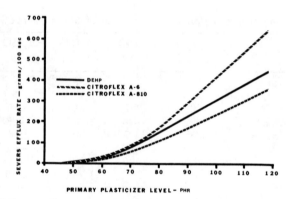

FIGURE 2. Severs efflux rate at varying plasticizer levels in GEON 178 system.

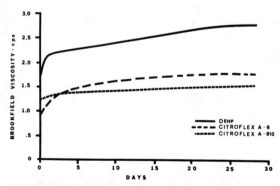

FIGURE 3. Effect of aging on viscosity of GEON 178.

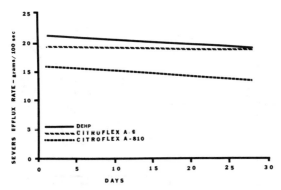

FIGURE 4. Severs efflux rate after thirty days (GEON 178 system).

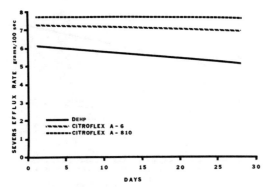

FIGURE 5. Severs efflux rate after thirty days (GEON 178 system, 15 PHR Albaglos USP).

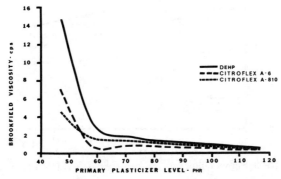

FIGURE 6. Brookfield viscosity at varying plasticizer levels in GEON 121 system.

195

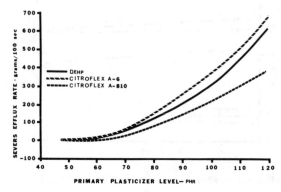

FIGURE 7. Severs efflux rate at varying plasticizer levels in GEON 121 system.

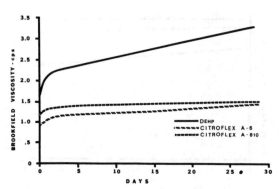

FIGURE 8. Effect of aging on viscosity of GEON 121.

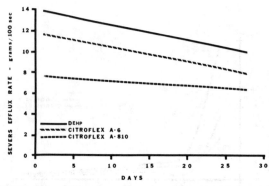

FIGURE 9. Severs efflux rate after thirty days (GEON 121 system).

Since ESO is less expensive than the citrates, a reduction in plasticizer cost would result if a higher ratio of ESO could be used. The results of tests with higher ESO/citrate ratios are shown in columns 2–5 of Tables 4 and 5. Interestingly, along with reduced plasticizer costs we find a significant improvement in properties up to, and perhaps beyond, a ratio of 20/80 ESO/citrate.

In another part of our investigation, two of the new citrate esters, A-6 and A-810 (the lowest and highest molecular weights respectively), were compared with DEHP in plastisols.

The citrate esters imparted lower Brookfield viscosities, which were very significant up to 80 PHR level (Figure 1).

The extrusion rates of these plastisols (Figure 2) are reasonably comparable up to the 70 PHR level. Some differences are seen above this level but, for most commercial applications, they will show equal performance.

Plastisols prepared through incorporation of the citrates with the medium-high molecular weight resin showed stable viscosities through the 30-day test period (Figure 3). Similarly, the extrusion rate was practically unaffected on storage for 30 days (Figure 4).

If opaque formulations are desired, U.S.P. Grade $CaCO_3$ can be employed as a filler to further lower the cost without sacrifice in the key processing properties (Figure 5).

Plastisols formulated with a medium molecular weight PVC resin also exhibit desirable rheological and stability propeties (Figures 6–9).

TOXICOLOGY

1. *Acute dermal toxicity and dermal and ocular irritation studies in rabbits for Citroflex A-6 and B-6.*

   The Citroflexes were evaluated for toxicity by dermal absorption and for dermal and ocular irritation in rabbits according to the Federal Hazardous Substances Act guidelines.

   The tests indicate that undiluted Citroflex A-6 and B-6 are not toxic substances, primary skin irritants, or ocular irritants to unrinsed eyes.

2. *Acute oral toxicity in mice and rats with Citroflex A-6, B-6 and A-810.*

   The purpose of these studies was to evaluate the effects in mice and rats following administration of single oral doses of Citroflex A-6, B-6 and A-810.

   The oral administration of maximum practical dose volumes (48 g/kg in mice and 20 g/kg in rats) of each of the samples produced no signs of systemic toxicity and no mortality in fasted mice or rats.

3. *The genetic toxicology on Citroflexes A-6, B-6 and A-810.*

Citroflexes A-6, B-6 and A-810 have been examined in a battery of genetic toxicology assays for detecting mutagenic activity at the gene or chromosomal level.

These studies demonstrate that at the levels tested these esters do not induce gene mutation in either microbial cells or in mammalian cells *in vitro* or chromosomal mutation *in vivo* or *in vitro*.

4. *Citroflex plasticizers—in vitro hydrolysis by serum, liver and intestinal enzymes.*

Citroflexes A-6 and B-6 were hydrolyzed upon incubation with rat sible three moles of hexanol for every Citroflex mole, only one hexanol mole was initially liberated. Hydrolysis proceeds faster in serum than in liver and is much slower in the intestinal preparation.

As is the case with other enzymatic reactions, the rate of Citroflex hydrolysis is concentration dependent and is much faster at lower concentrations. Since the realistic levels of human exposure to Citroflex plasticizers are likely to be much lower than the concentrations in the present study, it is possible that, under *in vivo* conditions, those esters are hydrolyzed rapidly and completely.

CONCLUSIONS

1. Compounded PVC plasticized with the Ciroflexes can be processed without difficulty by conventional extrusion, calendering or plastisol techniques.
2. The plasticized PVC meets all of the known requirements for physical properties needed in the medical area.
3. The incorporation of higher-than-usual levels of ESO appears to have a synergistic effect, resulting in an enhancement of properties at lower cost.
4. Opaque formulations can be compounded with U.S.P. grade $CaCO_3$ to realize cost savings without adverse effects on physical properties.
5. In biological studies conducted to date a low order of acute toxicity is indicated.
6. The Citroflex esters merit serious consideration as replacements of DEHP in medical plastics. It should be noted that these new esters would require regulatory approval before use.

REFERENCES

1. S. C. Kevy and M. S. Jacobson, *Environmental Health Perspectives,* 45, 57 (1982).

Visible Light Cured Biomaterials

HENRY LEE
Lee Pharmaceuticals
South El Monte, California

ABSTRACT

The development of tooth colored polymeric filling materials over the past 50 years is described. The earliest material was unfilled poly (methyl methacrylate). Due to its softness and other problems chemists evaluated numerous other classes of materials such as: filled poly(methyl methacrylate), filled polyesters, filled aziridino polyesters, filled amine-cured and Lewis acid-cured epoxy resins, and poly (urethanes). Eventually aromatic thermosetting acrylic resins derived from epoxy resins, and numerous analogs synthesized directly for this purpose, became popular. Fillers evaluated and adopted or rejected include whiskers, chopped fibers, powdered minerals (including diamond dust) and glasses ranging in particle size from 1 micron to 40 microns, precoated submicron aerosils, and sintered and porous fillers. Organo functional silanes are widely used to preserve resin-filler bonds for long service in wet fields. Set times must range from 60 seconds to 300 seconds, with 90% of full properties (such as compressive strengths of 45,000 psi and bond strengths to enamel and dentin and cementum of 2000 psi) being achieved within 1 hr or less. Cure mechanisms available to the dentist have evolved from two container resin-catalyst formulas to single container ultra violet light cured formulas, and more recently to visible light cured systems. The advantages and disadvantages of each cure method is reviewed.

INTRODUCTION

THE WIDESPREAD USE of sugar in the past few hundred years has led to a rapid increase in the number of carious teeth found in the mouth of the average teenager or adult in the civilized world. Although the introduction of various programs to make the tooth more resistant

Reprinted from *SAMPE Journal*, May/June 1985, courtesy of Society for the Advancement of Materials and Process Engineering, Covina, CA U.S.A.

to decay by converting normal hydroxy apatite to fluoro apatite through systemic or topical use of fluorides, has been reasonably successful in some countries, nevertheless there has been great demand for over 50 years for materials which could be used to fill cavities in teeth and which would survive the rigors of a wet field, rapid temperature changes from 4 to 40 C, abrasion from food, and abrasion from contact with the hardest biological substance, enamel, as well as the disruptive action of saliva, which is slightly basic, and regurgitated stomach fluids, which can be strongly acid.

For many years gold was the popular filling material. It could be introduced as foil, and condensed into a solid with proper mechanical working. It was both strong and durable. It was unfortunately too expensive as to both labor and materials. It also did not restore teeth to their natural color.

Hence, materials and process engineering concepts had to be applied. One less expensive material developed over 100 years ago was silver alloys, which are amalgams of silver, mercury, and minor elements such as copper and tin, etc. These alloys have served moderately well for posterior teeth and cements based on silicates for anterior teeth. Unfortunately the alloys are not cosmetic, and the silicates wash out in the alkaline saliva of the mouth.

INTRODUCTION OF POLYMER

In the late 1930's plastic or polymeric filling materials began to appear. These were based primarily on methyl methacrylate. To minimize shrinkage and to provide suitable viscosity for handling and application, the formula was divided into two parts. Part A was a liquid made of methyl methacrylate monomer, with perhaps a few percent of ethylene dimethacrylate to improve hardness and solvent resistance, and weak tertiary amine as part of a redox catalytic system. Part B was polymerized methyl methacrylate (PMMA) in powder form. The powder was coated with a peroxide as the catalyst of the redox curing system. When Part A and B were mixed together the monomer softened the surface of the polymer and a workable paste was achieved which could be placed in a cavity and which would then set in a few minutes. It could be finished or polished easily, and with a trace of pigments could match the pearlescence of the human tooth.

Unfortunately, methyl methacrylate has too high a polymerization shrinkage for filling teeth, even if some of the mass has been prepolymerized. As the material sets, it pulls away from the margins of the cavity, opening up microscopic leakage paths for further decay causing factors. This was offset to some degree by conscientious dentists who painted the material in layer by layer, sealing all shrinkage gaps by the application of the next coat.

However, the good work of these operators was undone by the introduction of the tooth brush with nylon bristles, which quickly wore their way into the filling material.

Of course, there were also other problems with these early PMMA formulas: (1) Some of the tertiary amines used as accelerators caused yellowing and browning of the restoration in the time, due to the action of sunlight entering the oral cavity. (2) Some of the minor formulating ingredients such as methacrylic acid, were of such a low viscosity and activity that they easily penetrated the tubules of the dentin and entered the pulp chamber and produced an inflammatory response to the tissue there, leading to tissue necrosis.

Thus, there were enough problems with PMMA to warrant further work and process development for anterior restorative materials. However, it was also a goal of the dental chemists to find a replacement for gold foil fillings and for silver alloy fillings. The posterior teeth, of course, where the occlusal (biting) surface is involved pose special problems of strength and wear resistance, making the formulation problems immensely more difficult.

INTRODUCTION OF COMPOSITES

During the 1960's a number of filled resin systems were tried. These included various polyesters, including the aziridino polyesters, epoxy resins, polyurethanes, and others. The thermosetting acrylic systems were also introduced for both anterior and posterior use. The early formulas used the reaction product of the diglycidyl ether of bisphenol A with methacrylic acid to produce a dimethacrylate. This dimethacrylate was then cured with the same general class of peroxides and amines used with the PMMA formulas.

The reader will recognize that when this adduct (see Bis-Gma in Table 1) is cured, it will be generally indistinguishable from an epoxy resin that has been cured with poly (methacrylic acid). In other words, the chemist has driven the epoxy-carboxylic acid reaction in a reactor, cooking the curing agent onto the epoxy resin with hear, as it were, and then letting the dentist polymerize the "curing agent" in the dental cavity at body temperature.

Thus, the cured resin has the molecular structure of a heat cured epoxy, with the full strength and chemical resistance inherent in the bisphenol moiety. It reveals somewhat higher shrinkage and thus

Table 1. Monomers in Use in Modern Dentistry for Cosmetic Restorative Materials, Enamel and Dentin Adhesives, and Fissure Sealants. Basic Epoxy Resin Monomer "Diglycidyl Ether of Bisphenol A," its Derivative Reaction Product with Methacrylic Acid, BIS-GMA, and Analogous Methacrylic Monomers, plus Specialized Methacrylic Monomers developed for Dental Applications.

Diglyclidyl Ether of Bisphenol A

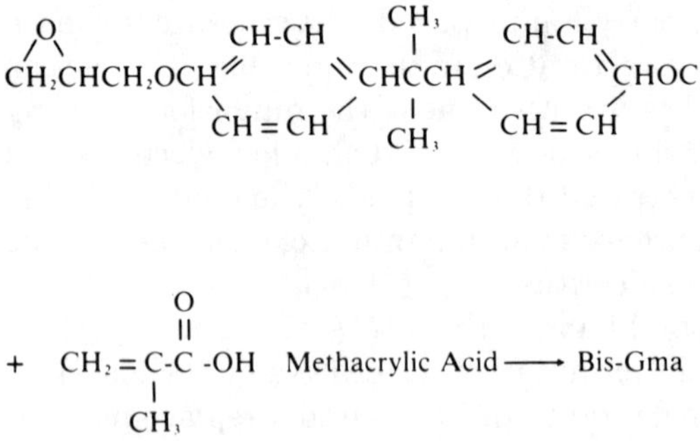

$$CH_2CHCH_2OCH \overset{CH-CH}{\underset{CH=CH}{\diagdown}} CHCCH \overset{CH_3}{\underset{CH_3}{\mid}} \overset{CH-CH}{\underset{CH=CH}{\diagdown}} CHOCH_2CHCH_2$$

$$+\quad CH_2=\underset{\underset{CH_3}{\mid}}{C}-\overset{\overset{O}{\parallel}}{C}-OH \quad \text{Methacrylic Acid} \longrightarrow \text{Bis-Gma}$$

1. Bis-Gma

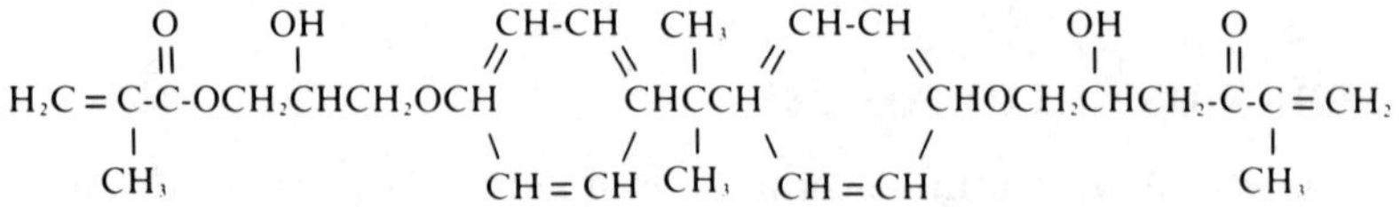

$$H_2C=\underset{\underset{CH_3}{\mid}}{C}-\overset{\overset{O}{\parallel}}{C}-OCH_2\underset{\underset{OH}{\mid}}{CH}CH_2OCH \overset{CH-CH}{\underset{CH=CH}{\diagdown}} CHCCH \overset{CH_3}{\underset{CH_3}{\mid}} \overset{CH-CH}{\underset{CH=CH}{\diagdown}} CHOCH_2\underset{\underset{OH}{\mid}}{CH}CH_2-\overset{\overset{O}{\parallel}}{C}-\underset{\underset{CH_3}{\mid}}{C}=CH_2$$

2. PBA (Bis-Gma without hydroxyl groups)

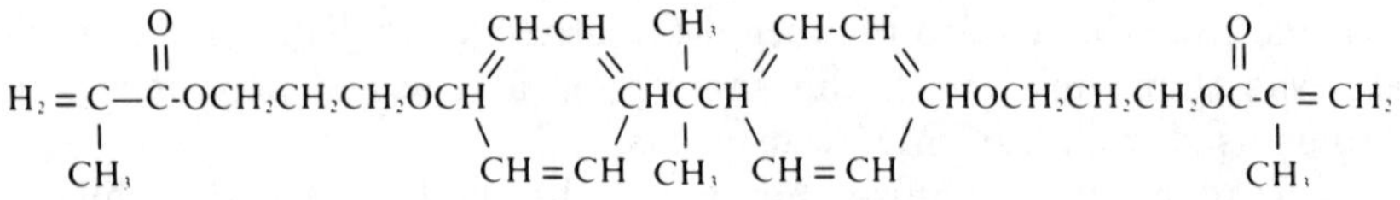

$$H_2=\underset{\underset{CH_3}{\mid}}{C}-\overset{\overset{O}{\parallel}}{C}-OCH_2CH_2CH_2OCH \overset{CH-CH}{\underset{CH=CH}{\diagdown}} CHCCH \overset{CH_3}{\underset{CH_3}{\mid}} \overset{CH-CH}{\underset{CH=CH}{\diagdown}} CHOCH_2CH_2CH_2OC-\underset{\underset{CH_3}{\mid}}{C}=CH_2$$

3. EBA (Bis-Gma without hydroxyl-methylene groups)

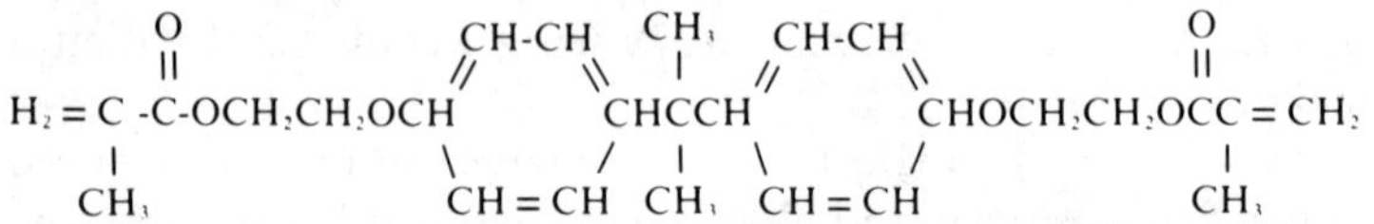

$$H_2=C-\overset{\overset{O}{\parallel}}{C}-OCH_2CH_2OCH \overset{CH-CH}{\underset{CH=CH}{\diagdown}} CHCCH \overset{CH_3}{\underset{CH_3}{\mid}} \overset{CH-CH}{\underset{CH=CH}{\diagdown}} CHOCH_2CH_2OCC-\underset{\underset{CH_3}{\mid}}{}=CH_2$$

(continued)

Table 1. (continued)

4. BADM (Bisphenol A Dimethacrylate — here the entire hydroxy propyl group of Bis-Gma has been eliminated.)

$$
\begin{array}{c}
\text{O} \qquad \text{CH-CH} \quad \text{CH}_3 \quad \text{CH-CH} \quad \text{O} \\
\;\;\;\overset{\cdot}{\|} \qquad /\!/ \quad \backslash\!\backslash \;\; | \quad /\!/ \quad \backslash\!\backslash \;\; \| \\
\text{H}_2 = \text{C -C-OCH} \qquad \text{CHCCH} \qquad \text{CHOCC} = \text{CH}_2 \\
\;\;\; | \qquad \backslash \qquad /\;\;|\;\;\backslash \qquad / \qquad | \\
\;\;\; \text{CH}_3 \qquad \text{CH}=\text{CH} \;\; \text{CH}_3 \;\; \text{CH}=\text{CH} \qquad \text{CH}_3
\end{array}
$$

5. Hydrogenated BIS-GMA (for better color stability).

$$
\begin{array}{c}
\text{O} \qquad \text{OH} \qquad\quad \text{CH}_2\text{-CH}_2 \;\; \text{CH}_3 \;\; \text{CH}_2\text{-CH}_2 \qquad \text{OH} \qquad \text{O} \\
\;\; \| \qquad | \qquad\quad /\!/ \quad \backslash\!\backslash \;\; | \;\; /\!/ \quad \backslash\!\backslash \qquad | \qquad \| \\
\text{H}_2\text{C} = \text{C-OCH}_2\text{CHCH}_2\text{OCH}_2 \qquad \text{CH}_2\text{CCH}_2 \qquad \text{CH}_2\text{OCH}_2\text{CHCH}_2\text{OCC} = \text{CH}_2 \\
\;\; | \qquad\qquad\qquad\quad \backslash \qquad /\;\;|\;\;\backslash \qquad / \qquad\qquad\qquad | \\
\;\; \text{CH}_3 \qquad\qquad\qquad \text{CH}_2\text{-CH}_2 \;\; \text{CH}_3 \;\; \text{CH}_2\text{-CH}_2 \qquad\qquad \text{CH}_3
\end{array}
$$

6. PH-BIS-GMA (Reaction of Bis-Gma with HOPO2Cl) for Enamel and Dentine Adhesives

$$
\begin{array}{c}
\qquad\qquad \text{cl} \qquad\qquad\qquad\qquad\qquad\qquad\qquad \text{cl} \\
\qquad\quad \text{O}\;\;|\;\;\text{O} \qquad\qquad\qquad\qquad\qquad \text{O}\;\;|\;\;\text{O} \\
\;\; \text{O} \qquad \backslash\!\backslash\text{P}/\!/ \qquad \text{CH-CH} \;\; \text{CH}_3 \;\; \text{CH-CH} \qquad \backslash\!\backslash\text{P}/\!/ \qquad \text{O} \\
\;\; \| \qquad | \qquad /\!/ \quad \backslash\!\backslash \;\; | \;\; /\!/ \quad \backslash\!\backslash \qquad | \qquad \| \\
\text{H}_2\text{C} = \text{C-OCH}_2\text{CHCH}_2\text{OCH} \qquad \text{CHCCH} \qquad \text{CHOCH}_2\text{CHCH}_2\text{OCC} = \text{CH}_2 \\
\;\; | \qquad\qquad\qquad\quad \backslash \qquad /\;\;|\;\;\backslash \qquad / \qquad\qquad\qquad | \\
\;\; \text{CH}_3 \qquad\qquad\qquad \text{CH}=\text{CH} \;\; \text{CH}_3 \;\; \text{CH}=\text{CH} \qquad\qquad \text{CH}_3
\end{array}
$$

7. Diethylene Glycol Dimethactrylate (Viscosity Reduction)

$$
\begin{array}{c}
\;\; \text{O} \qquad\qquad\qquad \text{O} \\
\;\; \| \qquad\qquad\qquad \| \\
\text{CH}_2 = \text{C-CO-CH}_2\text{CH}_2\text{OCH}_2\text{CH}_2\text{OCC} = \text{CH}_2 \\
\;\; | \qquad\qquad\qquad\qquad\qquad | \\
\;\; \text{CH}_3 \qquad\qquad\qquad\qquad \text{CH}_3
\end{array}
$$

8. Triethylene Glycol Dimethacrylate (Viscosity Reduction)

$$
\begin{array}{c}
\;\; \text{O} \qquad\qquad\qquad\qquad\qquad \text{O} \\
\;\; \| \qquad\qquad\qquad\qquad\qquad \| \\
\text{CH}_2 = \text{C-CO-CH}_2\text{CH}_2\text{-O-CH}_2\text{CH}_2\text{-O-CH}_2\text{CH}_2\text{-O- C-C} = \text{CH} \\
\;\; | \qquad\qquad\qquad\qquad\qquad\qquad\qquad | \\
\;\; \text{CH}_3 \qquad\qquad\qquad\qquad\qquad\qquad \text{CH}_3
\end{array}
$$

(continued)

Table 1. (continued)

9. Polyethylene Glycol Dimethacrylate (Viscosity Reduction)

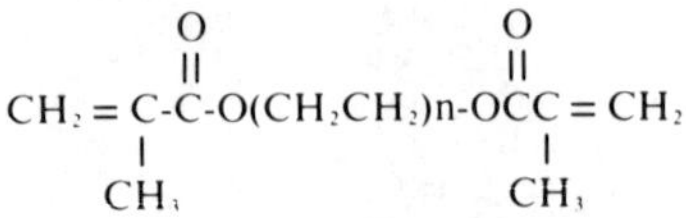

$$
\begin{array}{ccc}
\quad\ O & & O \\
\quad\ \| & & \| \\
CH_2 = C\text{-}C\text{-}O(CH_2CH_2)n\text{-}OCC = CH_2 \\
\quad\ | & & | \\
\quad\ CH_3 & & CH_3
\end{array}
$$

10. Phosponyl Dimethacrylate (for enamel and dentin adhesives)

$$
\begin{array}{ccccc}
O & & O & & O \\
\| & & \| & & \| \\
CH_2 = C\ \text{-}C\text{-}O\text{-}CH_2\text{-}\ P\ \text{-}\ CH_2\text{-}O\text{-}C\text{-}C = CH_2 \\
| & & | & & | \\
CH_3 & & OH & & CH_3
\end{array}
$$

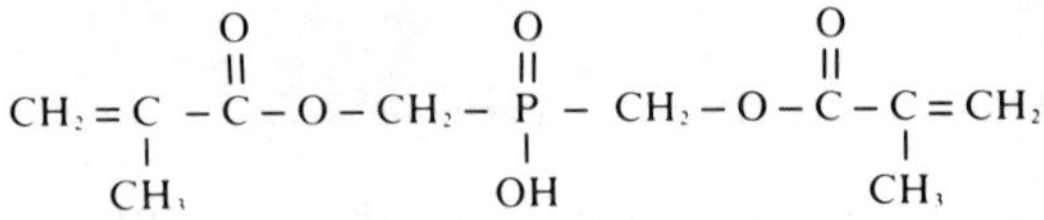

11. HHPA Diester Dimethacrylate (for better color resistance)

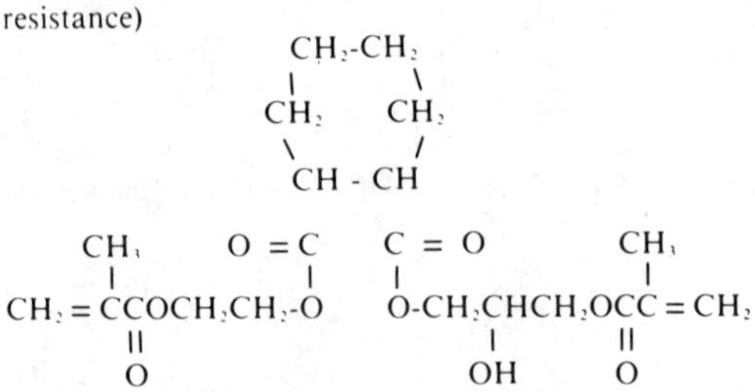

$$
\begin{array}{c}
CH_2\text{-}CH_2 \\
|\quad\quad\ \backslash \\
CH_2 \quad CH_2 \\
\backslash \quad\quad / \\
CH\text{ - }CH
\end{array}
$$

$$
\begin{array}{cccc}
CH_3 & O = C & C = O & CH_3 \\
| & | & | & | \\
CH_2 = CCOCH_2CH_2\text{-}O & & O\text{-}CH_2CHCH_2OCC = CH_2 \\
\| & & |\quad\ \| \\
O & & OH\quad O
\end{array}
$$

12. 4-META (for enamel and dentin adhesives)

$$
\begin{array}{cccc}
O & CH_2 & O & O \\
\| & /\!/\ \backslash & \| & \| \\
C\text{ - }CH_2\ CH_2\text{ - }C\text{ -}O\text{ - }CH_2CH_2\text{-}O\text{-}C\text{ - }C\ =CH_2 \\
/ & & | \\
O\text{-}C\text{ - }CH_2\ CH_2 & & CH_3 \\
\| \quad \backslash\!\backslash\ / \\
O \quad\ CH_2
\end{array}
$$

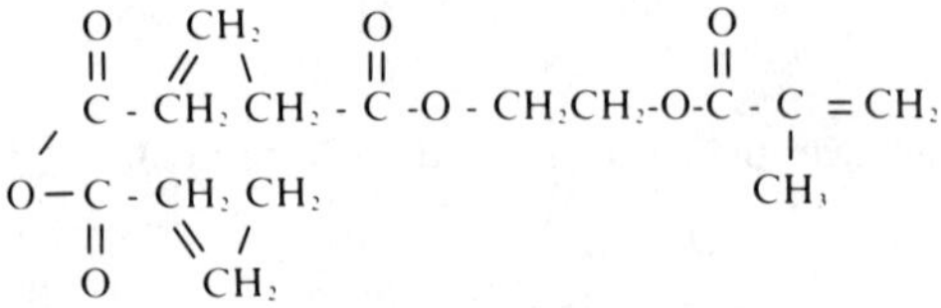

13. Brominated Resin (for Fissure Sealants)

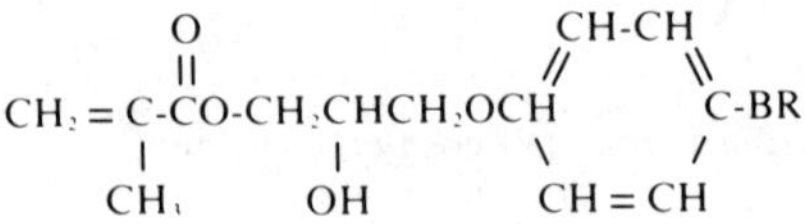

$$
\begin{array}{ccc}
O & & CH\text{-}CH \\
\| & & /\!/ \quad\ \backslash\!\backslash \\
CH_2 = C\text{-}CO\text{-}CH_2CHCH_2OCH & & C\text{-}BR \\
| \quad\quad | & & \backslash\quad / \\
CH_3 \quad OH & & CH = CH
\end{array}
$$

14. Polyurethanes (for cavity varnishes and dentin adhesives)

OCN-Ar-R-Ar-NCO

somewhat lower adhesion in theory, but overall its properties and structure resemble those of a cured epoxy resin. Because of this, there is some reference to the materials as epoxy-resin based, whereas, in general, the class of monomers are technically aromatic thermosetting acrylics, with a structure analogous to the popular aromatic epoxy resins.

RESEARCH DRIVING FORCES

The dental market is very small in terms of poundage, but the materials sell for rather expensive prices in terms of dollars per pound because of the high requirements placed on the material and the cost of supporting its sales to a demanding profession. Thus, a dentist will spend a half hour to an hour or more in preparing a cavity and placing a filling material. With equipment, office staff, and overhead, he must bill $50–$100/hr. The amount of materials he uses in a typical filling is about 0.1 cubic centimeter, or about 0.2 grams. Thus, if he pays $.50 or $1.00 or even $2.00 for this bit of material, and if it "offers" 20 years or a life time of good service, he does not mind the price, he wants to do the best he can for the patient, and its cost is almost lost in the overall cost of $30–$75 or so he must charge the patient. But at $.50 per 0.2 grams, the cost of the filling material works out to be $2.50 per gram and in the order of a thousand dollars per pound.

This price is cheap compared to gold at $350 per oz. or $11,000 per pound. Also, since composites have a lower specific gravity than gold, they are even less costly than implied by the per pound cost. Thus, since the dentist will buy the best material he can find, the cost of composites in the dental market is controlled by the same factors which control industrial markets: (1) manufacturing costs, (2) marketing costs, and (3) the price the application will bear. It is just that in the dental market the third factor is much higher than in the industrial situation, but on the other hand, the first two factors are correspondingly higher.

Thus, one must also recognize that several tens of thousands of pounds go a long way to meeting the entire world demand, and that there are aleady over 100 firms making such problems, all of whom feel that they alone could produce the entire world's needs if only given a chance. The result of such competition is a fierce price war combined with a fierce technical war in the laboratory and on the research clinic floor.

The net result of the churning of the industry has been the definite introduction of very modern and high tech research approaches to formulation and testing dental materials. Full scale laboratory testing of thirty or so mechanical and physical chemical properties has become the order of the day. Extensive clinical trials with controlled populations have become a standard.

In recent years, companies and dental schools started to publish the results of these studies to the dentists. Although there were arguments as to the exact significance of each laboratory property as regards durability in the mouth, of the significance of one small clinical group of patients to the adult or child community at large, there could be no argument with big improvements, generally, and the race was on. If one company claimed 30,000 psi compressive strength and everyone else was still at 18,000 or 22,000 psi, then the others had to respond. If one claimed lower water pickup and lower extractibles in water immersion tests, then the other competitors had to do more research. It would be hard to understand a trade war based on such factors, compared to papers on 20 year clinical studies, but 20 year clinical studies are hard to come by in a fast moving field.

UV & VISIBLE LIGHT CURE

In the past fifteen years, the field has moved from the very early offerings, which had compressive strengths of 12,000 psi, to some systems today which offer 55,000 psi, from materials which were cumbersome to dispense and mix in small quantities, that is, powder/liquid and paste/liquid systems and paste/paste systems which had to be dispensed in sub-gram amounts, to single container ultra violet light (UV) cured materials, to more recently, visible light cured materials.

UV curing systems were adopted by dentistry about the time the coatings industry looked at them seriously. The UV systems came first presumably because the high energy lamps were already available and the UV catalysts were available. But as is typical in each field, technical improvements found to be needed. Whereas the photo resist coatings industry has moved to shorter and shorter wave length UV light, so as to improve definition, the dental profession has moved to longer wave lengths.

The dental profession has moved to the visible range of light for curing many of its filling materials for a variety of reasons:

1. UV light offered the advantage of a single container formulation, which eliminated the need for careful dispensing and mixing of small amounts. It also freed the dentist from the pressure of time when he

was placing the restorative material in the cavity. The material was not setting up on him as he worked. However, there was concern that use of powerful UV radiation in the mouth—even in the case of the longer wave lengths that were used in comparison to the short wave lengths of UV used industrially—could have long-term effects of epithelial tissue, and back radiation from the lamps could have an affect on the dentist, who was using the lamps everyday. Thus, there was an impetus to move to the safer visible range.

2. Ordinarily one would feel that there was more energy available for curing the UV range. But the chemists soon found that since his formulations were highly transparent to visible light—which they had to be to permit a good match of the adjacent semi-translucent tooth structure—and as such he got better penetration in the visible range than he did in the UV range where the high concentration of aromatic monomers was absorbing much of his UV energy any way.

Of course, visible light cured filling materials require a special curing lamp, a device for checking its output, or a test to measure the light outputs. No matter which lamps are offered to the profession, there is not enough energy to cure a large filling in one shot and it must be cured in layers. Also, the extra bright lights require that precautions be taken to protect his eyes or those of the patient. Filling materials must also be packaged to dispense small amounts without the remainder of the package setting up in the jar or container due to the light.

CONCLUSIONS

Despite all the great progress, the big challenge remains—developing a composite material that can outperform alloy in terms of wear resistance. We need to match the wear resistance of human enamel before we can say that we have fully solved the problem. Also, the material must bond to dentin and enamel so that the filling material provides a seal against entry of oral fluids into the cavity and pulp, and ideally provide mechanical support to the adjacent tooth structure, such as tooth cusps, so that mastication does not introduce new shear planes which split the natural tooth.

Great progress has been made on adhesion. Bond strengths of 1500 to 2000 psi are now being achieved in actual dental practice, to both enamel and dentin. So the present race seems to boil down to wear resistance. Here, a great deal of work is going on in laboratories and dental clinics around the world, using a variety of wear testers, scanning electron microscopes or laser interferometers to measure wear resistance. Laboratory measurements can usually be made directly on the wear specimens. In the case of in vivo tests in patients, usually an impression is taken and a model is cast in the impression, and comparative measurement are made with reference to adjacent tooth structure.

Overall these are exciting times for the composite chemist in the dental field. And these new dental materials are expected to eventually provide materials and methods for bonding broken bones and other orthopedic applications far beyond the achievements that the medical profession has achieved with acrylic cements.

REFERENCES

1. Henry Lee and Kris Neville, *Handbook of Epoxy Resins,* McGraw-Hill Book Co., New York, p.800 (1967) (Classic Edition offered as of 1982).
2. H. Lee, *SAMPE Journal, 20* (4), 13 (1984).

Silicone Contact Lenses

JOHN K. FITZGERALD

Dow Corning Corporation
Midland, Michigan

1. INTRODUCTION

THE CONCEPT OF wearing a small lens on the surface of the cornea to provide optical correction was first developed by Leonardo Da Vinci in the sixteenth century. Many different methods were used to bring this concept into practice. In the late 17th through the 19th century lenses were made of glass. For many reasons, glass contact lenses proved to be impractical. Before they could be fit the lenses had to be blown into a plaster mold taken from the patient's eye. These lenses were also usually quite large and covered the entire eye. It wasn't until the 1940's when a new material was recognized to make contact lenses. Several eye surgeons noted during World War II that fighter pilots whose eyes had been invaded by slivers of Perspex from their shattered cockpit canopies were able to tolerate these shards in their eye. By the 1950's, the use of Perspex, chemically known as polymethylmethacrylate, had come into wide use as a contact lens material. The chemical and mechanical properties of polymethylmethacrylate (PMMA) allowed it to be made in a variety of designs.

While PMMA had excellent biological and optical properties, it tended to seal off the cornea from its supply of oxygen. A variety of strategies were used to try to get more oxygen to the cornea under a PMMA lens. Unfortunately, for the most part, these strategies proved inadequate.

Significant progress has been made in recent years which led to the development of new contact lens materials and improvement in the designs and performances of existing materials.

Reprinted from Vol. 30 SAMPE Proceedings, courtesy of Society for the Advancement of Materials and Process Engineering, Covina, CA U.S.A.

The trend in material and lens development during the 1970's was primarily (with a few exceptions) directed toward hydrogel materials. Hydrogel materials are a class of materials that are essentially a polymer matrix swollen with a percentage of water. These lenses were a quantum leap forward in material technology. Early hydrogel lenses were relatively thick, possessed a low water content and were reasonably durable. During the later half of the decade however, problems with these lenses, as well as a general awakening to what a hydrogel material could and could not accomplish resulted in the creation of materials with very high water contents (in excess of 70%) and the development of the manufacturing technology needed to lathe cut or mold very thin lenses, i.e., less than 0.10 mm in thickness.

The driving force behind these developments was the recognition that the original hydrogel materials and designs did not allow enough oxygen to reach the cornea to maintain a normal metabolism, particularly for extended wear.

At the time, this finding was unexpected as it was predicted that those materials and designs would be a significant improvement over the existing PMMA materials.

While this work with hydrogel lenses was going on, several corporations took a different tack. Most of the effort for improving the hydrogel lens oxygen performance was directed toward increasing the oxygen transmission rate across the contact lens. O_2 Transmission = $DK/L \times \Delta P$ where DK is the Oxygen Permeability coefficient, L is the lens thickness and ΔP is the O_2 concentration gradient across the lens. As noted before, this lead to tactics involving either extremely high water content gels, thereby increasing the oxygen permeability (DK) of the materials, or manufacturing very thin lenses out of lower DK materials. Dow Corning Corporation, as well as several other research oriented corporations throughout the world, decided to attempt to manufacture contact lenses out of materials with the highest possible permeability coefficients which also did not possess the disadvantage of hydrogels. These materials were the silicone elastomers.

2. CHEMICAL AND PHYSICAL PROPERTIES

Silicone elastomer has several physical properties that make it a very useful contact lens material. Silicone elastomer is as much as 6–10 times as permeable to oxygen as hydrogel materials. It is also an extremely durable material which can withstand a great deal of patient handling. This property is especially useful for aphakic lenses, which are worn by people who have had cataracts surgically removed.

These patients are usually older, and cannot handle small contact lenses easily. Because of their durability, silicone elastomer contact lenses are more appropriate for their use than a comparable hydrogel lens.

Silicone elastomer is also biologically inert. Silicone elastomers are used in an extraordinary range of biomedical applications for products such as catheters, implants, and orthopedic devices. Silicone elastomer lenses are chemically and physically stable over a wide range of temperatures, allowing them to be either chemically or thermally disinfected during use. Conversely, many hydrogel materials, especially the high water content materials, cannot be thermally disinfected. The ability to be thermally disinfected is an important characteristic since up to 30% of the lens wearing population is allergic to the preservatives that are commonly found in chemical disinfection solutions.

Silicone elastomer lenses are also stable in a wide range of chemical environments. Hydrogels are subject to dehydration, and many of the high water content hydrogel materials are sensitive to the pH of the surrounding solution. Changes in pH or in temperature can effect the hydration of the material, which affects its oxygen permeability. Changes in hydration of the hydrogel material also affect the physical shape of the lens, altering the lens-cornea fitting relationship. It is not uncommon for certain high water content hydrogel materials to lose as much as 30% of their water content when placed on the eye. Another consequence of containing water in their polymer matrix is that the hydrogel materials can act as media for bacteria and fungi.

The water in the matrix can also pick up various contaminants such as chemical preservatives or other debris and hold them like a reservoir. Silicone elastomer lenses, in comparison, contain no water are not subject to the same dehydration that affects hydrogels, and thus do not change their shape when they are placed in the eye. They will also not act as reservoirs for chemical contaminants, and will not support microbial or fungal growth.

Silicone polymers consist of a chain of alternating silicon and oxygen atoms with organic side groups attached to a significant portion of the silicon atoms. The silicone polymer which is the subject of this paper is known as elastofilcon A, whose chemical name is dimethyl diphenyl methylvinyl polysiloxane.

Permeability in its simplest form can be explained by visualizing the silicone polymer as a screen through which to pour a fluid. The alternating chemical structure of silicone elastomer prevents close packing of the molecules in the polymer, thus leaving a much more open structure than is usually found in materials such as PMMA and hydrogel

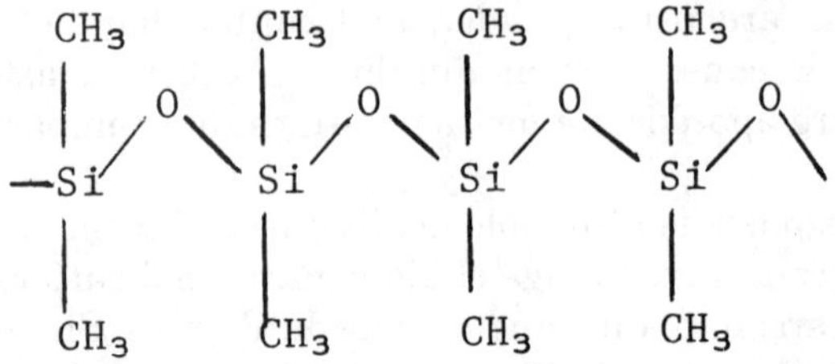

FIGURE 1. Schematic of a poly dimethyl siloxane polymer chain.

materials which have carbon-carbon backbones. The side group structures for the silicone elastomer contact lens material are primarily
methyl groups which are extremely small and nonpolar.

Conversely, in the organic PMMA and hydrogel materials, the side
groups tend to be highly polar and somewhat bulky compared to
methyl groups. Both the polarity and the bulk enhance the stiffness of
the polymer structure due to the carbon backbone close packing.
Because of this highly organized molecular structure, the organic
PMMA and hydrogen materials are therefore much less permeable
than the silicone elastomer material with its more open polymer
matrix and nonpolar side groups.

The same chemical properties that make it one of the most gas
permeable materials in existence make the silicone elastomer a highly
hydrophobic material. Contact lenses must have hydrophilic surfaces to
be useful in the eye. A brief examination of the interaction between the
contact lens surface and the tear film will illustrate this. The tear film
of the eye is made up of three layers. The layer closest to the cornea is
known as the mucin layer. This mucin layer contains biomaterials that

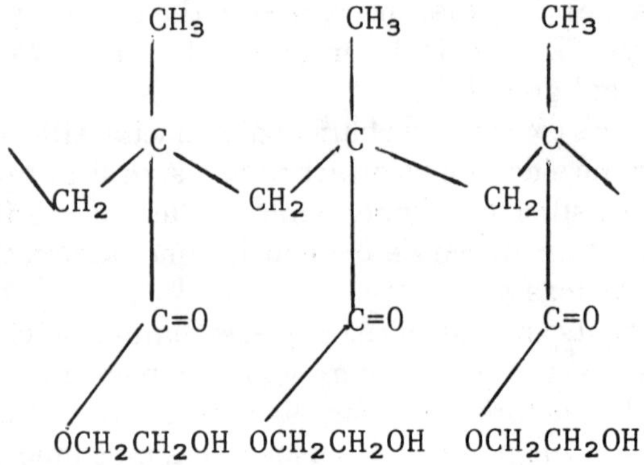

FIGURE 2. Schematic of poly hydroxyethyl methacrylate polymer chain.

Table 1. Elastofilcon A physical properties.

Specific Gravity:	1.13
Refractive Index:	1.44
Light Transmission:	Measures Greater than 85%-dry
Surface Character:	Hydrophilic
Water Content:	Approximately 0.2%
Oxygen Permeability:*	$340 \times 10^{-11} \dfrac{cm^3\text{-}cm}{cm^2\text{-}sec.\text{-}mmHg}$ at 21°C

*ASTM D1434-75 Method.

enhance the wettability of the surface of the cornea. The next and thickest layer is the aqueous layer. This layer is primarily water which contains various salts. The third layer is the lipid layer whose purpose is to retard the evaporation of the aqueous layer. A properly functioning tear film will remain spread across the corneal surface for a period of time longer than the time between a patient's blinks. When a contact lens is placed in this system, it is important that the contact lens surface be hydrophilic. This hydrophilicity will promote the spread and maintenance of the tear film across the lens surface. Failure to maintain an adequate tear film can lead to visual as well as mechanical stress to the eye. An unstable tear film can also promote the deposit of materials that exist in the tears. These deposits have been identified by various researchers as being proteins, lipids, salts, and various other constituents. The accumulation of deposits will eventually lead to failure and replacement of the lens.

3. MANUFACTURING

Silicone elastomer lenses are compression molded between two highly polished molds, thus replicating the lens design in the appropriate parameters. Because this is a compression molding process, and no mechanical modification of the lens curves can be made after molding, the mold inventory must be quite large, allowing for all the possible combinations of lens parameters such as lens diameter, lens base

Table 2. Material wetting characteristics.

Material	Contact Angles	
	Advancing	Receding
Untreated Silicone Elastomer	105	65
Treated Silicone Elastomer	65	15
PHEMA (35%H$_2$O) (blotted dry)	75	20

curve, and lens power. After molding, the lenses are post cured to remove any volatile residual materials. Because this lens is elastomeric, generation of an appropriate edge profile is very difficult. Many methods have been used in attempt to generate adequate edges on silicone elastomers. Currently, the edges are generated using mechanical processes, such as grinding and polishing. This process is particularly difficult, and is comparable to attempting to polish the edge of a rubber band. After edging, the lenses are then surface treated so that the surfaces are permanently changed from hydrophobic to hydrophilic using a proprietary process. The lenses are then placed in vials, filled with distilled water, autoclaved, and inventoried.

4. CLINICAL RESULTS

Extensive premarket clinical trials and in-vitro testing are required before the FDA will approve any new contact lens materials for marketing. The requirements for "extended wear" of a contact lens are especially stringent. This is necessary to ensure that the device can be put onto a patient's eye and left there for as long as 30 days with no ill effects. Over 200 patients have worn this lens for an extended period of time, some for as long as 5 years. The results of these clinical trials are presented in Tables 3–6.

Particular note should be paid to the fact that the incidence rates of edema and neovascularization are extremely low with this lens. This is a result of the extremely high oxygen permeability of this material. Because of these results, the SILSIGHT™ silicone elastomer contact lens was the first contact lens approved for a full 30 days of wear.

PMMA and hydrogel materials, by their chemical nature, are hydrophilic when placed in the eye. Unfortunately, silicone elastomers are hydrophobic and will not support the spread of an adequate tear film.

Table 3. Clinical population wearing time.

Months Wearing Silsoft Lenses	% of 218 Patients
24–29	35.8
30–35	10.5
36–41	26.6
42–47	13.8
48–53	8.3
54–59	5.0

Table 4. Demographics.

Age:	Range: 13–64 years	
	Median: 31 years	
Sex:	Male-28.9%	
	Female-71.1%	
Motivation:	Cosmetic	36.2%
	Recreative	2.5%
	Convenience	56.4%
	VA Improvement	4.9%
Occupation:	Office & Clerical	32.1%
	Homemaker	8.2%
	Professional	24.3%
	Student	21.8%
	Laborer	5.8%
	Other	5.8%
Previous VA Correction:	None	0.8%
	Glasses	40.0%
	Contact Lenses	59.1%

Table 5. Visual acuity results.

Visual Acuity Achieved	% of Patients
20/15	11.5
20/20	78.0
20/25	6.9
20/30	1.4
20/40	0.4
Not Indicated	1.8

Table 6. Slit lamp findings.

Slit Lamp Finding	Positive Findings	% (7434 Exams)
Edema	8	0.1
Neovascularization	15	0.2
Staining	241	3.3
Injection	146	2.0
Iritis	0	0.0

For this reason, silicone elastomer lenses must be treated by a proprietary process which changes some of the methyl (CH_3 groups on the siloxane backbone to hydroxyl (OH) groups. This change raises the surface energy of the silicone materials and allows the tear film to spread across it.

Since that time, there are hydrogel lenses that have been approved for 30 days of wear, but the silicone elastomer contact lens with its unique combination of material and chemical properties is acknowledged as the premium performer for extended wear.

Titanium Alloy Alumina Ceramics and UHMWPE Use in Total Joint Replacement

I. C. CLARKE
Bioengineering Research Institute
Los Angeles, CA 90025

INTRODUCTION

THE MODERN TOTAL hip replacement (THR) has undergone extensive research and development in the last decade but still suffers from three limitations: stem loosening, cup loosening and potential complications from undesirable tissue reactions to the wear products [12,25,39]. These complications are especially troublesome in younger patients [9]! To try to improve on this situation, material innovations for the heavily-loaded femoral stem have included multiphase Co-Ni-Cr alloy (MP35N), hot-isostatically pressed (HIPPED) cobalt-chrome, forged high-strength cobalt-chrome (FHS), and titanium-6-4. The high-strength metal alloys were introduced mainly because of the stem fracture problems in the U.S. and Europe. Semlitsch and Panic [53] have now demonstrated that in their experience, over 500,000 implants with stem alloys such as MP35N have had zero incidence of fracture in patients.

Ceramic's attributes include superior inertness, exceptional biocompatibility, high wear-resistance and considerable potential for bone ingrowth. In fact, *"Alumina is classified as one of the most biocompatible materials"* [40]. Current use of alumina ceramics in the total hip includes the femoral ball (by virtue of low friction, virtually zero wear and totally inert material) and a ceramic acetabular shell for direct anchorage in bone (uncemented, totally inert).

Reprinted from Vol. 30 SAMPE Proceedings, courtesy of Society for the Advancement of Material and Process Engineering, Covina, CA U.S.A.

217

Our aim is to review the applications of high strength alloy and ceramic THR designs to determine current progress, especially for the younger patient.

STATE-OF-THE-ART CEMENTED

Understanding of cemented THR successes and failures over the last decade is an important prerequisite. In other words, until you know where you've been, you can't tell where your going! Reviewing the long-term *cemented* THR results from Europe and the U.S., it is apparent that there are two quite separate groups of results. The group which included the Charnley prostheses and its progeny, e.g., Charnley, T28, STH, etc., had published success rates higher than 90 percent at last follow-up (Table 1).

Furthermore, it is interesting to note that in U.S. medical centers which have used both the Charnley and the Charnley-Muller THRs,

Table 1. Comparison of THR revision-operation rates in USA and Europe with respect to follow-up times (excluding infection where possible). Note that direct comparisons of data may be made difficult due to varied patient selection and evaluation criteria, e.g., elderly patients, varied netiology and lengths of follow-up, etc.

Author	THR	Years Followed	THR series[a]	THR	Retention[b] Primary RATING
Almby and Hierton, 82	Muller[c]	10+	63	57%	
Tillberg, 82	McKee-Farrar[c]	1–7	327	64%	
Dobbs and Scales, 82	Stanmore	10	(173)	58%	
Sutherland et al, 82	Muller	10+	53	68%	
Stauffer, 82	Charnley	10	231	92%	*
Reikeras, 82	Muller	9–12	107	75%	
Salvati et al, 81	Charnley	9.5–11.5	67	95%	*
Gruen et al, 81	STH	1–6	387	98%	*
Ling, 80	Exeter	5–9	228	86%	
Moreland et al, 80	Charnley/T-28	2–9	444	96%	*
Carlsson and Gentz, 80	Charnley[d]	8–12	288	92%	*
Gruen et al, 79	Charnley/T-28	0.5–6	389	92%	*
Beckenbaugh and Ilstrup, 78	Charnley	4–8.5	301	92%	*

*Greater than 90 percent success: a: number of THR reviewed; b: related to number of cases and follow-up; c: metal to metal; d: Study of femoral implant only (3 percent reoperations, 5 percent patients declined reoperation for pain, 8 percent minimum complications).

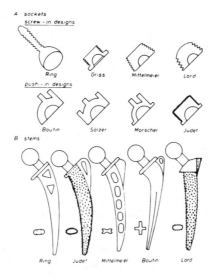

FIGURE 1. Illustration of interaction of three biocompatibility criteria: a) material, b) design and c) implant-bone interface.

the Muller stem design failed at a 6 to 12 times more frequent rate than the Charnley THR [23,28]. Griss [14] noted from the results of a German multicenter study (22 hospitals, representing 4,035 reviewed procedures) that there was an 11.4 percent reoperation rate in the first decade post-op but 19.2 percent (on average) beyond nine years post-op. Thus the results from multicenter studies show higher failure rates than from individual, specialized hospitals.

So, to examine the results of the major pioneers of *non-cemented* THRs (Drs. Bombelli, Boutin, Griss, Judet, Lord, Mittelmeier, Morscher, Ring, etc.), we must currently judge their short-term clinical data against the ten percent failure criteria of the cemented Charnley THRs, (bearing in mind any major differences in patient age-ranges).

NON-CEMENTED IMPLANT FIXATION

Reliable long-term clinical results for *non-cemented* total hip replacements will only be achieved when we can ensure consistently that they are anchored securely in the bone. Under this definition, the separation of implant from bone by a fibrous membrane would be construed as a potential failure. Our goal then must be to learn what combination of materials and design technology is most compatible with the implant-bone attachment concept.

For attachment criteria, we can consider four possibilities: a) direct bonding to bone, b) bone ingrowth into the implant's surfaces, c) bone apposition immediately adjacent to the implant and d) bone separated by a potentially unstable fibrous membrane (Figure 1). The key word in this process is *compatibility*.

1. *Material Biocompatibility:* i.e., the response of the cells to materials.

2. *Design Biocompatibility:* i.e., the stresses produced in the bone by virtue of prosthesis design (and function) must be within the tolerance levels of the bone to avoid either instability or possibly long-term disuse atrophy.

3. *Interface Biocompatibility:* The interaction of load transfer between implant and bone results in micromotion at the prosthesis-bone interfaces. Depending on the micro or macro geometry (2- or 3-dimensional) of the prosthetic surface, it is possible to create either fibrous or bone tissue immediately adjacent to the implant's surface (Figure 1).

The three biocompatibility concepts outlined above also interact with the expediency of obtaining immediate *short-term stabilization* to ensure that long-term support by bone can be a consistent reality.

SELECTION OF STEM DESIGN AND MATERIAL

To minimize yielding (plastic deformation) or fracture of the stems in U.S. and European patients, we need to use a high-strength alloy, preferably stronger than annealed stainless-steel or cast cobalt chrome.

With regard to materials technology, the ideal choice should be to always use the material with the superior biocompatibility. Titanium-6A1-4Va alloy (Ti-6-4) in fact has the best biocompatibility of our current orthopaedic alloys. It also has much higher fatigue strength than either cast cobalt-chrome or the standard 316-stainless-steel alloys.

With approximately 1200 Ti-6-4 stem implantations from three centers (spanning eight to eleven years in England, France and the U.S.), there have been *zero Ti-6-4 THR stem fractures reported* [4,15]. Thus, the Ti-6-4 femoral stem appears an excellent choice due to good biocompatibility, high strength and excellent fatigue behavior.

FIT OF THE FEMORAL STEM IN THE IM CANAL

Clinical studies of THR stem fit demonstrated that *Charnley stems in large canals loosened 1.8–2.5 times more frequently than the same size stem in small canals* [1,36]. The larger stems may fill the canal better, thereby minimizing loosening of cemented designs, but also very importantly, promoting better stability. Since some of the new stem designs are quite large and therefore much stiffer than the Charnley THR, the use of the more flexible Ti-6-4 alloy may be even more advantageous (with half the elastic modulus of cobalt chrome).

Opinion is divided as to whether the "press-fit" of the stem should be a wedging in the distal canal, in the proximal trochanteric region or even 100 percent overall. Possibly these different concepts will resolve with a few more years clinical experience.

SURFACE STRUCTURING FOR BONE FIXATION

Surface roughness is frequently characterized as "micro" or "macro" and 2-dimensional (2D) or 3-dimensional (3D). These terms are not defined in a precise fashion for orthopaedic device concepts, but may be used in the following manner:

Micro: Geometrical features up to the 500 or 600μm range.
Macro: Geometrical features greater than 500μm.
2D: Ridges, grooves, cavities and protuberances (or *single* layer of beads).
3D: Interconnecting channels for bone ingrowth (and interlocking), by surface porosity or *multiple* layers of beads or wires.

The principle of micro-interlock is being actively pursued by many U.S. centers, using materials as diverse as cobalt chrome and Ti-6-4 (Figure 2). Ti-6-4 coated with carbon, and various polymer coatings, e.g., polyethylene and polysulfone. Some of these surfaces have been used cemented as well as non-cemented. Such implant systems generally all share three criteria:

1) Exact preparation of bone bed to provide intimate contact of prosthesis to bone.
2) Adjunct anchoring system to provide immediate immobilization in bone.
3) Pore sizes somewhere in the range 100–450μm.

When these three criteria were achieved in animal experiments, it has been shown that immature bone ingrowth can begin at two weeks and by six weeks, mature bone growth has occurred throughout the implant [13]. For intermedullary implants, the resulting shear strengths improve with time and can vary from 2-10MPa which is *higher than those measured in cemented systems* [2].

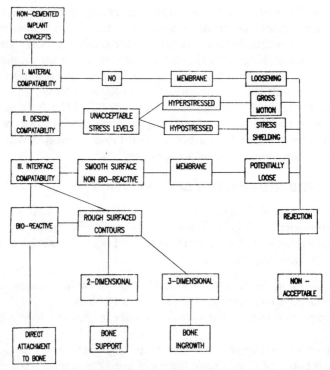

FIGURE 2. Overview of non-cemented acetabular and femoral prostheses with bone macrocontouring and micro-contouring. (Reproduced with permission from Griss [14]).

Advocates of 3D interlocking contours claim [12] that there is: a) greater resistance to tensile forces, b) better fixation, and c) more physiologic stress transfer.

To minimize stress shielding and also provide *easier revision* when necessary, the current trend is to provide for bone ingrowth *only on the proximal 30 to 50 percent of the stem length* rather than 100 percent as on the earlier designs.

CLINICAL RESULTS: NON-CEMENTED THRs

Boutin initiated his non-cemented press-fit Ti-6-4 stem concept in May 1975 with a conical, stepped, sleeve design [4]. In 40 cases he had only one stem loosening (2.5 percent) and four instances of femoral bone fractures (10 percent). However in 1978, he abandoned this design in favor of another with a large collar and lateral fenestrated flange (also press-fit type).

Lord and Bancel [21] reported on their *bone-ingrowth* Mad-reporic design in 1509 cases. *There have been no loosenings of the femoral stem!* Note that this was a relatively elderly patient series. Reviewing 933 stems radiographically at one year, only 2 percent showed partial or complete radiolucent zones and 17 percent had somewhat less than perfect bony stabilization. Review of a group of 235 cases beyond five years showed 74 percent remained stable, 23 percent demonstrated some "bony ingrowth" and 3 percent still retained their radiolucent lines. Thigh pain in the first and second years appeared to be associated with these radiographically loose stems. Note however that there is a radically new Lord prosthesis now being used without this type of bone-ingrowth surface. *Revision of this 100% porous-coated stem was a major technical undertaking!*

In the US, Lunceford [22] reported on the non-cemented clinical AML experience (multiple layers Co-Cr beads, $125\mu m$ average pore size). With 100 hips followed 3–5 years, *there were no revisions due to loosening.* Engh [12] reported on 300 THR's using the same non-cemented Co-Cr system with 100 hips followed more than two years. Detailed questioning of 77 patients revealed a 20 percent incidence of some thigh pain at one year, decreasing to 14 percent at two years. *None of the prostheses had evidence of loosening.*

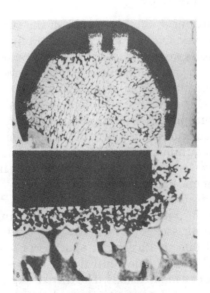

FIGURE 3. Illustration of growth of bone trabeculae into multi-layered (3-dimensional) 100–150μm dia. titanium beads (micro porosity) in femoral cup in a canine hip.

Mittelmeier [24] reported on more than 1500 cases involving his Series I and II *press-fit* Co-Cr stem designs. The incidence of early loosening was approximately 19 percent and 5 percent for Series I and the larger Series II design, respectively. The incidence of intraoperative complications involving femoral shaft and trochanteric fractures was 9 percent.

Bombelli [3] reported on 270 cases using three successive designs of the Isoelastic press-fit stem (polyacetal sheath, stainless steel core). In the first series, there was visible stem subsidence from one to 10mm (in virtually 100 percent of cases). In the second and third series with larger, modified stems, this subsidence was more or less eliminated.

Gustillo [16] used his long Ti-6-4 straight stem in 21 cases, with 11-19 (average 13) months follow-up. This design used anterior and posterior pads of porous titanium fiber mesh for ingrowth. There were no loosenings at this time.

It is interesting that in the desire the have a porous implant surface, a compromise has to be made between surface structure and implant strength. The endurance limit for sintered alloys can drop below 200 MPa [11], i.e., as low as cast stainless-steel which was abandoned around 1975 due to inadequate fatigue strength.

ACETABULAR CUP FIXATION

It is more difficult to get a firm estimate of the survival of cemented acetabular cups at, say, five and ten years follow-up. The Mayo Clinic's Charnley THR results were presented for their first 300 patients at five years [1] and then ten years [35]. The first review revealed radiographic evidence of 5.5 percent acetabular cups loose but only 1 percent required revision. The ten year review figures had almost increased to 11.3 percent radiographically loose and a 4 percent reoperations.

Current THR techniques in the U.S. now focus on metal-backed UHMWPE cups to minimize the stresses in the bone cement. Use of a porous backing layer is also considered advisable to increase the shear strength of the cement-implant bond.

The more rigid ceramic and metal-backed UHMWPE cups have been used non-cemented for many years in Europe. Boutin's first press-filled hemispherical ceramic socket (with central peg) was used from 1971 to 1974 but modified due to 12 percent short-term loosening complications [4]. A second design (one central and two peripheral pegs) experienced 6.5 percent complications. The third design (three peripheral pegs) was used since 1977 and initial complications were of the order 0.5 percent (Figure 2).

The screw-in Lindenhof ceramic:ceramic THR system was introduced in September 1974 and reported at review to have *zero cup failure rate* [17,30].

The press-fit Isoelastic UHMWPE cup (2-peripheral pegs) was introduced in 1976. Reporting on 150 cases with up to four years follow-up, Morscher and Dick [25] noted *neither revisions due to cup loosening nor any radiographic signs of loosening.*

Lord and Bancel [21] reviewed a series of 1509 Mad-reporic patients, of which 882 (since 1976) have used the *screw-in metal-backed* UHMWPE cups. There was a 4 percent dislocation rate due to poor cup positioning and 1.3 percent reoperation rate. *Cup loosening was not a problem and there was no radiographic evidence of late cup migration.*

Mittelmeier [24] presented the results of his Series II design with the screw-in ceramic sockets, totalling more than 400 cases. Incidence of cup loosening was approximately 1 percent (one cup was exchanged to obtain a better position).

Thus the non-cemented acetabular cups appear to have continuing good results in the short term, *at least as good if not better than cemented cups.* Note that in the U.S. the only THR approved for use by FDA is the press-fit Mittelmeier type with cobalt-chrome stem, ceramic ball and choice of UHMWPE or screw-in ceramic cups.

THR WEAR PERFORMANCE

Wear is generally considered to have not yet been a major problem in metal: UHMWPE joints. Average wear is generally estimated to be about 0.2 to 0.5mm range per year but there have been several reports of acetabular cups wearing out and fracturing, with the expectation of more to come [7,21]. However the continual shedding of wear debris into the joint has been implicated in the cement-bone interface loosening problem [40] and must be minimized, especially in the younger patients! Wear is an inevitable and continuous process and therefore for continued good long-term results, we have to provide the patient with the *best high-wear resistance materials available.*

Another practical and very useful trend is to incorporate the European concept of an *interchangeable femoral ball.* This allows the surgeon to select ball material and diameter to fit each patient's needs. With the increasing use of Ti-6-4 alloy for the stem, the next decision is whether to use a femoral ball of Ti-6-4, cobalt chrome or ceramic? The wear resistance of Ti-6-4 against UHMWPE has been criticized frequently but in fact there are contradictory reports [8,9]. As a result of this uncertainty, some designs use cobalt-chrome balls on Ti-6-4 stems.

Table 2. Summary of laboratory studies comparing superior wear resistance of ceramic THRs to metal:UHMWPE designs.

Study	Lubricant	Joint Load	Type	Wear Advantage of Ceramic
Huttinger (19):	Saline	2.5kN 6.6MPa	MP:CP	4:1, 7:1
Semlitsch (33):	Water	1.5kN	MP:CP/MP:CC	20:1, 56:1
Sieber (34):	Synovial Fluid	Patients	MP:CP	4:1
Walter (38):	Water	3kN	CC	(Large Sphericity changes)
Niederer (26):	Water	3.5kN	MP:CP	34:1
Wright (41):	Serum	1.4kN	MP:CP	1.3:1
Sieber (34)	Synovial Fluid Saline	2.8N	MP:CP/MP:CC	(Friction study only)

CC: Ceramic-Ceramic.
CP: Ceramic-UHMWPE.
MP: Metal-UHMWPE.
NS: Not Specified.

In terms of minimal joint friction, ceramic represents the optional material either bearing on UHMWPE or ceramic counterfaces (Table 2). To further minimize the friction torque, a small diameter femoral head is advantageous [6]. Most European ceramic femoral heads are at least 30 to 32mm diameter but the ceramic heads in use in Japan are currently 28mm and now smaller sizes are under development [27].

Alumina: UHMWPE and alumina: alumina bearing surfaces were introduced to reduce not only the volumetric rate of wear debris release but also reducing the toxicity shock to the tissues (since alumina has exceptional biocompatibility).

Initial ceramic:ceramic laboratory wear studies predicted an initial wear-in phase and then vitually zero wear [4,18,29,37]. However, Jager and Plitz [20] and Plitz and Hoss [31] expressed concern on a tribological basis. They analyzed 17 such removed THRs ex-vivo with wear-evident. Regardless of manufacturer and design, they suggested that excavation of a ceramic strain could occur due to any combination of a) contamination defects, b) large grains, c) excessive sphericity deviations, d) inadequate surface finish and/or e) ball-cup subluxation.

Walter and Plitz [38] ran ceramic-ceramic simulator studies with two standard THRs plus two with "artificial defects." They described surprising changes in sphericity with test duration. They also noted a progressive wear mode from: a) trans-crystalline laminar smooth erosion with separation of grain boundaries, b) trans-crystalline scratching by 0.1μm size particles, c) push-out of larger ceramic particles and d) "severe wear debris accelerating avalanche-like." The authors pointed out that this runaway wear was demonstrated in the laboratory where there was no possibility of subluxation, i.e., no rim fracture phenomenon. For confirmation, Plitz and Hoss [31] noted extreme wear in cases where the surgical procedure appeared faultless as evidenced by radiographs, ie., there was little reason to suggest subluxation as a necessary initiator for wear fragments on ceramic: ceramic THRs.

Regardless of the cause, Heimke and Griss [17] have noted wear on all removed ceramic:ceramic THRs they have examined.

Willert et al [39] have examined tissues from around *ceramic* THRs by optical, atomic absorption spectrometry and electron microprobe analysis. However, from *ceramic:ceramic THRs,* the ceramic particles resembled "fine grains, splinters or greater fragments in the range from 0.5 to 10um diameter, with the predominant size of about 1μm." Probably for these reasons, the ceramic:ceramic THR procedures represented only a small proportion of the THR procedures and have not increased to date. However in no case have they yet found any alumina wear particles *from removed ceramic:UHMWPE THRs!* The ceramic:UHMWPE THRs are now being used in increasing numbers (Griss, personal communication, 1984).

In conclusion, until there is more consistent information available on the relative success rates of ceramic:ceramic systems, the judicious choice would appear to be ceramic:UHMWPE. There seems little doubt that the wear improvement has been achieved because the wear advantage of ceramic:UHMWPE over metal:UHMWPE has varied from 1.3 to 34 times improvement in the laboratory and from three to four times improvement clinically [14,20]. Thus the combination of Ti-6-4 stem, ceramic ball and UHMWPE cup bearing surface currently appears to offer the best features of fatigue strength, wear resistance and excellent biocompatibility.

MECHANICAL FAILURES OF CERAMIC FEMORAL BALLS AND CUPS

The all-ceramic designs have experienced a very small incidence of cup fractures. Boutin [4] had four acetabular cup fractures (0.8 percent) in his early 1970 series. Plitz and Griss [30] also described three fractured Mittelmeier cups. Acetabular positioning for the all-ceramic THR appears to be critical [17].

To be fully responsive to all the indications for surgery in the total-hip population, femoral ball sizes of 22, 26, 28 and 32mm diameter are required. However, the smaller the alumina ceramic ball, the higher the risk of fracture. The Lindenhof ball design of 26mm was abandoned early on [17,30]. Boutin [4] reported six ball breakages (0.8 percent) of his design in the first year but with no subsequent failures beyond 1971. Plitz and Griss [30] reported on 23 fractured ceramic femoral balls; Mittelmeier (5 THRs), Salzer [8] and Lindenhof [10] designs. Out of such ceramic:ceramic experiences has come a large body of test data for quality control and design testing [11].

While there is no record of any fractures of ceramic:UHMWPE combinations [42], the test data is needed to verify quality control and survivorship data as well as provide background data for comparing new designs and new ceramics. Human gait studies have demonstrated that peak joint loads can vary from 2–10 and 2–4 times in selected small samples of normal volunteers and total-joint patients, respectively. Therefore, allowing for a general factor of safety of three times in a laboratory text, it should be expected that a THR ball should be able to withstand more than 1,950kg (19kN) cyclic loading for possibly 10 million cycles or more without failure.

Following the German example [11], we have now studied the mechanical strength of 28 and 32mm alumina ceramic femoral heads as well as developing a suitable test for evaluation of potential new ceramic applications (for even smaller diameter balls). The implants were received from Kyocera, Japan, with the 28mm balls already fitted. The balls were loaded at a physiological angle of 20° to the vertical by means of 48mm OD UHMWPE Bio-ceram cups mounted in a two-station fatigue machine. The cyclic load frequency was 16.3Hz for a minimum of 10 million and maximum of 30 million cycles duration. Minimum load values were progressively step raised incrementally from 15 to 30kN during these tests.

Overall, the successful tests produced in excess of 100 million cycles at loads above 20kN which is 27 and 15 times higher than a) average American patient weight and b) heaviest American patient, respectively. The state of the badly distorted UHMWPE cups after the tests was further convincing evidence that we were testing the implants well above the normal patient range.

Such tests can now be used very effectively to evaluate improvements such as new stem materials, stem cone designs and new ceramic materials suitable for the younger, more active American patients. We have also modified the text fixtures so that the problem of the UHMWPE distortion does not affect subsequent tests.

DISCUSSION AND CONCLUSIONS

The first series of cemented Charnley THRs have achieved a remarkable success of about 90 percent in basically the "elderly" patient population at ten years follow-up. The evolution of the THR design has basically been to 1) address the stem and cup fixation problems and 2) improve the wear resistance of the hip joint so that there would be no ensuing complications due to tissue reactions to wear debris.

The phenomenon of wear is insidious, unrelenting and consistent. It is therefore important to minimize the production of wear debris whenever possible, otherwise there may be more loosening complications, especially in younger patients. With the clinical wear results of the ceramic:ceramic THR wear resistance uncertain, *the optimal clinical choice currently is the ceramic balls: UHMWPE cup combination.* Clinical reports show *four to five times decrease in UHMWPE wear compared to metal: UHMWPE, with the added advantage that there is no metallic wear debris or ion release and no ceramic wear products detectable in the tissues. The decreased frictional torques with ceramic balls may also reduce the incidence of cup loosening.*

On the acetabular side, the screw-in ceramic and metal backed cups appear to have experienced virtually zero loosening with up to six years clinical experience. However, we known from results of the cemented cups that late loosening becomes *more* evident at 8–11 years follow-up. Thus the non-cemented acetabular cups appear to be doing very well but need to be followed closely for several more years to be sure.

On the femoral side, the clinical results are less well defined. Each pioneer has generally changed stem designs two or three times, gener-

Table 3. Overall summary of complications involving press-fit and bone-ingrowth THR prostheses.

| Type | Reops (loose) | | Bone FX | New THR Pain Max Fu (years) |
	Stem	Cup		
Boutin	2.5%	12%, 6.5%, 0.5%	10%	—	4
Lord	0	0	5%	20%	8
Lindenhof	cemented	0	—	—	—
Mittelmeier	19%, 5%	1%	11%	16%	8
Isoelastic	Subsid.	0	—	—	4
Gustillo	0	cemented	—	—	2
AML/Lunceford	0	0	—	—	5
AML/Engh	0	0%	1%	20%	5

ally making them bigger and longer. Press-fitting these larger stems has resulted in one to 11 percent complications of femoral shaft fractures and 16–20 percent thigh pain during the first one or two years. Stem loosening in European press-fitted stem has varied from one to 19 percent. The Lord bone-ingrowth stem had apparently zero stem loosening per se but provided major technical problems at revision if such was required for other clinical reasons, i.e., infection, dislocations, fractured femur, etc.

The first three studies of bone-ingrowth stem designs from the U.S. quoted *zero stem loosening* with follow-ups from two to five years (Table 3). There was however up to 20 percent thigh pain recorded in the first one or two years. Thus, these early results are encouraging but need to be followed carefully for continuing supporting information. More data is required on the fatigue strength of both the stem device and for the bonds between implant and textured surfaces if such are actually contributing to load-support of the prosthesis.

The role of the ceramic material in femoral ball designs appears to have made a lasting improvement in low friction improvement in low friction and wear of ceramic:UHMWPE components. Future improvements will come from a more complete range of ball sizes, introduction of new high-strength ceramics and eventually a better polymeric bearing.

For acetabular fixation, the screw-in ceramic cups appear to have the potential for such improved results over the cemented UHMWPE cups. Whether micro porous-ingrowth ceramic surfaces or the bioreactive coatings, e.g., hydroxylapatite, tricalcium phosphate or bone morphogenetic protein, will prove additionally useful remains to be determined.

REFERENCES

1. R. D. Beckenbaugh and D. M. Ilstrup, *J. Bone Jt. Surg., 60-A;* 306 (1978).
2. J. L. Berry, J. J. Brems, D. L. Peterson, J. S. Schuster, W. S. Berg, and A. S. Greenwald, *Trans. Orthop. Res. Soc., 8,* 132 (1981).
3. R. Bombelli, "Isoelastic Total Hip Replacement." *Scient. Meeting AAOS,* Atlanta, Feb. (1984).
4. P. M. Boutin, *Orthop. Ceramic Implants, 1,* 11 (1981).
5. H. P. Chandler and R. L. Wixson, "A Five Year Review of Total Hip Replacements in the Young Patients Under the Age of 30 with Emphasis on Loosening." *Scientific Presentation, AAOS* (1979).
6. J. Charnley, "Low Friction Arthroplasty of the Hip: Theory and Practice" (1979).

7. I. C. Clarke, "Wear of Polymeric Prosthesis—Clinical Reality, Retrieved Implants and Laboratory Predictions," *Implant Retrieval: Material and Biological Analysis* (1981).

8. I. C. Clarke, *CRC Bioengineering J.,* 8, 29 (1982).

9. I. C. Clarke, H. A. McKellop, P. A. McGuire, R. Okuda, and A. Sarmiento, "Wear of Ti-6A1-4V Implant Alloy and UHMW Polyethylene Combinations," *Titanium Alloys in Surgical Implants* (1983).

10. S. D. Cook, F. S. Georgette, H. B. Skinner, and R. J. Haddad, Jr., *J. Biomed. Mat. Res., 18,* 497 (1984).

11. E. Dorre and W. Dawihl, "Ceramic Hip Endoprosthesis." *Mechanical Properties of Biomaterials,* 113–127 (1980).

12. C. A. Engh, *Clin. Orthop., 176,* 52 (1983).

13. J. O. Galante, W. Rostoker, R. Luek, and R. D. Ray, *J. Bone Jt. Surg., 53A,* 101 (1971).

14. P. Griss, "Assessment of Clinical Status of Total Joint Replacement," *Functional Behavior of Orthopaedic Biomaterials II,* Ch. 2, 1984.

15. T. A. Green, A. Sarmiento, E. T. Espiritu, C. R. Barnhart, D. Hull, and P. McGuire, "Clinical Reality of a Titanium Alloy Total Hip Replacement," Sci. Exhibit, #12101981, AAOS (1981).

16. R. Gustillo, "Short Term Follow-Up of a Non-Cemented Porous Ingrowth Femoral Stem," Scient. Meet. AAOS, Atlanta, (Feb. 1984).

17. G. Heimke and P. Griss, *Arch. Orthop. Traumat. Surg., 98,* 165 (1981).

18. G. Heimke , W. Beisler, H. von Andrian-Werburg, P. Griss, and B. Krempien, *Ber. Dt. Keram. Ges., 50* (1), 408 (1973).

19. K. J. Huttinger and H. J. Maurer, "Tribological Properties of Carbon Materials in Artificial Joints," *Biomaterials 1980,* Ed., G. D. Winter, D. F. Gibbons, and H. Plenk, Jr., John Wiley & Sons, Ltd. (1982).

20. M. Jager and W. Plitz, "Tribology of Aluminum Ceramics," Symposium of Biomaterials, 114–122, 1981.

21. G. Lord and P. Bancel, *Clin. Orthop., 176,* 67 (1983).

22. E. M. Lunceford, "The Use of Porous Chrome Cobalt Alloy Prosthesis for Total Hip Arthroplasty," Scient. Meet. AAOS, Anaheim, CA (March 1983).

23. A. A. McBeath and R. N. Foltz, *Clin. Orthop., 141,* 66 (1979).

24. H. Mittelmeier, "Fixation of Total Hip Replacement without Cement," Scient. Meet. AAOS, Atlanta, (Feb. 1984).

25. E. W. Morscher and W. Dick, *Clin. Orthop., 176,* 77 (1982).

26. P. G. Niederer, M. Semlitsch, E. Doerre, and C. Dietsch, "Total Hip Arthroplasty with Ceramic-Polyethylene Articulation," *Scientific Exhibit Handout,* XIV SICOT World Congress, Kyoto, Japan (Oct. 1978).

27. H. Oonishi, "Experience in Prosthetic Operation with Bioceram Total Hip Prosthesis," 1st Meet. Ceramic Implant Investigation Committee, Paper 5 (1981).

28. P. M. Pellicci, E. A. Salvati, and H. J. Robinson, *J. Bone Jt. Surg., 61A,* 28 (1979).

29. W. Plitz, "Simulator Studies of Ceramic-Ceramic THR," Report #9/80 FF,

Biomechanical Laboratory, Orthopaedic University Hospital, Munich. Report quoted by Heimke and Griss (1981).

30. W. Plitz and P. Griss, "Clinical, Histo-Morphological and Material Related Observations on Removed Alumina Ceramic Hip Joint Components," *Implant Retrieval: Material and Biological Analysis,* Ed., A. Weinstein, D. Gibbons, S. Brown, and W. Ruff (1981).

31. W. Plitz and H. V. Hoss, "Wear of Alumina-Ceramic Hip Joints: Some Clinical and Tribological Aspects," *Biomaterials, 3,* 187 (1982).

32. M. Semlitsch, M. Lehmann, and H. Weber, *J. Biomed. Mat. Res., 11,* 537 (1977).

33. R. Semlitsch and B. Panic. "Corrosion Fatigue Testing of Femoral Head Prostheses Made of Implant Alloys of Different Fatigue Resistance," *Mechanical Properties of Biomaterials,* Ch. 25, 323–335, Ed., G. W. Hastings and D. F. Williams, John Wiley & Sons, Ltd. (1980).

34. H. P. Sieber and B. G. Weber, "HDPE Ceramic Total Hip Replacement: The St. Gallen, In Vivo and In Vitro Experience, *Ceramics in Surgery,* 287–294, Ed., P. Vincenzini, Elsevier Scient. Pub. Co., Amsterdam (1983).

35. R. N. Stauffer, Ten-Year Follow-Up Study of Total Hip Replacement, *J. Bone Jt. Surg.,* 983 (1982).

36. C. V. Sutherland, A. H. Wilde, L. S. Borden, and K. E. Markes, *J. Bone Jt. Surg., 64-A,* 970 (1982).

37. M. Ungethum and H. J. Refior, *Arch. Orthop. Unfall-Chir., 79,* 97 (1974).

38. A. Walter and W. Plitz, "Wear Mechanism of Alumina-Ceramic Bearing Surfaces of Hip-Joint Prostheses," *Biomaterials and Biomechanics,"* Ed., P. Ducheyne, G. Van der Perre, and A. E. Aubert (1983).

39. H. G. Willert, G. Buchhorn, and U. Bucchorn, "Tissue Response to Wear Debris in Artificial Joints," *Implant Retrieval: Material and Biological Analysis,* Ed., A. Weinstein, D. Gibbons, S. Brown, and W. Ruff (1981).

40. D. F. Williams, *Biomaterials, 2,* 133 (1981).

41. K. W. J. Wright and J. T. Scales, "The Use of Hip Joint Simulators for the Evaluation of Wear of Total Hip Prostheses," *Evaluation of Biomaterials,* 135–146, Ed., G. D. Winter, J. L. Leray, and K. de Groot (1980).

42. K. Zweymuller and M. Semlitsch, *Arch. Orthop. Trauma Surg., 100,* 229 (1982).

PART III

Testing

The Biostability of Various Polyether Polyurethanes Under Stress

KENNETH B. STOKES, ANTHONY W. FRAZER, AND ELIZABETH A. CARTER

Medtronic, Inc.
3055 Old Highway 8
Minneapolis, MN 55418

INTRODUCTION

PACING LEADS ARE insulated wires with electrodes that carry stimuli to tissues and biologic signals back to implanted pulse generators. The use of polyether polyurethanes as insulation on such leads offers several advantages over silicone rubber. Because of the significantly higher tear strength and elastic modulus of polyurethane, it can be used to make smaller, tougher devices (1). A low wet coefficient of friction allows relatively easy use of two polyurethane leads in one vein for dual-chamber pacing. Reoperation rates on cardiac leads due to previously common complications such as electrode dislodgment have dropped from 4 to 5% for state-of-the-art silicone leads to ≤1% with polyurethane designs [2,3]. A two-year long animal study of injection-molded specimens and many shorter-term lead implants in canines revealed no untoward effects on the materials [4]. Permanent polyurethane leads were first implanted in humans in 1975 (neurologic) and in 1977 (cardiac). In 1981, a relatively short-term cardiac implant was discovered with insulation failure due to a previously undiscovered cracking mechanism. As of October 1983, <.1% of over 220,000 cardiac pacing leads distributed have been returned with similar insulation failures. The primary failure mechanism has been determined to be environmental stress cracking (ESC), although secondary mechanisms

Presented at ANTEC '84, The Society of Plastics Engineers, Inc. 42nd Technical Conference, April 30–May 3, New Orleans, LA have also been identified [5,6,7]. Process changes have been shown to be effective in reducing the number of failures. Meanwhile, studies on other polyurethanes reveals that most may be subject to ESC to widely varying degrees. A short-term screening test has been developed which may help in selecting improved materials and processes for future implantable devices.

MATERIALS

Most implantable polyurethane leads are made from Pellethane 2363-80A (P80A). This is apparently a composition of polytetramethylene ether glycol (PTMEG) and methylene bis (diisocyanatobenzene) (MDI) extended with butane diol (BDO). Isocyanate end groups are intended to react with urethane to form allophonate cross-links. A harder version, Pellethane 2363-55D (P55D) has also been used extensively in cardiac and neurologic leads. P55D is made from the same components, but with a higher ratio of MDI/BDO hard segment compared to soft-segment PTMEG. Tecoflex EG 80A and 60D (T80A and T60D, respectively) are cycloaliphatic analogs. These polymers replace MDI with methylene bis (diisocyanatocyclohexane). The number designation used with the above polymers (such as 80A or 60D) refers to their Shore hardness.

A number of other materials have been tested, but will only be briefly mentioned. These include a block copolymer of polyether polyurethane and polydimethyl siloxane, (Cardiothane-51, C51); a water-extended polyether polyurea urethane (extruded Biomer, EB) and various thermoplastic polyurethanes including Cardiomat 610 (C610) and proprietary compositions.

METHODS

Analytical methods include optical microscopy (OM), scanning electron microscopy (SEM), infrared spectroscopy (IR), and gel permeation chromatography (GPC). All explanted specimens are evaluated by OM at up to 30X magnification. Occasionally surfaces are scraped with a scalpel blade to determine if features are body residues. If there is any doubt, specimens are soaked in 0.5% pepsin solution. Specimens selected for SEM are dissected free with microsurgical instruments, then mounted on aluminum stubs with silver or carbon-loaded adhesive. A light sputter coating of gold is applied prior to study on an ISI-40 scanning electron microscope. A Perkin-Elmer grating infrared spectrophotometer with a frustrated multiple internal reflectance attachment (FMIR) was used for surface studies. A Micromeritics 750 HPLC pump was used for GPC with separation by a pair of Shodex columns and detection by a Perkin Elmer LC-55 UV detector at 254 nM. Standards were polystyrenes from Waters Associates.

Tubing specimens were prepared on a 2.5 cm Killion extruder with a 24:1 length to diameter ratio usinga custom-made "urethane" screw. Prior to extrusion, all materials were vacuum dried for 48–72 hours at 60 ± 5°C.

Two types of specimens were used in experiments to evaluate the in vivo effects of fixed strain. Extruded tubing 2.0 × 2.25 mm or 1.38 × 1.63 mm diameter was placed over 7.5 cm lengths of stylet-reinforced conductor coils, 0.90 or 0.75 mm outside diameter respectively. The tubing was strained to approximately 300% elongation (%E), then firmly ligated at both ends with 2-0 polyester suture material. A very firm ligature was placed in the center using as much tension as possible just short of breaking the suture material. Three such specimens were tied end to end in strings. After cleaning, ethylene oxide sterilization and aeration, four strings were implanted subcutaneously in dogs under general anesthesia. Specimens were recovered 12 weeks postimplant for analysis by OM, SEM, and FMIR. While much interesting data were obtained from these specimens, control of strain was not always accurate. Thus, a second version was developed. Stainless-steel wire 0.50 mm diameter was bent into staple or figure-8 shapes, 12.5 mm long. Extruded tubing 2.0 × 2.25 mm diameter was placed over the mandrel and strained to elongations ranging from 0–500% in increments of 100%. Firm ligatures were placed over the tubing at each end of each mandrel to fix the strain. Specimens were tied in strings of three or four, depending on animal size, ethylene oxide sterilized, aerated, and implanted subcutaneously in rabbits under general anesthesia. Explants were made weekly for 12 weeks. Material showing superior results by OM, and SEM, were prepared in the same manner and have been implanted in canines for long-term studies.

RESULTS

Extensive analytical studies on failed and unfailed leads explanted from humans and canines have been reported in detail elsewhere [5–9]. In review, these studies show that cracks are preceded by crazes in oriented patterns, not the random smooth (brittle) faced cracks that occur on oxidized P80A surfaces [5]. Sequential canine explants do not show that microscopic surface cracks propagate deeper with time, but tend to form early and stabilize [5]. Failures are always associated with

sources of residual strain [5,6,9]. Tensile strength and elongation are
essentially unaffected in cracked areas [5,8]. There is no evidence of
chemical changes in cracked outer surfaces by techniques including
FMIR, bulk IR, ESCA, Auger spectroscopy, etc. [5,6,8]. These data
implicate residual stresses and strains as primary sources of failure.
Thus, studies were initiated to evaluate the effects of fixed strain in
vivo.

Using small specimens from rabbit experiments, the effects of fixed
strain on P80A as a function of extrusion process were determined. For
example, when a relatively hot melt and a hot cooling tank were used
during extrusion, no changes were observed at ≤214% elongation over
12 weeks. At ≥330% elongation, a mixture of undamaged surfaces,
shallow surface cracking and cracks to failure were observed four
weeks postimplant. From that time on, all but three of forty-seven specimens with elongations ≥332% failed. Thus, an induction period of
four weeks and a strain threshold (ST) of >214, <332% appears to
exist for P80A extruded by this process. GPC molecular weight of
undamaged and failed specimens over the time course of the experiment showed no appreciable changes ranging from about 250,000 to
300,000 (Mw). When stress relaxation was accelerated with a thermal
treatment, most specimens with greater than 300% elongation broke.
Those that survived were implanted. Such "stress relieved" specimens
resulted in no ESC failures throughout the 12-week experiment. Thus,
a thermal treatment can raise ST to >300%E. When a cooler melt was
used, induction time decreased slightly to three weeks, and ST <200,
≥100%E. When a very cold cooling tank was used, the induction
period decreased to one week, and ST decreased to 100% elongation.

Similar studies on T80A resulted in failure at 200%E (the lowest
elongation studied) in one to two weeks. In contrast, T60D appears to
require a 9-week induction and ST ≥ 400%E in order to fail. P55D had
no evidence of cracking at all over the entire 12-week experiment at
elongations up to 400%. EB had ≤ one week induction period and
ST ≤ 100% elongation. These data are summarized in Table 1.

Larger specimens strained to about 300% elongation over coils gave
relatively poor control of strain. Tubing could neck-down enough to
grip coils before elongation was completed. Nonetheless, the observed
data on cracking was in agreement with the above. The larger specimen size allowed us to do FMIR testing. As summarized in Table 1,
surface spectra of strained cracked, unstrained uncracked, and
unimplanted P80A tubing were virtually identical. In similar 12-week
studies, 13 of 16 T-80A specimens suffered severe cracking to failure
(even when unstrained). FMIR spectra of cracked surfaces showed a

Table 1. *In vivo resistance of various polyether polyurethanes to stress cracking when implanted under fixed strain.*

Polymer (Extrusion Process)	Induction Time Before Failure (Weeks)	Strain Threshold Before Failure (%E)	FMIR Analysis
P80A (Hot melt temperature, hot cooling tank)	4	>214 <332	No changes
P80A (Cooler melt)	3	>200 ≤100	
P80A (Cold cooling tank)	1	100	
P80A (Thermal stress relaxation treatment)	>12	>300	
P80A—oxidized	—	—	Loss of aliphatic ether at 9.0 μ with gain of carbonyl at 5.75 μ.
T80A	1–2	≤200	Loss of 9.0 μ aliphatic ether, gain of carbonyl at 5.75 μ.
T60D	9	≥400	Slight loss of 9.3 μ amide ether relative to 9.0 μ aliphatic ether.
EB	<1	<100	—

definite loss of aliphatic ether with a concomittant gain in carbonyl compared to unimplanted material. Unstrained T-60D was uncracked only when not previously exposed to certain solvents used in device assembly. Thus, the effects of such solvents must be carefully considered. When strained to 300% elongation, cracking to failure occurred. Uncracked surfaces had normal FMIR spectra, similar to unimplanted material, but cracked surfaces appeared to lose some amide ether (urethane) compared to aliphatic ether.

Similar tests on strained and unstrained materials have shown cracking to various degrees of severity in other polyurethanes, including Cardiothane 51 (cracks visible only under SEM at 500X), Cardiomat 610 and proprietary compositions. P55D did not appear to be cracked at lower magnifications, although some surface features at >5000X did resemble extremely shallow cracks.

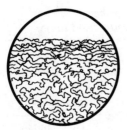 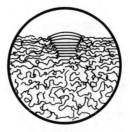 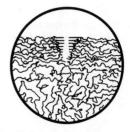

FIGURE 1. Polymer surface with amorphous skin molecules in slight tension and more ordered core molecules in slight compression (left). A chemical agent penetrates the skin plasticizing it to reduce its tensile strength. Residual skin stress pulls the surface molecules into fibrils to form a craze (center). The tensile strength of craze fibrils is exceeded, resulting in a crack (right).

When a polymeric device is implanted, body fluids immediately begin to penetrate it. It is well known that water, per se, and saline do not result in appreciable chemical attack or cracking [1,10]. Some components of body fluid (so far unidentified) soak into the surface layer (skin) of the implant. This plasticizes the surface to reduce its tensile strength. When the plasticized surface tensile strength drops below the residual skin-core stress, a craze forms, which then rapidly degenerates into a crack (Figure 1). This plasticization requires time and is dependent upon the molecular morphology—thus, an induction period is observed on in vivo strain studies. In many stress-cracking situations, the chemical penetrates the craze. It plasticizes the highly stressed craze tip, propagating the defect to failure. This is not always the case, however. By SEM, we find that P80A surfaces strained to greater than 300%E develop ripples in a vector normal to the strain. An amorphous biologic material attaches itself to the ripples surface in parallel rows.

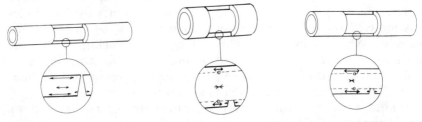

FIGURE 2. A crack has formed in the surface of an unstrained section of tubing. It propagates to a neutral axis where, under certain conditions, it can stabilize (left). With the application of some strain, surface molecules have more tension and core molecules are under less compression. The neutral axis can move inward and the crack propagates deeper (center). With application of enough strain, all molecules are in tension, the neutral axes disappear and cracks propagate to failure (right).

Cracks initiate under the biologic deposits which subsequently disappear. Thus, we hypothesize that in the absence of an applied strain the biologic plasticizer is too large or too viscous to penetrate the P80A craze tip. The craze/crack, therefore, can stabilize at a neutral axis without propagating to failure. Alternatively (or additionally) binding of such biologic residues at sites of hard segment/soft segment phase separation may reduce surface energy enough to initiate the craze [10].

When a residual strain is built into the device, however, cracks propagate deeper. This occurs because the applied strain drives the neutral axis deeper into the bulk (Figure 2). In addition, this opens the crack to allow easier penetration of body fluids. With enough strain the neutral axis can disappear entirely. During device assembly, processes have been used that stretch tubing which has been softened in swelling solvents [5,9]. This constitutes one of the many differences between certain early lead models with higher percent failures and those with no failures. One early lead, Medtronic Model 6991U had an assembly process which stretched solvent softened tubing. Obviously, if the ESC mechanism is correct, one way to reduce Model 6991U failures would be to change the assembly process. This was done in October and December of 1981. Twenty-four months later, none of the newer Model 6991U devices made by the revised assembly process are known to have failed. An example of a lead that has no known insulation failures is Model 6957. This device uses thicker tubing, no solvent stretching, and thermal post treatments.

It must also be pointed out that at least one other failure mechanism exists, which is beyond the scope of this paper [7]. For example, if insulation failure occurs by ESC or any other mechanism, an oxidation reaction can be initiated inside the lead. But this secondary failure mechanism can occur only in the presence of certain metal ions from the lead's metallic components with half-cell potentials $>.7V$ and body fluids from an insulation breach. Changes to preclude this mechanism have also been made. While the efficacy of preventative measures has been verified experimentally in animals and on the bench, it will require several years to establish a clinical improvement. This is especially true since the verifiable failure percentage is so small to begin with.

DISCUSSION

Are polyether polyurethanes biostable or not? Do they degrade over time due to oxidation or hydrolysis? The answer to this may depend upon which polyurethane is being discussed. The analytical findings on P80A lead explants simply do not fit a biodegradation mechanism. They do fit an environmental stress cracking mechanism per the following theory. When tubing is extruded, the hot (amorphous) melt is suddenly exposed to a cooling medium. The surface of the tubing freezes in its amorphous state. Since its tempeature is above its glass transition, intermolecular voids appear and the surface can expand slightly. Meanwhile, the bulk or core cools more slowly, allowing time for at least some degree of molecular order to form. In segmented polyurethanes this order is generally thought to include crystalline-amorphous mycells. The inner core, therefore, tends to shrink slightly. These differing conformations result in skin core stresses with neutral axes between them [5]. Thicker tubing will cool at slower rates minimizing amorphous skin, maximizing more ordered core. The use of a hot melt and hot cooling temperature can also slow the rate of heat transfer allowing low skin-core stresses with neutral axes close to the surface. Cold tanks give more efficient heat transfer, hence, maximize the amorphous skin. Thus, the molecular morphology of the tubing and the magnitude of its residual skin-core stresses are dependent primarily upon extrusion processes.

Why not just change to a more ESC resistant, less process sensitive material? The data presented here indicates that while most (if no all) polyether polyurethanes may be susceptible to stress-related in vivo cracking, P55D and T60D appear to be superior to P80A, which appears to be superior to everything else we've tested so far. Indeed, P55D has been used with success in implantable devices for over eight years with no known failures. It has a high elastic modulus, however, which is not easily adapted to certain lead designs. If the lead is too stiff, for example, it can perforate the heart. T60D is also a stiff polymer, with the same design considerations. In addition, however, we find that it has a high degree of susceptibility to the above-mentioned oxidative reaction, whereas P55D is only minimally affected. Of the softer polymers necessary for certain device designs, P80A (properly extruded) is so far the most stable. On the other extreme, T80A appears to undergo significant oxidative degradation. EB also cracks severely. The other polymers tested all fall somewhere in between. It has not yet been established whether or not process changes can improve the performance of these other materials. Thus we are reluctant to change polymers to solve a known problem at the risk of discovering a more severe complication. This is especially true since neither ESC nor the secondary oxidation failure mechanism were discovered in our detailed long-term animal studies. We are, therefore, concentrating on improving P80A and P55D processes while we very thoroughly test new polymers.

CONCLUSIONS

In a series of over 220,000 human cardiac pacing leads made from Pellethane 2363-80A, a small percentage (less than 0.1%) have been explanted and returned because of insulation failure. Extensive analysis led to the conclusion that the primary failure mechanism is environmental stress cracking. Thus, a short-term animal test was devised to evaluate the effects of fixed strain on in vivo stability. In these studies the propensity for shallow surface cracks is related to extrusion thermal profiles as they in turn control molecular morpohology. The propensity for surface cracks to propagate to failure is related to device assembly and implant processes, particularly those that result in strain induced orientation. At least one assembly process change to reduce strain-injduced orientation has been proven effective in reducing failures over two years clinical experience in one lead model. Numerous other improvements have been made and await the proof of time.

Based in vivo fixed strain tests, the stability of Pellethane 2363-55D > Tecoflex EG-60D > Pellethane 2363-80A (properly extruded) > Pellethane 2363-80A (improperly extruded) ≥ Cardiothane 51, Cardiomat 610, ≫ extruded Biomer and Tecoflex EG-80A. Some aromatic diisocyanate-based resins do not appear to undergo chemical changes in conjunction with in vivo cracking whereas some cycoaliphatic diisocyanate-based resins do.

REFERENCES

1. K. Stokes, K. Cobian, and T. Lathrop, "Polyurethane Insulators, a Design Approach to Small Pacing Leads," *Proceedings of the VI World Symposium on Cardiac Pacing,* C. Meere (ed.), Montreal, Pacesymp, 28—2 (1979).
2. T. Lathrop, "Transvenous Ring-Tipped Tined Ventricular Leads Models 6961 and 6962," *Medtronic Product Performance Verification Report* (May 1978).
3. N. L. Stephenson, "Spectraflex® Transvenous Leads, Models 6971 and 6972, *Medtronic Clinical Study Report* (May 1980).
4. K. Stokes and K. Cobian, *Biomaterials, 3,* 225 (1982).
5. K. Stokes, *Stimucoeur Medical, 10,* 205 (1982).
6. K. B. Stokes, W. A. Frazer, and R. A. Christopherson, "Environmental Stress Cracking in Implanted Polyurethanes," Submitted for the Second World Congress on Biomaterials (April 1984).
7. A. J. Coury, P. T. Cahalan, E. L. Schultz, and K. B. Stokes, "In Vitro Aging of Implantable Polyurethanes in Metal Ion Solutions," Submitted for the Second World Congress on Biomaterials (April 1984).

8. G. C. Timmis, D. C. Westveer, R. O. Martin, and S. Gordon, *PACE, 6,* 845 (1983).

9. C. L. Byrd, W. McArthur, K. Stokes, M. Sivina, W. S. Yahr, and J. Greenberg, *PACE, 6,* 868 (1983).

10. G. S. Pande, *PACE, 6,* 858 (1983).

Testing Methods in Biomaterials

WESLEY D. JOHNSON
MTS Systems Corporation
Minnneapolis, Minnesota

ABSTRACT

In defining the behavior of materials and structures used in implant devices, it is important for test system specifications to address the application of controlled loads and displacements, environmental conditions, and monitoring of test parameters. Since the early 1800's, materials have been implanted in the human body to stabilize fractures, reconstruct articular joints, or enhance biological tissue. The demands placed on implant materials from a chemical and mechanical standpoint are severe. Advances in implant technology require the development of improved biomaterials.

Biochemical evaluation of biomaterials provides a qualitative estimate of biocompatibility. The physical properties of biomaterials are attained through mechanical testing. Evaluation of the mechanical interaction between implant device, supporting material, and supporting biological tissue may be done through the application of physiological loads and displacements to an implant device/host bone specimen.

The use of orthopedic implants has significantly improved the treatment of severely traumatized patients, and provided relief and mobility for arthritic patients. The use of biomaterials in implant devices is ever-expanding. Test specifications have been defined for various implants, and will be developed for new devices. In the future, testing methods and equipment will have to be versatile and expandable to meet the requirements of this developing and growing arena.

INTRODUCTION

MATERIALS TEST SYSTEMS such as those designed and built by our company are created to perform exacting tests to a wide range of

---

Reprinted from *SAMPE Journal*, July/August 1984, courtesy of Society for Advancement of Material and Process Engineering, Covina, CA U.S.A.

245

Table 1. Implant devices in use or being tested, their function, and the biomaterials used.

Device	Function	Biomaterial
	Sensory and neural systems	
Artificial vitreous humor	Fill the vitreous cavity of the eye	Silicone Teflon sponge; polyglyceryl methacrylate (PGMA)
Corneal prosthesis	Provide an optical pathway to the retina	Polymethyl methacrylate (PMMA); hydrogels
Intraocular lens	Correct problems caused by cataracts	PMMA (lens); nylon, polypropylene, Pt, Ti, Au loops
Artificial tear duct	Correct chronic blockage	PMMA
Artificial eustachian tube	Provide clear ventilation passage	Silicone rubber, Teflon
Nerve tubulation	Align severed nerves	Silicone membrane, porous surgical metals
Middle ear prostheses	Replace diseased bones of the middle ear	PMMA; metallic wire, Proplast (PTFE + carbon fiber); Bioglass; Ceravital
Percutaneous leads	Conduct power to electrical sensory devices	Nylon or Dacron velour, PMMA
Auditory prostheses, visual prostheses	Restoration of hearing and vision	Pt and Pt-Ir wires and electrodes, Ta-Ta$_2$O$_5$ electrodes, stainless steel, Elgiloy wires; silicone rubber; PMMA
Electrical analgesia	Eliminate chronic pain	Pt and Pt-Ir wires and electrodes, Ta-Ta$_2$O$_5$ electrodes, stainless steel, Elgiloy wires; silicone rubber; PMMA
Electrical control of epileptic seizures	Conduct electrical signals to brain	Pt and Pt-Ir wires and electrodes, Ta-Ta$_2$O$_5$ electrodes, stainless steel, Elgiloy wires; silicone rubber; PMMA
Electrophrenic stimulation	Control breathing electrically	Pt and Pt-Ir wires and electrodes, Ta-Ta$_2$O$_5$ electrodes, stainless steel, Elgiloy wires; silicone rubber; PMMA
Bladder control	Stimulate bladder release	Pt and Pt-Ir wires and electrodes, Ta-Ta$_2$O$_5$ electrodes, stainless steel, Elgiloy wires; silicone rubber; PMMA

(continued)

Table 1. (continued)

Device	Function	Biomaterial
Heart and cardiovascular system		
Myocardial and endocardial stimulation (heart pacer)	Maintain heart rhythm	Stainless steel, Ti cans; silicone rubber, was epoxy encapsulants; Pt or Pt-Ir alloy electrode, Eligiloy wire
Chronic shunts and catheters	Assist hemodialysis	Polyethylene, hydrophilic coatings
Cardiac heart valves	Replace diseased valves	Co-Cr alloys; low-temperature isotropic carbon; porcine grafts; Ti alloy with Silastic or pyrolytic carbon disks or balls
Arterial and vascular prostheses; artificial heart components; heart-assist devices	Replace diseased arteries and blood vessels; replace the heart augment diseased heart	Segmented polyurethanes; silicone rubber or pyrolytic carbon mandrels with Dacron mesh sheaths; heparin [S] GBH or TGBH coupled coatings on Teflon or silicone rubber PHEMA-coated polymers; Dacron velours, felts, and knits; textured polyolefin (TP), TP with cross-linked gelatin surface; Teflon (PTFE) alone
Skeletal system repair and replacement		
Artificial total hip, knee, shoulder, elbow, wrist	Reconstruct arthritic or fractured joints	Stems: 316L stainless steel; Co-Cr alloys; Ti and Ti-Al-V alloy; Co-Cr-Mo-Ni alloy cups: high-density, high-molecular-weight polyethylene; high-density alumina; "cement" PMMA; low-density alumina; polyacetal polymer; metal-pyrolytic carbon coating; metal-Bioglass coating; porous polytetrafluoroethylene (PTFE); and PTFE-carbon coatings on metal; PMMA-carbon fibers, PMMA-Ceravital powder composite; porous stainless steel; Co-Cr; Ti and Ti alloys

(continued)

247

Table 1. (continued)

Device	Function	Biomaterial
Bone plates, screws, wires	Repair fractures	316L stainless steel; Co-Cr alloys; Ti and Ti alloys; polysulfone-carbon fiber composite; Bioglass-metal fiber composite; polylactic acid-polyglycolic acid composite
Intermedullary nails	Align fractures	316L stainless steel; Co-Cr alloys; Ti and Ti alloys; polysulfone-carbon fiber composite; Bioglass-metal fiber composite; polylactic acid-polyglycolic acid composite
Harrington rods	Correct chronic spinal curvature	316L stainless steel; Co-Cr alloys; Ti and Ti alloys; polysulfone-carbon fiber composite; Bioglass-metal fiber composite; polylactic acid-polyglycolic acid composite
Permanently implanted artificial limbs	Replace missing extremities	316L stainless steel; Co-Cr alloys; Ti and Ti alloys; polysulfone-carbon fiber composite; Bioglass-metal fiber composite; polylactic acid-polyglycolic acid composite; plus nylon or Dacron velours on Silastic for soft tissue ingrowth
Vertebrae spacers and extensors	Correct congenital deformity	Al_2O_3
Spinal fusion	Immobilize vertebrae to protect spinal cord	Bioglass
Functional neuromuscular stimulation	Control muscles electrically	Pt, Pt-Ir electrodes; silicone; Teflon insulation

(continued)

Table 1. (continued)

Device	Function	Biomaterial
Dental		
Alveolar bone replacements mandibular reconstruction	Restore the alveolar ridge to improve denture fit	PTFE carbon composite (Proplast); porous Al_2O_3; Ceravital: HEMA hydrogel-filled porous apatite; tricalcium phosphate; PLA/PGA copolymer; Bioglass dense apatite
Endosseous tooth-replacement implants (blades, anchors, spirals, cylinders—natural or modified root form)	Replace diseased, damaged, or loosened teeth	Stainless steel, Co-Cr-Mo alloys, Ti and Ti alloys, Al_2O_3 Bioglass, LTI carbon, PMMA, Proplast, porous calcium aluminate, $MgAl_2O_4$ spinel, vitreous carbon, dense hydroxyapatite
Subperiosteal tooth replacement implants	Support bridge work or teeth directly on alveolar bone	Stainless steel, Co-Cr-Mo alloy, LTI carbon coatings
Orthodontic anchors	Provide posts for stress application required to change deformities	Bioglass-coated Al_2O_3; Bioglass-coated Vitallium
Space-filling soft tissue prostheses		
Facial contouring and filling prostheses (nose, ear, cheek)	Replace diseased, tumorous, or traumatized tissue	Silicone rubber (Silastic), polyethylene, PTFE, silicone fluid, dissolved collagen fluid, polyrane mesh
Mammary prosthesis	Replace or augment breast	Silicone gel and rubber, Dacron fabric; hydron sponge
Cranial boney defects and maxillofacial	Fill defects	Self-curing acrylic resin; stainless steel, Co-Cr alloy, Ta plates; polyethylene and polyether urethane-coated polyethylene terephthalate-coated cloth mesh
Artificial articular cartilage	Replace arthritis deterioration cartilage	Crystallized hydrogel-PVA and polyurethane polymers; PFTE plus graphite fibers (Proplast)

(continued)

Table 1. *(continued)*

Device	Function	Biomaterial
Miscellaneous soft tissues		
Artificial ureter, bladder, intestinal wall	Replace diseased tissue	Teflon, nylon-polyurethane composite; treated bovine pericardium; silicone rubber
Artificial skin	Treat severe burns	Processed collagen; ultrathin silicone membrane polycarprolactone (PCA) foam-PCA film composite
Hydrocephalus shunt	Provide drainage and reduce pressure	Silicone rubber
Tissue patches	Repair hernias	Stainless steel, Marlex, Silas, Dacron mesh
Internal shunt	Provide routine access to dialysis units	Modified collagen; Silastic
External shunt	Provide routine access to dialysis	Silastic-Teflon or Dacron
Sutures	Maintain tissue contact to aid healing	Stainless steel, silk, nylon PGA, Dacron, catgut, polypropylene
Drug delivery systems	Release drugs progressively; enzymes	Silicone rubber; hydrogels ethylene-vinyl acetate copolymer, PLA/PGA polysaccharides-vinyl polymers
Artificial trachea	Reconstruct trachea	Porous Dacron-polyether urethane mesh, Ta mesh, Ivalon sponge and polypropylene mesh

stringent, varying specifications. Nevertheless, there is a common thread running through these applications and that is their focus on purpose. Each test application has three key factors which help the material researcher gain insight into the behavior of materials and structures.

1. Accurate simulation of service loads, displacements, and strains.
2. Testing in controlled environments.
3. The accurate and timely monitoring of test parameters.

In medicine, the requirements concerning materials and structures to be implanted in the human body are stringent, and rightfully so. Early surgical procedures in which metals were implanted to stabilize fractures were marred by high incidence of material failure and degradation combined with wound infection.

In the early 1800's, Bell [1], Levert [2], and Malgaige [3] reported on the effects implanted metals have on living tissue. Metals studied included gold, silver, lead, steel, and platinum. Early procedures involving implantable devices were complicated by pain, infection, and device failure.

A major surgical breakthrough occurred in the 1860's which dramatically increased the number of surgical procedures and frequency of implanted devices. This was the introduction of aseptic surgical techniques by Joseph Lister [4]. In these early applications, implant materials were used for fracture fixation, either internal or external. For internal fixation of fractures, plates, screws, nails, and wires were, and still are, commonly used. For external fixation, metal pins link bone fragments to an external frame to stabilize the fracture.

In addition to fracture fixation, biomaterials are often used for repair or reconstruction of human joints. During 1891, Theophilus Gluck [5] reported on implanting artificial joints for the hip, finger, and thumb. The implants were constructed of various metals and ivory. In some cases, Gluck used cements comprised of californium, pumice, and plaster of Paris to secure the implant in host bone.

During these early stages, surgeons used readily available materials to repair or enhance biological tissue. As complications ensued, materials with improved biocompatibility and physical properties were sought out. With new materials research, the frequency and variety of implants increased.

A comprehensive list of implant devices used in medicine and dentistry was comprised by Hench [6] (Table 1). Biomaterials used in these devices may be classified in four basic types [7]:

Type 1. Nearly inert, smooth surface.
Type 2. Nearly inert, microporous surface.
Type 3. Controlled reactive surface.
Type 4. Resorbable.

With each type, there is some tissue reaction due to the implant material. In general, the body will work at encapsulating the implant in fibrous tissue. For Type 1 biomaterials, minimal tissue response is desired. For Types 2, 3, and 4, varying levels of tissue response are desired. In Types 2 and 3, tissue reaction is promoted to improve the "bond," either chemical or mechanical, between implant and host tissue, thereby increasing implant life. In Type 4, the implant is designed to dissolve, and gradually transfer the one stabilizing structure from the implant to the bone.

Type 1 biomaterials are used for articulating surfaces of total joint replacement prostheses to minimize tissue growth. Type 2 biomaterials are used for soft tissue reconstruction such as tendon or ligament repair. Type 3 biomaterials are used in contact with hard tissue, for example, a porous coated femoral component of a total hip replacement prosthesis. And Type 4 biomaterials are used in trauma fixation devices.

At present, the majority of total joint replacement prostheses for the hip and knee are anchored to the host bone using polymethyl methacrylate (PMMA). This "cement" provides a uniform medium to transfer force from an implanted total joint to the irregular contour of the reamed intramedullary canal of the host bone. Numerous porous coated total hip and total knee prostheses are being tested and used in hopes of establishing a direct mechanical and/or chemical bond between the implant device and supporting tissue.

As Table 1 shows, the use of biomaterials in implant devices spans numerous medical and dental disciplines. Orthopedic implant devices will be used here in describing testing methods for biomaterials. Test specifications for orthopedic implant devices, in general, will apply to biomaterials and devices used in other disciplines.

Test specifications encompass two areas: material testing and struc-

Table 2. Material properties deduced
through biochemical testing.

1. Biocompatibility
2. Toxicity
3. Corrosion resistance
4. Material degradation

*Table 3. Material properties deduced
through mechanical testing.*

1. Modulus of Elasticity
2. Poisson's ratio
3. Yield and ultimate strength
4. Creep and viscoelastic characteristics
5. Fracture mechanics and fracture toughness
6. Wear characteristics
7. Coefficient of thermal expansion
8. Fatigue characteristics

tural testing. Material testing involves determining the properties of the biomaterial under study. Structural testing is the evaluation of the implant device independent of, or in conjunction with supporting tissue.

MATERIAL TESTING

The design and application of implant devices is founded on a sound data base of material properties for biomaterials and supporting tissue. This data base is generated through testing, and will be expanded through testing, Material properties of concern are determined through a combination of biochemical testing (Table 2) and mechanical testing (Table 3).

Biochemical Testing

In a biochemical approach, toxicity and metabolic responses of surrounding tissue to a biomaterial are evaluated. Such tests may be conducted in vivo or in vitro. In each method, the biocompatability of the material, the potential wear debris, and the corrosion residue is qualitatively defined.

In vivo evaluation involves implanting a sample of the material in test animals. The geometry of the test sample should simulate that of the implant device. Surface textures and relative size should be similar. If there is a possibility of wear debris in adjacent tissue, then particles of the material similar in size and shape to wear debris should be implanted with the implant specimen. The implant specimen may be placed in muscular structures, or cortical bone.

In vivo evaluation also includes the testing of the implant device. In the case of a total hip replacement prosthesis, a custom prosthesis may be designed and implanted in a test animal. After a period of use, the device and surrounding tissue are removed and studied for adverse tissue response and device degradation.

In vitro evaluation offers, in some cases, a more controlled test. The evaluation involves simulating in vivo conditions. A test protocol proposed by Homsy [8] utilizes tissue culture tests for evaluation of polymer toxicity. The biocompatibility of the material is qualitatively defined based on a comparison between changes in behavior of testing cultures compared to control cultures.

Other in vitro tests may involve subjecting a biomaterial to solutions simulating body chemistry and temperature. The biomaterial may also be exposed to irritants typical of surgery, such as radiation, gas sterilization, or thermal sterilization. Degradation of the material resulting from such factors is evaluated independently, or in conjunction with in vivo, in vitro, or mechanical tests.

MECHANICAL TESTING

In applying biomaterials to implant device design, an engineer must match material properties of the biomaterial with those of the supporting tissue. In orthopedics, implant devices are attached to bone. The devices can be grouped as trauma fixation devices or joint reconstruction devices. Fixation devices are designed to stabilize fractures or realign the spine. Joint reconstruction devices have been developed to enable replacement of virtually every joint in the body. The complexity of joint replacement prostheses ranges from devices which provide new articular surfaces to devices which replace the entire joint and majority of supporting tissue.

Bone is in a continuous state of remodeling, and reacts to applied stresses by adding or removing bone. In highly stressed areas, bone will resorb if its yield strength is exceeded. However, if bone is not stressed past its yield point and the applied stress is varied from normal, new bone will be put down to decrease these stresses and enhance load carrying capability. And in cases where bone is shielded from stress, it will resorb due to disuse. This phenomenon, the remodeling of bone as a result of altered stress distribution, is known as Wolff's Law. Therefore, whenever an implant is used to stabilize a fracture or resurface an articular joint, the remodeling characteristics of the supporting bone need to be considered to ensure the desired results.

The material properties of biological tissue and biomaterials such as modulus of elasticity, Poisson's ratio, yield and ultimate strength, creep, and fracture toughness are typically determined through application of an axial or axial/torsional load to standardized specimens. The specifications defined by the American Society of Testing Materials (ASTM) cover a broad range of material types, standardized specimen geometries, and test protocols. Similar specifications exist in Germany (DIN), United Kingdom (BS), and Japan (JIS).

Material properties of biomaterials attained from standard specimen geometries are based on measured load and specimen deflection, or in the case of thermal expansion, temperature and specimen deflection. Load is measured using an axial load cell, or a multi-axial forced-moment transducer. Specimen deflection may be measured using contacting or non-contacting extensometers or linear variable displacement transducers (LVDT). To optimize the resolution of load and displacement transducers, and associated electronic, the transducers should be matched with expected specimen loads and deflections.

In testing the structural properties of implant devices, the anatomical loads typically experienced by the device are reproduced by a test system. For trauma fixation devices, such as internal plates, the plate may be subjected to flexion, compression, or torsion, or a combination of these. In stabilizing a fracture, the plate spans the fracture site and is secured to the bone fragments with screws. Potential failures of the plate include screw pull out, fatigue fracture, or bending.

Mechanical testing of joint replacement prostheses involves evaluation of the fatigue, wear, and stress distribution characteristics of the device. Hip (Figure 1) and knee prostheses (Figure 2) are typically anchored to the host bone using stems which extend into the medullary canal of the femur or tibia. The stems support a metal structure that

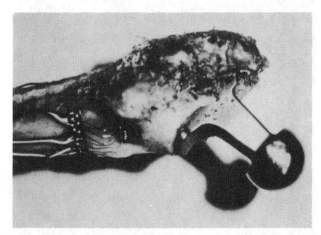

FIGURE 1. Femoral component of a total hip prosthesis implanted in a cadaver femur. Strain gages are applied for strain distribution measurement. (Courtesy of David Hoeltzel, Orthopaedic Biomechanics Laboratory, Metropolitan Medical Center, Minneapolis, MN.)

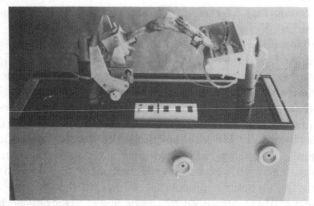

FIGURE 2. Knee Joint Tester. (Courtesy of Paul McLeod, G.I.T., University of Arkansas, Little Rock, AR.)

provides an articular surface for the joint. Mating articular surfaces of a joint prosthesis are typically a metal surface riding on an ultra-high molecular weight polyethylene (UHMWPE) surface. To improve stress distribution and reduce cold flow, UHMWPE components of total joint prostheses are sometimes metal-backed.

Measurement of applied loads and displacements are typically made with uniaxial or multi-axial transducers. Fatigue characteristics are

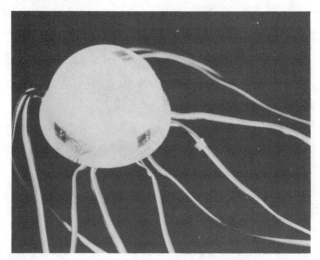

FIGURE 3. Acetabular component (UHMWPE) of a total hip prosthesis. Strain gages are applied for strain distribution measurement. (Courtesy of David Hoeltzel, Orthopaedic Biomechanics Laboratory, Metropolitan Medical Center, Minneapolis, MN.)

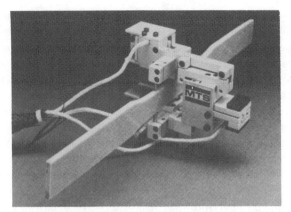

FIGURE 4. Biaxial strain extensometer.

attained by applying sinusoidal or physiological load profiles to the prosthesis while monitoring crack initiation and propagation in the metal stem or backing, in the UHMWPE, in the supporting PMMA cement, or in the supporting tissue. Stress distribution along interfaces between metal, UHMWPE, PMMA, and bone may be evaluated using imbedded and surface mounted strain gages (Figure 3). Settling of a prosthesis in supporting bone may be measured using multiple extensometers (Figure 4) or LVDT's. It should be noted that in vitro testing of implant device/bone specimens neglects the remodeling characteristics of supporting bone. Bone remodeling may enhance or degrade the integrity of the prosthesis fixation. In addition, in vitro tests typically do not account for the fibrous tissue layer separating the implanted material from living tissue. In some cases, bone remodeling and the fibrous tissue layer are accounted for by using implant device/bone specimens retrieved after a period of use.

Total joint prostheses are subject to wear. The articular surfaces are typically metal on plastic. The wear debris is primarily UHMWPE particles. The dominant wear mechanisms in total joint replacements are adhesive wear, abrasive wear, and fatigue wear.

In a review by Clarke [9], a classification for wear machines was proposed in which test machines were grouped by complexity:

Class 1—Wear-screening devices. These are non-physiological in design, and are used for first-level comparison of material wear characteristics.

Class 2—Wear-screening devices which approximate physiological contact stress, frequency, and stroke amplitude. These wear testers typically do not simulate the complex load profiles of an articular joint.

Class 3—Joint simulators. Here, the in vivo biochemical and biomechanical conditions of an articular joint may be simulated.

In this review, there were significant variation in measured wear rate
of polymers used in implant devices. The variations were attributed to
differences in test equipment and test protocol between researchers.
The most dramatic differences were attributed to the lubricating fluid
used. Other factors included reproduction of physiological loads and
displacements, specimen temperature, pretest conditioning of the specimen, and wear measurement technique.

In Class 1 and Class 2 wear testing systems, the wear measurements
method is simplified due to the uniform shape of the specimen. Typically the specimen is a disk on flat, or pin on flat in which wear is fairly
uniform over the specimen surface. Wear is measured as the loss of
material relative to applied pressure and sliding distance. The measurement of material loss due to wear is complicated by the creep characteristics of polymers. Dimensional changes in an UHMWPE specimen appearing as a wear facet may be attributed to a combination of
wear and creep (cold flow). To minimize the influence of creep on wear
measurements, researchers have used gravimetric approaches to determine material loss based on weight changes. Difficulties here include
errors due to fluid absorption.

MECHANICAL TESTING SYSTEMS

The most widely used testing systems are designed to apply an axial
compression/tension load to a specimen. The primary components of a
test system include a load unit, control electronics, data display and
recorders, and function generator. Such systems are suitable for a wide
variety of tests including tension and compression, fatigue, fracture
mechanics, strain rate sensitivity, flexure, creep, and service life
simulation.

In biomechanics, body movement is the result of muscle contraction
and relaxation. The movement is dynamic and carried out under a complex combination of load and displacement control. The resulting forces
on the skeletal system are dynamic and complex. The load profiles in
articular joints and supporting bones are multi-dimensional, varying
through six degrees of freedom. The simulation of such loads and
displacements requires a test system with a high level of dynamic
response. This requirement is met with the use of servohydraulics.

The heart of a servohydraulic test system (Figure 5) is a servovalve
which transforms an electrical signal into a fluid pressure. The pres-

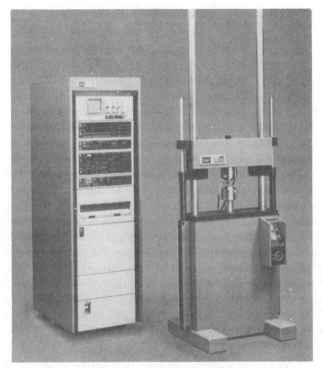

FIGURE 5. Automated universal servohydraulic test system.

sure reacts through an actuator to apply load to a specimen. The servo-hydraulic system is under closed loop control. Options for control mode are load, strain, or stroke. The desired wave shape is generated by a function generator and fed into the control electronics for the servo-valve. The signal from the control transducer (load cell, extensometer, or LVDT) is compared to the control signal and the error summed into the control signal. This closed loop control of the load unit provides accurate, dynamic reproduction of the desired control signal.

Using servohydraulic technology, load units comprised of a linear actuator and a rotary actuator may be oriented to enable simulation of the complex load and displacement profiles typical of an articular joint. In simulating an articular joint to track its own center of rotation, rather than that of the load unit. A single axis test system may accomplish this through proper fixturing to the specimen [10]. How-ever, with two channels of control, only two degrees of freedom may be controlled. The other degrees of freedom are either constrained or unconstrained. A direct approach to simulating articular joints would involve active, closed loop control of each degree of freedom. The base system would be a standard servohydraulic axial/torsional load unit. To this, additional channels of control would be added in conjunction with linear and rotary actuators to provide multi-degree of freedom capability.

Combining active closed loop control of a multi-axial servohydraulic system with computer control enables programming the system to apply physiological loads and displacements to an articular joint. Specific load and displacement profiles may be attained through modeling techniques or gait analysis. In evaluating an implant device in conjunction with supporting and connective tissue, the specimen may be used to establish the range of motion for the joint in the test system.

For a six-degree of freedom system, six independent channels of control would be synchronized under a combination of load and displacement control to simulate physiological loads and displacements. The articular joint, or the replacement prosthesis, would track its own center of rotation throughout its range of motion. Through imbedded or surface mounted strain gages, the strain distribution between host bone and implant may be measured under complex physiological loading conditions. Multi-degree of freedom extensometers may be used to monitor relative motion of joint surfaces. And multi-degree of freedom load and moment sensors would be used to monitor forces applied to the articular joint.

In addition to applying loads to a specimen, a testing system should provide an environment similar to in vivo conditions. The chemistry and temperature of the solution should be variable at the researchers discretion.

REFERENCES

1. B. A. Bell, *A System of Surgery*, Penniman, Troy, N.Y., p. 22 (1804).
2. H. S. Levert, *Am. J. Med. Sci.*, 4:17 (1829).
3. C. S. Venable and W. G. Stuck, *The Internal Fixation of Fractures*, Charles C Thomas, Springfield, Ill., p. 5 (1947).
4. C. Singer and E. A. Underwood, *A Short History of Medicine*, Clarendon Press, Oxford, p. 352 (1962).
5. P. S. Walker, *Human Joints and Their Artificial Replacements*, Charles C Thomas, Springfield, Ill., p. 253 (1977).
6. L. L. Hench, *Science*, *208*, 826 (1980).

7. L. L. Hench and E. C. Ethridge, *Biomaterials: An Interfacial Approach,* Academic Press, Inc., New York, NY, p. 3 (1982).

8. C. A. Homsy, *J. Biomed. Mater. Res., 4,* 341 (1970).

9. I. C. Clarke, *Crit. Rev. Biomed. Eng., 8*(1), 29 (1982).

10. T. Fukubayshi, P. A. Torzilli, M. F. Sherman, and R. F. Warren, *J. Bone and Joint Surg., 64A*(2), 258 (1982).

Evaluating Dental Restorative Materials with an Automated Servohydraulic Test System and Artificial Oral Environment

WESLEY D. JOHNSON
MTS Systems, Corp.
Minneapolis, Minnesoata

SUMMARY

The ability of automated servohydraulic systems to replicate the complicated, multi-dimensional motions of biomechanical movement is demonstrated by the MTS artificial oral environment. This system is designed for evaluation of dental materials or restoration techniques, dynamically, in a relatively short period of time. Developed jointly by MTS Systems Corp., and University of Minnesota School of Dentistry researchers, it can subject materials to five years of wear in a matter of weeks. During tests, the system replicates the masticatory motions and forces in an environment which simulates actual conditions of corrosion and temperature variability. The system, thus, enables researchers to measure wear, roughness, and integrity of restorative materials.

INTRODUCTION

SIMULATION OF THE three dimensional masticatory motion, as well as loading, is accomplished through use of a servohydraulic system with closed loop control (Figure 1). Closed loop means the system has the capacity to dynamically make adjustments while a test is in progress, based on sensed changes in the test or test specimen to make certain that the desired control values are maintained.

A transparent environmental chamber, as shown in Figure 2, is used for duplicating the oral environment. Volumetric measurement of

Reprinted from *SAMPE Journal*, July/August 1984, courtesy of Society for Advancement of Material and Process Engineering, Covina, CA U.S.A.

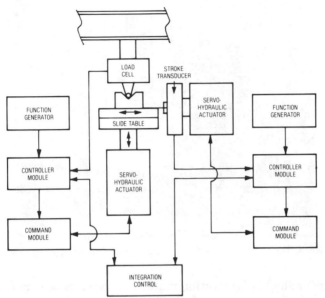

FIGURE 1. Control logic for horizontal and vertical mechanical closed-loop systems.

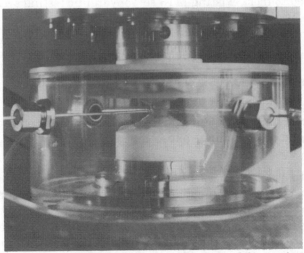

FIGURE 2. Environmental chamber during resynthesis of the masticatory cycle.

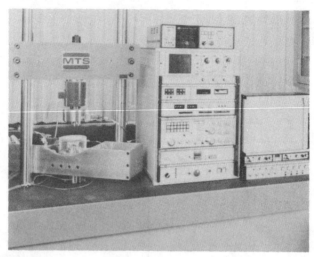

FIGURE 3. The test system without the artificial oral environment chamber.

removal of enamel or restoration material by wear is obtained through a computerized profiling system. Roughness and integrity are measured using a displacement sensitive stylus. Because MTS servohydraulic test systems are modular (Figure 3), the capabilities described in this application, including the MTS Artificial Oral Environment can be adapted to most existing MTS servohydraulic testing systems. Or, a complete system for dental or orthopaedic testing can be configured.

RESYNTHESIS OF THE MASTICATORY CYCLE

The masticatory cycle is characterized by three phases:

1. The preparatory phase during which the mandible is positioned.
2. The crushing phase during which the molars compress the bolus.
3. The gliding (grinding) phase during which the bolus is ground between the molars.

The preparatory and crushing phases are carried out under muscular or load control. The gliding phase is carried out under displacement or stroke control defined by tooth anatomy.

During the gliding phase, the motion of mastication is described by an eccentric contact of the mandibular buccal cusps with the inner inclines of the maxillary buccal cusps followed by a working movement to centric occlusion. This three dimensional movement can be described by motion in two planes: the horizontal and frontal planes. Horizontal

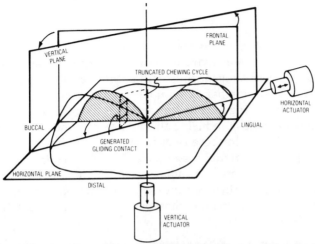

FIGURE 4. Cross-sections through the maxillary first molar inverted on the testing unit. This illustration shows the reduction of three dimensional movement to two dimensional control.

movement is approximated by straight line motion, whereas frontal plane movement is defined by occlusal anatomy.

A two dimensional simulation of three dimensional masticatory motion is accomplished by aligning linear actuators with the appropriate planes of motion (Figure 4). Motion in the frontal plane is provided by a linear actuator directed vertically. Motion in the horizontal plane is provided by a linear actuator directed horizontally, and aligned with the straight line approximation of horizontal motion.

Loading during the glide phase is accomplished by inputting the desired electronic waveform into the servohydraulic closed-loop control of the vertical actuator. The electronic waveform may be programmed to provide a constant contact load during the glide phase, or a haversine contact load which closely simulates anatomical loading. The contact load during the glide phase is controllable from 1 pound (4.45 N) to 1,000 pounds (4,450 N).

Motion throughout the chewing cycle is dictated by movement in the horizontal plane which is under stroke control at all times. The vertical actuator is in load control during the gliding phase, and movement is defined by occlusal anatomy. The glide phase may have duration of 0.25 to 0.33 seconds. Control of the vertical actuator switches to stroke control for the preparatory and crushing phases. The servohydraulic control loops for the vertical and horizontal actuators are synchronized to ensure accurate resynthesis of the chewing cycle of frequencies up to 4 Hertz.

RESYNTHESIS OF AN ORAL ENVIRONMENT

The wear characteristics of tooth enamel and restorative materials are highly dependent on environmental conditions. An environmental chamber has been developed which will bathe the test specimen in synthetic saliva. The chamber is equipped with a temperature control system to enable testing at body temperature. The temperature control system is also capable of inducing thermal shocks and gradients in the test specimen similar to those seen in everyday activities.

Specimen preparation and installation is facilitated through the use of an articulator to ensure anatomically correct alignment of the teeth. Once potted in polyethylene fixtures, the test specimen is easily installed in the environmental chamber without loss of alignment.

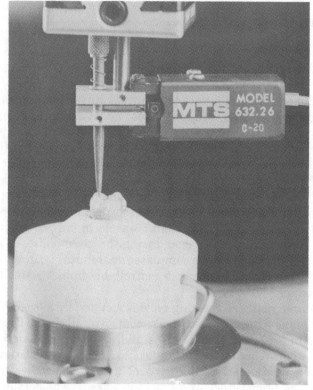

FIGURE 5. Profiling a specimen prior to a test. The strain sensitive stylus controls vertical actuator; data is fed to programmable data acquisition system. Many passes result in a three dimensional profile. "Before" and "after" test profiles are matched in the computer to measure wear.

THREE DIMENSIONAL TOOTH PROFILING

In evaluating wear characteristics of restorative materials, it is necessary to have a method to determine the volume of removal material. This is accomplished by profiling the tooth surface before and after testing as shown in Figure 5.

The profiles are then overlapped, and the volumetric change calculated.

A tooth profile is generated using the test system along with a precise displacement stylus and programmable data acquisition system. The stylus is drawn across the tooth via the horizontal actuator. Movement of the vertical actuator is controlled by the stylus which traces the contour of the tooth. Displacement data from the horizontal and vertical actuator's linear variable displacement transducers (LVDT) is gathered providing a contour line of the tooth in the plane of stylus motion. The stylus is then moved over to trace another contour line parallel to the first. This is repeated until a three dimensional profile of the chewing surface is obtained.

Profiles of "before" and "after" testing are overlapped to align areas of the tooth not subjected to wear. The volume between these profiles is then calculated and attributed to wear. This technique may be used on both the restored specimen to evaluate wear rate of the restoration, and on the opposite tooth to evaluate wear of enamel against the restoration.

The stylus is capable of measuring enamel and restoration roughness with an accuracy of ±5 microns. Integrity of the restoration and enamel interface at the surface of the tooth may also be evaluated with the stylus.

CONCLUSION

While this report describes a dental system, the technology is applicable to simulation of other biomechanical resynthesis. Systems like this are well suited for determining wear and loading characteristics of permanent implantable orthopaedic prostheses, and temporary orthopaedic devices such as fixators.

PART IV

Reliability

Durability Prediction and Testing of Elastomeric Biomaterials

J. L. KARDOS, K. GADKAREE, AND A. P. BHATE
Materials Research Laboratory and
Department of Chemical Engineering
Washington University
St. Louis, Missouri

INTRODUCTION

SYNTHETIC POLYMER BIOMATERIALS are often asked to perform under conditions of large cyclic deformations for long lifetimes. Typical of such applications are Left Ventricular Assist (LVA) pump bladders, heart valve components, and vascular grafts. In designing with these materials and eventually qualifying them for clinical usage, it is necessary to be able to predict the fatigue lifetimes accurately and reliably. To be sure, these materials must be biologically compatible; but even the most perfectly biocompatible material will not be qualified for structural use in humans unless its mechanical longevity can be proven from an accurate data base.

The nature of the fatigue problem is complicated by the statistical spread of cycles-to-failure data at any one stress level. If fatigue life is to be reliably predicted, the statistical nature of the failure must be examined. Curiously, there has not been much effort to do this for polymers [1,2], although fatigue laws involving two-parameter Weibull distributions have often been employed in describing fatigue of metals and reinforced plastics [3].

Usually, the problem of life prediction is treated in a deterministic way by experimentally determining a flaw growth law and then integrating it to a limit of the number of cycles in the lifetime. This has been the approach adopted in the studies on elastomers [4–7] and most

---

Presented at ANTEC '85, The Society of Plastics Engineers, Inc., 43rd Technical Conference, April 29–May 2, Washington, DC U.S.A.

investigations of plastics [2] and reinforced plastics [8]. This does not help in explaining the scatter observed in the lifetime of specimens which look exactly the same and are subjected to the same conditions.

PREDICTIVE FORMAT

Uniaxial Deformation

The calculational format for predicting fatigue lifetimes under cyclic uniaxial deformation was developed recently by Gadkaree and Kardos [9]. Very briefly, the failure process is viewed as initiating when a population of flaws begins to grow in a material under cyclic loading. The statistical nature of these flaw sizes dictates that a spectrum of failure lifetimes results as the population of growing flaws reaches a critical size for failure. To describe this process mathematically, we proceed as follows. First, a sample population of specimens (~ 20) is tested in tension. The resulting ultimate strengths are fitted to the normal distribution function

$$ f(\sigma_b) = \frac{1}{\sigma\sqrt{2\pi}} \exp\left\{ -\frac{1}{2}\left[\frac{\sigma_b - \mu}{\sigma} \right]^2 \right\} \tag{1} $$

where μ and σ^2 are the mean and variance of the distribution and σ_b is the breaking strength. It is a theoretical and experimentally verified fact that the ultimate or breaking strength of elastomers depends on the flaw size according to

$$ \sigma_b = \frac{M}{c^N} \tag{2} $$

A second population (~ 20) of specimens having purposely introduced sharp flaws of known critical size is then tested in uniaxial tension and the constants M and N evaluated. Equation (2) is substituted into 1 and, after a variable transformation, we obtain

$$ f(c) = \frac{MN}{\sigma\sqrt{2\pi}\; c^{1+N}} \exp\left\{ -\frac{1}{2}\left[\left(\frac{M}{c^N} - \mu\right)\bigg/ \sigma \right]^2 \right\} \tag{3} $$

Thus, the distribution of hypothetical flaw sizes in a given specimen population is obtained. A similar procedure can be used for any other distribution function.

The growth of this flaw distribution is governed by a tearing energy concept [10].

$$\frac{dc}{dn} = AT^b \tag{4}$$

where A and b are constants depending on experimental conditions and the material. T, the tearing energy, is given for an edge crack by $T = 2KUc$ where K is a numerical constant and U is the area under the stress–strain curve. Integrating this equation between the limits c_o to c (initial flaw size and flaw size after n cycles, respectively) and 0 to n, where n is the number of cycles, and substituting into Equation (3) yields the probability distribution of crack sizes after n cycles.

Assuming that the final flaw size is much greater than the initial flaw sizes, c_o, the probability distribution of fatigue lives can be directly derived [9] as

$$f(n) = \frac{MN}{\sigma\sqrt{2\pi}} \left(\frac{1}{b-1} \right) \frac{n^{(N+1-b)/(b-1)}}{\left(\dfrac{1}{A(b-1)(2KU)^b} \right)^{N/(b-1)}} \tag{5}$$

$$\exp\left\{ -\frac{1}{2}\left\{ \left[\frac{M\,n^{N/(b-1)}}{\left(\dfrac{1}{A(b-1)(2KU)^b} \right)^{N/(b-1)}} - \mu \right] \Big/ \sigma \right\}^2 \right\}$$

Thus, Equation (5) can provide the fatigue lifetime distribution functions under given experimental conditions without carrying out any fatigue tests at all, if the six constants (M, N, μ, σ, A, b) are known.

Three independent, short-term experiments provide the necessary values of the constants; namely determination of the breaking strength in uniaxial tension with and without an introduced critical flaw, and a flaw propagation experiment in which the flaw growth is measured as a function of a small number of cycles.

Biaxial Deformation

The same format can be used to predict biaxial fatigue lifetime distributions. Determining the six constants under biaxial stress becomes experimentally much more difficult because the stress is usually hydraulically applied. Nonetheless, this technique has been developed by Bhate and Kardos [11] using a Swanson tuned fluid oscillator system

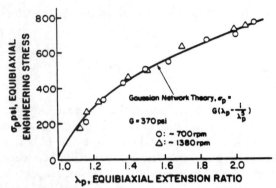

FIGURE 1. High frequency equibiaxial stress-deformation relation for Biomer.

[12]. Figure 1 shows the biaxial stress–strain relation for Biomar,[1] which must be used to calculate the tearing energy for the flaw growth rate experiments. Figure 2 shows the effect of tearing energy on the flaw growth rate for Avcothane 51[2] at a frequency of 26.5 Hz. The slope and intercept of this plot provide the values for the constants b and A of Equation (4). The tuned fluid oscillator may also be used in a static mode to determine the biaxial strength distribution and the effect of a

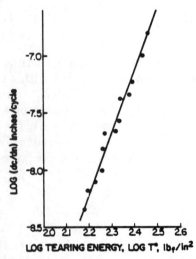

FIGURE 2. Cyclic biaxial flaw growth relation for Avcothane 51 at 26.5 Hz.

---

[1]Trademark of Ethicon, Inc., Somerville, NJ.
[2]Trademark of Avco Everett Research Labs, Inc.

flaw on that distribution. The six constants determined from these three biaxial experiments can be used with Equation (5) to predict the biaxial fatigue lifetime distribution.

EXPERIMENTAL RESULTS

A detailed description of the testing procedures and materials may be found elsewhere [9,11]. We briefly present here some of the pertinent experimental results.

Fatigue Lifetime Distributions—Predicted vs. Measured

At a 90% confidence level, the predicted uniaxial fatigue lifetime distribution accurately described the experimentally determined distribution for Biomer for three different maximum cyclic stress levels [9]. The two distributions were compared using a Kolmogoroff statistical goodness-of-fit test [13] for small numbers of samples.

Figure 3 shows the cumulative uniaxial fatigue lifetime distribution for Avcothane 51 at a frequency of 0.1 Hz and maximum tensile stress of 1800 psi. At a 90% confidence level, the predicted curve accurately represents the experimental data points (using Kolmogoroff statistics). The prediction is extremely good at the low lifetime region and is conservative throughout and at the longer lifetime end of the distribution; both of these trends are desirable in designing the material for life-sustaining applications.

As can be seen from Equations (2) and (4), a material's resistance to fatigue failure depends on both the effect of flaw size on static strength as well as its resistance to flaw growth during dynamic loading. Table 1 displays the uniaxial values for M and N in Equation (2) for a variety of potential elastomeric biomaterials. High values of M and low values

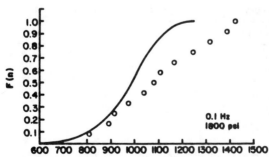

FIGURE 3. Cumulative fatigue lifetime distribution for Avcothane 51 at 0.1 Hz and 1800 psi maximum stress.

Table 1. Effect of frequency on constants in flaw growth equation, $dc/dn = At^b$.

Frequency, cps	A	b
0.01	1.778×10^{-8}	2.50
0.1	40×10^{-8}	1.58
1.0	2.511×10^{-8}	2.12

for N indicate an intrinsic resistance of the material to initiation of flaw growth. Clearly, Biomer, Goodyear Polyolefin[3] and NBS butyl rubber[4] all have better resistance than Avcothane 51 and Pellethane[5].

The effect of frequency on the fatigue lifetime distribution is not obvious. Table 2 shows the values for the constants A and B in Equation (4) over two orders of magnitude in frequency for Biomer. There is not much effect at room temperature. If the tearing energy T, is not affected by strain rate (which is true in this case), then one might expect to be able to safely extrapolate high frequency test results to lower frequency in this range. However, the frequency range covered is much too limited and higher frequency testing (at, say, 30 Hz) may exhibit totally different results. Clearly more high frequency data is vitally needed before any conclusions can be drawn.

CONCLUSIONS

It is now an accepted fact that fatigue failure initiates at pre-existing flaws. These flaws grow due to fatigue loading and catastrophic failure takes place as the critical size is reached. Thus, knowing the distribution of initial flaw sizes and the fatigue law for flaw propagation, the distribution of flaw sizes after n cycles can be determined and the probability of failure calculated.

Table 2. Parameters M and N for the flaw size—strength relation, $\sigma_b = M/c^N$.

Material	M	N
Biomer	608	0.39
Avcothane 51	14	1.28
Goodyear Polyolefin	167	0.35
Pellethane	11	1.24
NBS Rubber	211	0.44

[3]Trademark, Goodyear Tire and Rubber Co., Akron, OH.
[4]National Bureau of Standards reference material 388j.
[5]Trademark, Upjohn Co., Torrance, CA.

ACKNOWLEDGEMENT

We are grateful for the support of this work by the National Heart, Lung, and Blood Institute, Division of Heart and Vascular Diseases, Devices, and Technology Branch under Contract No. N01-HV-02910.

REFERENCES

1. J. A. Manson and R. W. Hertzberg, *Crit. Rev. Macromol. Sci.*, *1*, 433 (1973).
2. R. W. Hertzberg and J. A. Manson, *Fatigue of Engineering Plastics*, Academic Press, NY (1980).
3. J. M. Whitney, *Fatigue of Fibrous Composite Materials*, ASTM STP 723, American Society for Testing and Materials, Phila., p. 133 (1981).
4. A. N. Gent, P. B. Lindley, and A. G. Thomas, *J. Appl. Pol. Sci.*, *8*, 453 (1974).
5. G. J. Lake and P. B. Lindley, *J. Appl. Pol. Sci.*, *8*, 107 (1974).
6. J. P. Berry, *J. Poly. Sci.*, *50*, 107 (1961).
7. R. E. Whittacker, *J. Appl. Pol. Sci.*, *18*, 2339 (1974).
8. A. T. DiBenedetto and G. Salee, *Proc. 34th Antec, Soc. Plastics Engineers*, Atlantic City, p. 103 (1976).
9. K. P. Gadkaree and J. L. Kardos, *J. Appl. Pol. Sci.*, *29*, 3041 (1984).
10. R. S. Rivlin and A. G. Thomas, *J. Pol. Sci.*, *10*, 291 (1953).
11. A. P. Bhate and J. L. Kardos, *Pol. Eng. Sci.*, *24*, 862 (1984).
12. A. P. Bhate, W. M. Swanson, and J. L. Kardos, *J. Biomed. Mat. Res.* (submitted).
13. K. V. Bury, *Statistical Models in Applied Science*, John Wiley, NY (1975).

Implantable Titanium
Feedthrough Reliability

D. E. DIXON*

Kyle Technology Corporation
Roseburg, Oregon

ABSTRACT

Implantable titanium feedthrough reliability was characterized by hermetic integrity, optimum mechanical design and critical process requirements.

Hermetic integrity of a titanium electrical feedthrough depended upon the coefficients of linear thermal expansion (CLTE) of the titanium, the sealing material, the center conductor metal and upon the degree of bonding obtained at seal to metal interfaces. Microscopic examination of the bond interface between titanium and the sealing material indicated fusion of the titanium oxide with the polycrystalline ceramic. Dilatometer measurements of titanium, a polycrystalline ceramic, and pure platinum (center conductor metal showed similar CLTE was less, assuring some degree of compression in the sealing mechanism.

Optimum mechanical design was determined by thermal stress methods, which stressed designs through increasing thermal shocks until loss of hermeticity occurred to 50% or more of the sample population. Two designs, one with mechanical reinforcement, the other without, were subjected to thermal shock ranges as severe as 755 K (482 C) to 78 K (−196 C). The plotted data indicated the design with mechanical reinforcement sustained higher levels of thermal shock without loss of hermeticity.

In vitro experiments on titanium feedthroughs with various surface configurations were conducted at low applied voltages (constant and pulse). Data indicated minimal electrochemical degradation at surfaces with maximum electrical leakage paths obtained by addition of ceramic standoff. Electrochemical degradation was measured in terms of insulation resistance between

Reprinted from *SAMPE Journal,* July/August 1984, courtesy of Society for Advancement of Material and Process Engineering, Covina, CA U.S.A.
*Mr. Duane E. Dixon has left Kyle Technology Corporation and is now residing in Tucson, Arizona.

the titanium housing and the platinum pin and correlated to accelerated battery depletion of a cardiac pulse generator. The battery life was observed to decrease rapidly as the electrical resistance across the titanium feedthrough decreased from 100,000 ohms.

Certain levels of temperature were shown to affect grain size of titanium. Titanium (grade 4) feedthrough housings were exposed to different temperature levels for the same one hour duration. SEM photomicrographs verified by ASTM grain size determinations indicated substantial grain growth above the 1255 K (982 C) temperature level. Conservative sealing conditions were recommended at less than the titanium beta transus temperature, 1158 K (885 C), and less than one hour exposure.

INTRODUCTION

TO PREVENT THE detrimental effects of moisture seepage into cardiac pulse generators (CPG) as discussed in NBS Special Publication 400–50 [1] necessitates that the external feedthrough maintain a high degree of hermeticity and electrical integrity throughout the life of an implanted device. Regarding a CPG encapsulated with titanium, the feedthrough housing, if not already an integral part of the encapsulating material, needs to be titanium to facilitate hermetic attachment by welding and to avoid dissimilar metal groupings with potentials for galvanic corrosion reactions [2].

Inherent factors affecting any type of hermetic feedthrough are the interface bonds and the relative coefficients of linear thermal expansion of materials. For analysis purposes, a titanium feedthrough with a pure platinum center conductor axially sealed by means of a polycrystalline ceramic, KRYOFLEX [3] was considered due to its flawless reliability record to implanted devices.

To ensure optimum titanium feedthrough reliability, mechanical design for each implantable application must be optimized. One method of design characterization is stressing the titanium configuration through temperature shock ranges while monitoring the hermetic integrity throughout the thermal aging cycles. Most implantable device manufacturers utilize some program of thermal stress to determine reliability or confidence in particular titanium configurations. One such program is discussed involving two design approaches to a titanium feedthrough requirement.

Moisture penetration of the titanium encapsulated CPS is eliminated by the hermetic titanium feedthrough and encapsulation and although there is an epoxy or silicone rubber covering, the external surface of the titanium feedthrough is susceptible to moisture. As evidenced by D. J. Debney [4], all organic materials absorb water to some greater or lesser degree, therefore, we must assume the moisture penetration of the epoxy or silicone rubber of critical potential. *In vitro* testing of titanium feedthroughs was peformed to determine the degree of electrochemical degradation developed across the feedthrough surface when exposed to moisture.

The final objective was to determine titanium grain size at various temperature levels as substantial grain growth may have an effect on feedthrough reliability in terms of mechanical strength and corrosion resistance. Due to the existence of three basic sealing technologies, each of which expose the titanium housing to certain temperatures for sealing, e.g., glass to metal seals and metallized ceramic seals, ~4000–4800 K [~3727–4527 C] and polycrystalline ceramic seals, ~800–3200 K [~527–2927 C] test conditions included these temperatures.

SPECIMEN PREPARATION

Titanium feedthrough construction of specimens for bondline examination, thermal aging comparison and *in vitro* experiments included a titanium (grade 4) bushing, a pure platinum center conductor axially located and a KRYOFLEX™ polycrystalline ceramic seal hermetically sealing the center conductor within the bushing inside diameter.

In the case of the thermal aging comparison, the two bushing designs differed while the other materials were consistent. Design 1 represented a bushing without a mechanical stiffener, whereas Design 2 included the stiffener.

Specimens tested under *in vitro* conditions in some cases included the addition of an alumina ceramic standoff to a relatively flat seal surface between pin and bushing that increased electrical leakage path and in all cases included a hermetic enclosure on the opposite end for protection from testing environments.

EQUIPMENT

1. Hermeticity measurements were made with a Du Pont Type 120 SSA leak detector calibrated to helium standards.

2. Photomicrographs were produced by either scanning electron microscopy techniques (SEM) or color microscopy apparatus.

3. CLTE measurements were recorded by an Orton automatic recording dilatometer.

4. The *in vitro* voltage measurements were made with a Tektronic Model 5111 storage oscilloscope.

5. The *in vitro* test apparatus consisted of individual glass containers filled with either deionized H_2O or isotonic saline (0.9% NaCl) maintained at 310 K (37 C) by means of a temperature controlled silicone oil bath. Application of voltage to the feedthrough test specimens was made by either a constant VDC power supply or a pulse generator, each of which applied power through a 6000 ohm current limiting resistor.

6. Electric furnaces were utilized as basic heat sources for thermal stress comparison and titanium grain growth studies.

PROCEDURE

CLTE Measurement

Automatic dilatometer graphs were generated from 25.4 mm long specimen rods of titanium (grade 4), KRYOFLEX™ Type 313 and KRYOFLEX™ Type 6002B in terms of percent linear thermal expansion versus degrees centigrade. The data was translated into CLTE versus degrees Kelvin and plotted in Figure 1.

Thermal Stress Testing

Eight consecutive batches each of titanium feedthrough Design 1 and Design 2 were sampled at the rate of 2%. The quantity tested per batch is shown in parenthesis in Figure 3. Each sample population was exposed to the same set of conditions as shown in Table 1. Hermeticity measurements were made and recorded after exposure to particular temperature shock level.

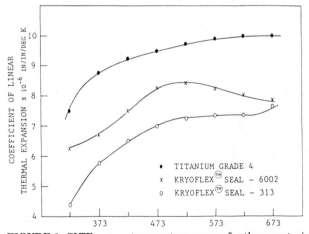

FIGURE 1. CLTE versus temperature curves for three materials.

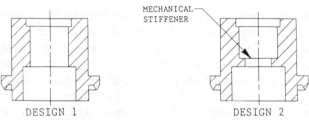

FIGURE 2. Two bushing configurations.

Feedthroughs with hermeticity of less than or equal to 2×10^{-9} cc/sec He at one atmosphere differential were exposed to the next higher temperature level, until 50% or more of each sample population measured more than 2×10^{-9} cc/sec He at one atmosphere differential. The maximum temperature level reached by 50% or more of the feedthroughs of each batch meeting the hermeticity requirement was plotted for both Design 1 and Design 2 in Figure 3.

In Vitro Testing

Titanium feedthroughs with and without alumina ceramic standoffs were subjected to the same set of voltage (i.e., 5VDC or 5V pulse amplitude, 3ms pulse width and 1ms rest) and chemical conditions (i.e., deionized H_2O or isotonic saline, 0.9% NaCl). In all cases each test was run continuously for one week minimum. Voltage drop measurements

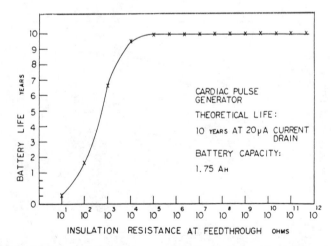

FIGURE 3. Temperature level versus consecutive batches of two different designs.

Table 1. Thermal stress test conditions at each temperature level.

Cycle	Time At Temperature Level	Rest Time	Time At 78 deg K (−196 deg C)	Rest Time
CYCLE 1	15 min	None	15 min	None
CYCLE 2	15 min	None	15 min	None
CYCLE 3	5 min	5 min	5 min	5 min
CYCLE 4	5 min	5 min	5 min	5 min
CYCLE 5	5 min	5 min	5 min	5 min

Temperature Level	deg K	(deg C)
LEVEL 1	478	(205)
LEVEL 2	533	(260)
LEVEL 3	589	(316)
LEVEL 4	644	(371)
LEVEL 5	700	(427)
LEVEL 6	755	(482)

across the titanium feedthroughs were monitored initially once every hour up to twelve hours, after which every twelve hours. Voltage drop data was translated into circuit currents which are plotted versus time for three sets of conditions in Figure 4. Various feedthrough resistances versus battery life are plotted in Figure 5.

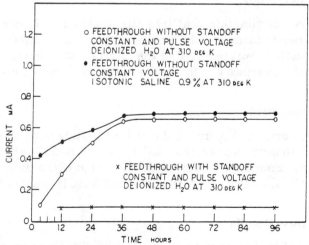

FIGURE 4. Circuit current versus time curves of titanium feedthroughs with construction and exposure variables.

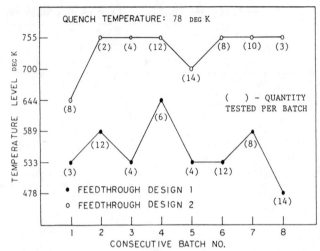

FIGURE 5. Battery life versus feedthrough electrical resistance curve.

Titanium Grain Size Determination

Table 2 lists ASTM grain size determinations of titanium (grade 4) at various temperature levels.

RESULTS AND DISCUSSION

Bondline Microscopy

A study of the titanium seal interface revealed a darkened area extending some distance into the polycrystalline ceramic. Heavy crystalline activity was observed at the interface with traces of micro-porosity as the interface was left in the direction of the polycrystalline ceramic.

CLTE Measurements

The CLTE curves in Figure 1 indicated the sealing materials have a lower CLTE than titanium (grade 4). The seal Type 313 rate of CLTE increase with temperature closely resembled that of the titanium rate increase of CLTE up to its softening point indicated by a sharp increase in CLTE.

Thermal Stress Results

As indicated by Figure 3, titanium feedthrough Design 2 with the mechanical stiffener added exhibited a higher temperature threshold attained than Design 1 without the stiffener. Design 2 maintained more consistent temperature level than did Design 1.

In Vitro Test Results

Figure 4 indicates consistent low circuit current, thus high titanium feedthrough resistance to moisture in the configuration with a standoff ceramic. The two feedthrough conditions without the alumina standoff in both deionized H_2O and isotonic saline show higher circuit currents attained with 36 hours; therefore, a relatively low titanium feedthrough resistance to moisture. Figure 5 shows rapid battery life decrease when a theoretical titanium feedthrough loses resistance past 100,000 ohms and pulse current drain and battery capacity are as stated.

Grain Size Determinations

ASTM grain size numbers in Table 2 show the largest grain size attained in the range of 1255 K (982 C) to 1366 K (1093 C). Grain size numbers are similar when comparing the titanium control (no temperature exposure) to titanium exposed in the temperature range of 866 K (593 C) to 1144 K (871 C). Rate of grain growth is accelerated at exposures beyond the beta transus temperature of 1158 K (885 C).

CONCLUSIONS

1. The dark band area adjacent to the titanium seal interface was determined to be the diffusion of titanium oxide into the sealing mate-

Table 2. *ASTM grain size number of titanium at various temperature exposures.*

ASTM Grain Size No.	Temperature Exposure of Titanium Grade 4	
	deg K	(deg C)
9	Control Specimen at Room Temp.	
9	866	(593)
9	1033	(760)
9	1144	(871)
8	1200	(927)
2	1255	(982)
2	1367	(1094)

rial. The diffusion mechanism is directly related to the hermeticity of the titanium feedthrough.

2. Due to a lower CLTE of the sealing material in respect to titanium and platinum, known to have a similar CLTE to titanium, the seal is in compression to some degree. The compression mechanism augments the diffusion mechanism to provide hermetic reliability.

3. Thermal stress tests were found to be useful in design optimization as well as an indicator of consistent or inconsistent performance of a titanium feedthrough on a continuum.

4. *In vitro* testing of titanium feedthroughs, although dramatized with the exclusion of epoxy encapsulation, has shown that the incorporation of additional electrical leakage path of ceramic standoff resisted direct contact of moisture (deionized water) of a much higher conductivity than moisture seepage through an epoxy covering found *in vivo* environments. In the case of epoxy covers splitting or delaminating completely, thus allowing direct saline solution contact with the titanium feedthrough, accelerated battery depletion of the CPG is almost certain.

5. To avoid potential mechanical and corrosion degradation of titanium, temperature exposure during the sealing process should be as low as possible to minimize grain growth.

ACKNOWLEDGEMENTS

I wish to thank James C. Kyle and Carol A. Kyle for their financial support of the project and D. F. Cook for the initial source of stimulation. I also acknowledge the cooperation of J. H. McMullin and N. M. Hodgkin who have contributed to the general development of the project.

REFERENCES

1. H. A. Schrafft, *Reliability Technology for Cardiac Pacemakers III,* NBS Special Publication 400–50, National Bureau of Standards, Gaithersburg, MD (June 1979).
2. F. L. La Que and H. R. Copson, *Corrosion Resistance of Metals and Alloys,* Reinhold, New York, Chapter 23, p. 648 (1963).
3. KRYOFLEX™, U.S. Patent No. 1,114,452.
4. D. J. Debney,. *Cardiac Pacemaker Encapsulation Investigation,* Biomedical Engineering (Oct. 1971).

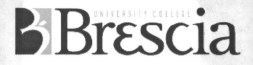

Inside the Mosaic

Edited by Eric Fong

UNIVERSITY OF TORONTO PRESS
Toronto Buffalo London

© University of Toronto Press Incorporated 2006
Toronto Buffalo London
Printed in Canada

ISBN-13: 978-0-8020-8834-5
ISBN-10: 0-8020-8834-1

Printed on acid-free paper

Library and Archives Canada Cataloguing in Publication

Inside the mosaic / edited by Eric Fong.

ISBN-13: 978-0-8020-8834-5
ISBN-10: 0-8020-8834-1

1. Immigrants – Ontario – Toronto – Social conditions.
2. Immigrants – Cultural assimilation – Ontario – Toronto.   3. Toronto
(Ont.) – Emigration and immigration – Social aspects.   4. Toronto
(Ont.) – Social conditions.   5. Multiculturalism – Ontario – Toronto.
I. Fong, Eric

FC3097.9.A1I57 2006   305.9'06912'09713541   C2005-905868-4

University of Toronto Press acknowledges the financial assistance
to its publishing program of the Canada Council for the Arts and the
Ontario Arts Council.

University of Toronto Press acknowledges the financial support for
its publishing activities of the Government of Canada through the
Book Publishing Industry Development Program (BPIDP).

Contents

Acknowledgments

The editor and contributors are grateful for the generous financial support for the publication of this book from the Department of Sociology, the Robert F. Harney Ethnic, Immigration and Pluralism Studies program, and the S.D. Clark Chair of Sociology at the University of Toronto.

INSIDE THE MOSAIC

1 Introduction: Immigration, Social Structures, and Social Processes

ERIC FONG

How is recent immigration shaping the structures and processes inside the Canadian mosaic? This is the major question addressed in this volume. Most people agree that major Canadian cities have become more diversified racially and ethnically – mainly the result of a large influx of immigrants. Although high levels of immigration are not uncommon in Canadian history, the recent wave is unique because of the disproportional representation of immigrants from non-European countries. This new immigration wave has brought both quantitative and qualitative changes to major Canadian cities. In quantitative terms, proportions of various racial and ethnic groups have grown considerably. In qualitative terms, growing diversity has transformed group relations within the mosaic. These changes are challenging researchers to explain the relationship between immigration and social structures and processes in Canadian cities today. In particular, they are challenging our understanding of racial and ethnic relations in Canadian society as presented in *The Vertical Mosaic* (Porter 1965), a book published forty years ago that has guided discussions of Canadian racial and ethnic relations ever since. Yet Porter's book was never intended to explore group relations in the context of high levels of racial and ethnic diversity in major Canadian cities half a century later.

Toronto vividly reflects changes in the Canadian mosaic. It is the most popular destination for Canadian immigrants and has experienced the most rapid population growth of all Canadian metropolitan areas, largely because of the increase in immigration. Because of this growing proportion of recent immigrants, Toronto provides an ideal location for the study of immigration and the exploration of the relationship between immigration and social structures and processes in modern Canadian cities. Although this book focuses on Toronto, the issues addressed herein do not arise only in that city. Toronto's experience is reflected in other Canadian cities, which are also growing in diversity in the new millennium.

Immigration in Canada and Toronto

Canada is one of the major immigrant-receiving countries, and immigrants are a large component of the Canadian population. Immigrants consituted 18 per cent of the Canadian population in 1941 (Li 2003), 16 per cent in 1960, and about 18 per cent in 2001 (Statistics Canada 2003a). Although the percentage of immigrants in Canada has remained fairly steady, the actual numbers of immigrants have increased over the years. The immigrant population was about 2,018,847 in 1941, 2,844,263 in 1961, and 4,342,890 in 1991. Between 1991 and 2001, close to two million immigrants came to Canada (Li 2003; Statistics Canada 2003a). Given these numbers, it is not surprising that immigration has become a major topic of public discussion.

Furthermore, the composition of the immigrant population in Canada has changed dramatically over the past two decades, mainly in response to changes in Canadian immigration policies. At the beginning of the twentieth century, immigration policies focused primarily on maintaining the existing ethnic composition. Most immigrants were of British or northern or western European origin. For instance, in 1921 about 44,000 immigrants of British origin constituted 48 per cent of total immigration (McVey and Kalbach 1995). Blacks and Asians were a very small proportion of the immigrant population throughout these years.

In 1976 changes in the Immigration Act placed more emphasis on market demand, and this has significantly altered the composition of the Canadian population over the past three decades (Dirks 1995). Between 1968 and 1974, 70 to 75 per cent of immigrants to Canada were in the categories of 'independent' or 'assisted relatives' (Reitz 1998). These immigrants entered Canada under the point system, which emphasized skills and market demand. For each applicant, occupational demand, occupational skills, an existing job offer, and educational level accounted for up to 55 of 100 points (Hawkins 1989). Some researchers contend that this strong bias towards skills has prevented a decline in immigrants' skill levels of the sort the United States is experiencing (Borjas 1999). However, it has also been argued that the point system does not guarantee that highly skilled immigrants will be selected, because too much leeway is given to immigration officers' subjective opinions (Reitz 1998).

After the introduction of the point system, new immigration was no longer dominated by Europeans. Greater numbers of immigrants came from Africa, Asia, and the Caribbean (Badets and Chui 1994). In 2001, immigrants from African countries constituted 5.2 per cent of the total immigration population in Canada; 11.0 per cent were from the Caribbean and Central and South America; and 36.5 per cent were from Asian countries (Statistics Canada 2003a). Most new immigrants are highly educated; only about 15 per cent of those admitted between 1999 and 2001 had fewer than nine years of education (Citizenship and Immigration 2002). About 38 per cent of immigrants admitted to Canada between 1999 and 2001 had earned a college degree or higher, and 44 per cent knew English and/or French (Citizenship and Immigration 2002).

Immigrants have not settled evenly throughout Canada. Most have settled in large cities, and Toronto is one of the preferred destinations. In 2001 about 39 per cent of all immigrants in urban Canada lived in Toronto, where they constituted 44 per cent of the total population of that city (Statistics Canada 2003a). That percentage is far higher than in other large cities in North America, such as Los Angeles (31 per cent in 2000) and New York (24 per cent) (Statistics Canada 2003a). The impact of immigrants on the ethnic and racial composition of Canada – especially in the large cities, where most immigrants choose to reside – is substantial. In 1971 the black population in Toronto was less than 1 per cent and the Asian population was about 3 per cent (Lemon 1985).[1] By 2001 about 7 per cent of Torontonians were black, and 24 per cent were Asian[2] (Statistics Canada 2003b).

Overview of the Volume

In the following sections I highlight the major findings of this volume. First I discuss the main findings of each chapter. Then I relate those findings to the relationship between immigration and social structures and processes. Finally, I suggest directions for further study.

With two exceptions, all of the chapters were written by researchers at the University of Toronto. One of the two exceptions is a scholar who was invited to contribute a chapter during a visiting year there. The close proximity of these researchers has allowed for constant dialogue and debate. Each chapter reflects different ideas and an ongoing dialogue about immigration and race and ethnic relations. Although each chapter can be read independently, the various topics are related.

Before the discussion of the chapters, a few terms should be clarified. The City of Toronto includes six 'regions': East York, Etobicoke, North York, Scarborough, Toronto, and York. These were separate municipalities before they were amalgamated in 1998. Toronto Census Metropolitan Area (CMA) is a term used by Statistics Canada and includes the City of Toronto and twenty-three other municipalities around the city, which are all socially and economically integrated. Also, the Greater Toronto Area (GTA) includes the City of Toronto and the surrounding regions of Durham, York, Peel, and Halton. In most of the discussion, when census data are used, Toronto will refer to the Toronto CMA.

Urban Structures/Processes and Immigration

Individuals and families come to Canada to attain their dreams and to achieve better lives. However, the urban structures and processes in the new society provide both opportunities and constraints. Gradually, the immigrants adjust their behaviour. While doing so, they do not realize that they are contributing to social forces that are altering existing urban structures and processes. In the next four chapters of the book, these complex relationships will be explored.

In chapter 2, Jeffrey Reitz and Janet Lum focus on race and ethnic relations with regard to immigration in contemporary Toronto. Despite the rapidly increasing diversity in that city, relations among racial and ethnic groups remain calm. They suggest that these dynamics show how the immigration adaptation processes are shaped by existing institutions and structures. The authors argue that this relative calm is not due to multiculturalism policies or immigrant selection policies, but rather to the delayed expansion of postsecondary education in Canada. Immigrants with limited education competed successfully in the labour market during the postwar years because their educational levels were not so different from those of native-born Canadians. However, Reitz and Lum point out that this advantage for immigrants has been diminished in recent decades by a drastic increase in postsecondary education in Canada.

In Chapter 3, Eric Fong examines the racial and ethnic residential patterns of visible minority groups in Toronto. He focuses on visible minorities because they have been the fastest-growing immigrant groups in Toronto in recent decades. His research is an attempt to capture the complexity of multiethnic group contexts by comparing the residential segregation patterns of visible minority groups with those of old and new European immigrant groups. The results suggest that although the residential segregation of visible minorities lessens as their socio-economic resources increase, at the same time their integration is strongly hampered by their social distance from other groups. Among the various visible minority groups, this is especially true for South Asians and blacks.

Although most earlier studies of the relationship between immigration and urban spatial structures focused heavily on the demand side (that is, the socio-economic and demographic backgrounds of immigrants), some more recent studies have argued for the importance of the supply side (Light 2002) – that residential mobility is also affected by property values and housing availability set by government through zoning (Logan and Molotch 1987). William Michelson in chapter 4 analyses residential patterns with respect to the role of government. He shows that all groups – including immigrant groups – experience similar levels of suburbanization and that all have low levels of residential concentration. To explain this pattern, Michelson emphasizes political processes. Using time series data, he argues that the development of a metropolitan government to oversee the growth of Toronto has been critical to obtaining equal levels of suburbanization and relatively low levels of residential concentration among groups, even though the city has experienced increased racial and ethnic diversity due to immigration.

Immigration is related not only to urban social patterns, but also to physical contexts. A change in population density or the introduction of a new population is associated with a change in the physical environment of existing groups. In chapter 5, John Veugelers explores the impact of immigration on the physical environment of the city – specifically, biodiversity and the quality of air, soil, and water. Few studies have explored this important topic. Contrary to the arguments of right-wing extremists who claim that immigration causes environmental degradation, Veugelers argues that immigration is just one of many factors that affect the environment.

Groups' Structures and Processes

One of the most widely discussed issues in immigration literature is the relationship between integration and immigrant groups' structures and processes. The integration process, whereby immigrants learn about and adapt to the new country, is multifaceted. It encompasses every-thing from shifts in individual values to transformations of immigrant family structures. This process is not always smooth (Zhou 1997). As immigrants adapt themselves to the wider society, disorganization within the immigrant group may occur.

Chapters 6 and 7 explore the relationship between integration and group structures, with the focus on immigrant family dynamics. For chapter 6, Nancy Howell interviewed immigrant families of Jews, Ital-ians, Caribbeans, Ghanaians, and Sri Lankans in Toronto. She examines how the social structures of the host society shape immigrant family structures and dynamics. Her research is based on detailed case studies of six recent immigrant groups. It points to both commonalities and differences among groups. Existing social structures, such as the legal and educational systems, affect traditional couple and parent–child relationships in immigrant families. As immigrant family structures are modified, family-related problems can be exacerbated.

In chapter 7, Joe Darden observes that Caribbean family structures have been shaped strongly by immigration policies. His work suggests that any study of the relationship between integration and the social structures of immigrant groups should consider the effects of govern-ment policies. Here he is echoing findings by Portes and Rambaut (2001). Using census data, Darden shows that a high proportion of black Caribbean families are headed by women. This is largely the consequence of immigration policies relating to Caribbean immigrants. His study highlights the crucial influence of contextual factors – espe-cially government policies – that affect the family structures of immi-grant groups. His findings point out that changes in immigrant families are not simply the consequences of accommodating the norms and values of the new society.

Group Differences in Integration Processes

The literature of group differences in integration processes has taken two major directions. The first stream considers the social structures and processes that emerge from the various adaptation stages of im-migrant groups. The second explores group differences in resource utilization.

In chapter 8, Jacinth Tracy and Blair Wheaton illustrate an important stream of research: newly emerging processes that reflect differences in adaptation stages among immigrant groups. They explore the mental health of immigrants with that of the native-born population. They show that the mental health of immigrant groups is better than that of the native-born population. The difference can be related to the institutional structures of immigration policies and to structural changes in society arising from immigration. Because of immigration policies, immigrants are a highly select group, and they are prepared to persevere through hardships in order to adjust to the new environment. By contrast, the native-born population faces increased competition in various aspects of life because of the structural changes arising from massive immigration.

As suggested by Alba and Nee (2003), ethnic networks are important resources in the adaptation process. In chapter 9, Emi Ooka and Barry Wellman extend the understanding of the role of ethnic networks by considering the socio-economic resources of various immigrant groups. Building on the work of Granovetter (1973), they show how groups utilize existing ethnic relations to overcome possible limitations. Their study is based on data collected in Toronto in the early 1980s, when that city was beginning to transform itself into a multiethnic city as a consequence of changes in Canadian immigration policies. They explore factors that affect ethnic members' use of interethnic and intra-ethnic ties to obtain job information as well as the consequences of those factors. The benefits of ethnic ties in job searches are related to ethnic resources. Interethnic ties with groups of high economic status are more likely to help members of groups with few economic resources obtain jobs. Interethnic ties with groups with low economic status do not help members of groups with high economic resources. Job searches through intra-ethnic ties are associated with higher incomes for those from high-status groups. This demonstrates that immigrants use existing social processes to overcome barriers in the integration process.

In the book's final chapter, Janet Salaff uses in-depth interviews to explore how the socio-economic backgrounds of immigrants shape their use of ethnic networks. She focuses on the role of intra-ethnic resources in helping immigrants find jobs. In her interviews with immigrants from three areas of the Pacific Rim (China, Hong Kong, and Taiwan), she found that middle-class immigrants were most likely to use their own ethnic resources to find jobs. Immigrants from areas with labour market structures similar to those in the West are more likely to retain their social networks at home and to maintain the option of returning if immigration does not work out as expected. Immigrants from areas with labour market structures different from those of the West are less likely to maintain networks back home; they are also less likely to return home if the immigration adjustment does not succeed. Salaff's study indicates that immigrants' adjustment processes in the labour market can be shaped by their own ethnic resources.

Concluding Thoughts

These studies suggest that the relationship between immigration and social structures and processes is multifaceted. Collectively, they argue that studies of cities with high immigrant populations should pay closer attention to immigrant adaptation processes. Three possible relationships must considered. The first is the one between urban structures and group adaptation. The second is the one between groups' internal structures and social processes arising from adaptation. Third and finally, there are differences in integration processes among groups. Collectively, all the studies in this volume demonstrate that the relationship between immigration and social structures and processes should be explored at three levels: individual, group, and city. Without doubt, these studies have painted a complex and 'colourful' picture of the relationship between immigration and social structures and processes.

It is not a new observation to say that the relationship between immigration and social structures and processes is multifaceted and multilevel. But, it is important to realize that the relationships become more complex as immigrant groups become more diverse racially. The relationship of immigration to social structures and processes is intertwined with race and ethnic relations. Together, these chapters forcefully demonstrate the reality.

Also, most of the chapters offer overwhelming evidence that the integration of new immigrant groups into today's Canadian mosaic is more complicated than has long been described in the literature. These integration patterns sometimes seem to follow the path of earlier immigrant generations suggested in the literature, especially by assimilation perspectives. Fong's chapter shows clearly that the residential patterns of visible minority groups are related to socio-economic resources and to duration in the country, as documented in the literature. Howell's chapter comes to a similar conclusion: these new immigrant groups, like past immigrant generations, adapt their family dynamics and structures to the wider society. Immigrant groups still utilize ethnic networks to smooth the adaptation process, as reported by Ooka and Wellman.

Yet often, the findings suggest paths of integration that diverge from those found in the literature. Some contributors highlight 'unexpected' patterns of immigrant adaptation. For example, Reitz and Lum show that the job attainments of recent immigrants do not gradually catch up with those of average Canadians over time. This marks a departure from the experiences of previous immigrant generations. To go one step further, Tracey and Wheaton point out that assimilation does not always benefit immigrants.

Although some studies indicate that integration does not necessarily follow the processes described in the literature, this does not amount to a call for us to immediately abandon previous models, which still have some validity. More studies are needed in order for us to identify factors that result in different integration paths. Some studies, such as those on segmented assimilation, have proposed a 'revised version' of the assimilation perspective; most of these proposals, however, are in response to the unique American urban context and the recent American immigrant population. How well these suggestions apply to Canada's new immigration wave in the urban context remains to be seen.

Some Challenges

Given the findings about the relationship of immigration to social structures and processes in this volume, what is the next step for research? Without doubt, the studies in this book raise some important issues. First, they point out the importance of individual characteristics, group resources, and urban contexts in shaping the integration processes of immigrants. Further studies will be required to link these three factors. Specifically, it is important to learn precisely how these factors interact with one another to produce different paths of integration. This will not be an easy task because a considerable number of paths can be produced from the interactions of various factors at these three different levels. But having succeeded, we will have produced a detailed picture of the integration patterns of immigrants. Although some work has been done in this area, there is still a need for detailed theorizing about the relations of various possible factors at these three levels. Such discussion will provide a larger and more comprehensive framework for understanding the complexity of immigrant adaptation.

Second, partly related to the first suggestion, these studies indicate that more specific discussion is required on how various city context factors affect integration. Although in recent years a number of theories have pointed to the significance of city context factors, such as government policies and labour markets, the discussion has been relatively general (Portes & Rumbaut 1996). For example, government policies can be related to various aspects of society, such as immigration, housing, and education. Without a clearer and more elaborate delineation of contextual factors and a detailed discussion of how these are related to immigrant adaptation, our understanding of the topic will still be limited.

Finally, the chapters highlight that social structures and processes are interrelated with the adaptation processes of immigrants. In other words, social structures and processes shape the adaptation process, and at the same time the adaptation process modifies existing structures and processes. Furthermore, this two-way process changes over time. However, most studies of the relationship are cross-sectional and focus on a single directional effect. Future studies should explore the dual dynamic across time.

Although these studies explore some theoretical issues and provide empirical findings related to immigration and social structures and processes, they also have important policy implications. Further studies should explore how these findings can be related to public policies. For example, what is the government role in immigrant settlement patterns? What policies should be developed so that groups with limited resources will be able to overcome their socio-economic limitations through social networks? How should policies be implemented so that social support is provided to alleviate the difficulties of immigrant families as they adapt to the new environment?

Any attempt to address the relationship between social structures and processes and immigration in this new century soon reveals that the reality is far more complicated than the theoretical discourse suggests. Drawing from the data collected in Toronto, which has the highest proportion of immigrants of any Canadian city, the results clearly and strongly recommend a hard evaluation and a careful rethinking of the theoretical frameworks for encompassing this complexity. Consequently, the study of Toronto with respect to immigration is important and timely.

This book provides diverse analyses of how immigration is related to social structures and processes. It is just a start. It covers only some of the many issues of race and ethnic relations with respect to immigration in Toronto. I hope it will attract the attention of researchers to the diverse and increasingly complex dynamics of this very important topic.

NOTES

1 In Lemon, blacks referred to people of African origin; Asians included only Chinese and Japanese.
2 In the Statistics Canada data, blacks include those individuals reporting Caribbean and African origins. Asians include respondents of Chinese, Filipino, Korean, Japanese, South Asian, and Southeast Asian origin.

REFERENCES

Alba, Richard, and Victor Nee. 2003. *Remaking the American Mainstream: Assimilation and Contemporary Immigration.* Cambridge: Harvard University Press.
Badets, Jane, and Tina W.L. Chui. 1994. *Canada's Changing Immigrant Population.* Ottawa and Scarborough: Statistics Canada and Prentice Hall.
Borjas, George J. 1999. *Heaven's Door: Immigration Policy and the American Economy.* Princeton, NJ: Princeton University Press.
Citizenship and Immigration Canada. 2002. *Facts and Figures 2001: Immigration Overview.* www.cic.gc.ca/english/pub/facts2001/1imm-06.html.
Dirks, Gerald. 1995. *Controversy and Complexity: Canadian Immigration Policy during the 1980s.* Montreal: McGill-Queen's University Press.
Gibson, Campbell J., and Emily Lennon. 1999. *Historical Census Statistics on the Foreign-born Population of the United States.* Washington, DC: US. Bureau of Census. www.census.gov/population/www/censusdata/hiscendata.html.
Granovetter, Mark S. 1973. 'The Strength of Weak Ties.' *American Journal of Sociology* 78:105–30.
Hawkins, Freda. 1989. *Critical Years in Immigration: Canada and Australia Compared.* Kingston and Montreal: McGill-Queen's University Press.
Lemon, James. 1985. *Toronto since 1918.* Toronto: James Lorimer and National Museum of Man, National Museums of Canada.
Li, Peter. 2003. *Destination Canada: Immigration Debates and Issues.* Toronto: Oxford University Press.
Light, Ivan. 2002. 'Immigrant Place Entrepreneurs in Los Angeles, 1970–1999.' *International Journal of Urban and Regional Research* 26:215–28.

Logan, John R., and Harvey L. Molotch. 1987. *Urban Fortunes: The Political Economy of Place*. Berkeley: University of California Press.

Lollock, L. 2001. *The Foreign-Born Population in the United States: Population Characteristics*. January (Current Population Report No. P20-534). Washington, DC: U.S. Census Bureau.

McVey, Wayne W., Jr., and Warren E. Kalbach. 1995. *Canadian Population*. Scarborough, ON: Nelson Canada.

Porter, John. 1965. *The Vertical Mosaic: An Analysis of Social Class and Power in Canada*. Toronto: University of Toronto Press.

Portes, Alejandro, and Ruben G. Rumbaut. 2001. *Legacies: The Story of the Immigrant Second Generation*. Berkeley: University of California Press.

– 1996. *Immigrant America: A portrait*. Berkeley: University of California Press.

Reitz, Jeffrey. 1998. *Warmth of the Welcome: The Social Causes of Economic Success for Immigrants in Different Nations and Cities*. Boulder, CO: Westview Press.

Rumbaut, Ruben G. 1997. 'Assimilation and Its Discontents: Between Rhetoric and Reality.' *International Migration Review* 31(4):923–60.

Statistics Canada. 2003a. *Canada's Ethnocultural Portrait: The Changing Mosaic* (2001 Census: Analysis Series). Ottawa: Ministry of Industry.

Statistics Canada. 2003b. 2001 Profile Series: Citizenship, immigration, birthplace, generation status, ethnic origin, visible minorities and aboriginal peoples (95f0489xcb01005). Canada Census.

Zhou, Min. 1997. 'Segmented Assimilation: Issues, Controversies, and Recent Research on the New Second Generation.' *International Migration Review* 31(4):825–58.

JEFFREY G. REITZ AND JANET M. LUM

One of Toronto's most striking characteristics today is the great ethnic diversity of its population. And because of Canada's aggressively expansionist immigration policy, this diversity keeps increasing. No longer the staid and inward-looking British enclave – Northrop Frye called it 'a good place for minding your own business' – Toronto is now Canada's largest metropolis and one of the North America's most heterogeneous cities. Toronto's population had passed 4.6 million by 2001, making it larger than all but ten American urban centres, and is now 44 per cent foreign-born – more than New York, Los Angeles, or San Francisco. Many of these foreign-born are European immigrants, who arrived in large numbers in the 1950s and 1960s, but most recent immigrants are of Asian, African, or Latin American origin. The founding British-origin population has been reduced to the status of one minority among many.

On the surface, intergroup relations in Toronto seem fairly positive. As the composition of the population has shifted from predominantly European to increasingly multiracial, local commentary on intergroup relations has shifted from a focus on cultural diversity to greater concern with equity and discrimination (Municipality of Metropolitan Toronto 1993). Yet although intergroup tensions have surfaced from time to time, the most publicly visible local discourse on race and ethnic relations emphasizes harmony and accommodation. There has even been a tendency to celebrate Toronto as a model for others. Thus, a June 1996 *National Geographic* article heralded ethnic diversity as Toronto's major attraction: 'With its sizzling cultural mix and a stylish new personality, this once bland metropolis breaks into the urban major leagues' (Conniff 1996, 121). *Fortune* magazine, in a comparative index evaluating the 'workability' and 'livability' of cities outside the United States, ranked Toronto first (followed by London, Singapore, Paris, and Hong

Kong), citing its 'safety' and 'nearly 2000 ethnic restaurants' (Precourt and Faircloth 1996, 145). Relatively positive attitudes towards immigration in Toronto are reflected in opinion polls as well. Canadians in general are more favourable to immigration than Americans, Britons, or Australians (Simon and Lynch, 1999, 416), despite proportionally higher immigration, and attitudes in immigrant-intensive Toronto are little different (Reitz 2004). From a comparative perspective, it appears that Torontonians by and large have accepted massive immigration and rapid population change with considerable equanimity.

How accurate is this generally positive assessment of race relations in Toronto? What are the underlying reasons for the differences between Toronto and other cities? What are the prospects for the future? Answers to these questions are critical to an assessment of the impact of massive immigration on social structures and processes in the metropolitan Toronto region. Experience in race relations suggests that the gap between perceptions and reality may be quite wide. Racial tensions may surface slowly, in a variety of scenarios (Reitz 1988). The following discussion identifies some issues arising in the analysis of race relations in Toronto from a comparative perspective. After briefly describing immigration and settlement, we suggest that understanding emerging race relations in Toronto requires attention to two sets of social forces. One is the extent of *opportunity for successful participation by minority groups within a range of institutions,* including economic, political, social, and cultural institutions. Is Toronto different from other North American cities regarding minority-group inclusiveness? A second set of forces is created by *rapid change in the structures of these institutions* themselves. Increased ethnic and racial diversity in Toronto has occurred during a time of rapid institutional change. New economic structures have arisen in the context of national and international trade liberalization. Governments have implemented changes in education, health, and social services, and metropolitan government itself has been restructured through the amalgamation of local municipalities into a new 'megacity.' There have been related changes in the media and in community organization. What is the impact that these institutional changes have had, or are having, on changing race relations in Toronto?

Multiracial Immigration and Settlement in Toronto

Expansionist immigration has been transforming Toronto for many decades. In the years just after the Second World War, huge numbers of Italians, Poles, Greeks, Hungarians, and others swelled the population.

When immigration policies changed in the 1960s to eliminate the preference for Europeans, Canada continued its expansionist policies, making it a leader among Western industrial nations in overall population growth. The impact on Toronto has been dramatic because nearly half of all immigrants to Canada settle in Toronto.[1] About 70 per cent of these more recent immigrants have come from Asia, the Caribbean, Central and South America, and Africa. Toronto is now home to more than one hundred different ethno-racial groups (see the historical overview by Troper 2003).

The changing face of Toronto, a result of immigration between 1971 and 2001, can be seen in the census data reported in Table 2.1, covering the Toronto metropolitan area (Census Metropolitan Area, CMA).[2] This includes the City of Toronto (formerly the Municipality of Metropolitan Toronto, comprising six constituent municipalities, the largest of which were the old city of Toronto, North York, Etobicoke, and Scarborough) and surrounding suburban areas such as Mississauga in the west, Richmond Hill in the north, and Pickering–Ajax to the east. In 1971, of 2.6 million Torontonians, over 95 per cent gave their ethnic origin as either British or other European. Over the ensuing thirty years, as the overall population grew by 77 per cent to 4.6 million, the proportion of Asian origin increased from 2.6 to 24.6 per cent. By 2001 the Chinese, with 8.2 per cent of Toronto's population, and the South Asians, with 9.0 per cent, both had displaced the Italians as the largest groups after the British. Over the same thirty years, Torontonians of African or Caribbean origin increased from 1.1 per cent of the population to 6.8 per cent. In contrast, those naming British as their ethnic origin declined from a majority to a minority. Those naming another European origin (single origin only) declined from 34.9 to 21.9 per cent. Most of these groups did not decline in absolute numbers, only in relative terms. The growth of new groups reduced the relative size of the older groups.

These 'ethnic origins' data provide a rough indication of the racial composition of the population, but there are significant ambiguities. These include the increased tendency to identify with a 'Canadian' ancestry and the growing prevalence of multiple-origins categories.

Racial groups in Toronto can be identified more directly since the 1996 census data, using a new 'race' question asked for the first time that year.[3] Table 2.2 shows how Torontonians responded in 1996 to this question, overall and within each of the various ethnic-origins groups. A substantial majority across the Toronto metropolitan area – 68 per cent – described themselves as 'white.' This included the great majority

Table 2.1. Population of Toronto (CMA) by ethnic origins, 1971–2001

Ethnic origins	1971* Population	%	1981* Population	%	1986 Population	%	1991 Population	%	1996 Population	%	2001 Population	%
Canadian (Sing. & Mult.)	–	–	–	–	–	–	430,196	11.1	707,868	16.7	1,449,246	31.2
British	1,495,355	56.9	1,390,005	46.7	1,311,100	38.6	1,024,690	26.5	694,908	16.4	385,160	8.3
French	91,935	3.5	74,800	2.5	66,100	1.9	52,399	1.4	34,668	0.8	26,472	0.6
British & French	–	–	44,425	1.5	115,600	3.4	87,266	2.3	66,924	1.6	–	–
British & other	–	–	109,825	3.7	304,100	8.9	323,530	8.4	275,544	6.5	–	–
French & other	–	–	8,830	0.3	26,350	0.8	29,333	0.8	26,496	0.6	–	–
British, French & other	–	–	11,175	0.4	60,650	1.8	63,299	1.6	42,444	1.0	–	–
British or French (sing. & mult.)	1,587,290	60.4	1,639,060	55.1	1,883,900	55.4	1,580,518	40.9	1,140,984	27.0	411,632	8.9
Dutch	44,500	1.7	34,220	1.2	31,750	0.9	30,500	0.8	28,224	0.7	27,204	0.6
German	116,610	4.4	82,930	2.8	71,300	2.1	68,766	1.8	54,576	1.3	50,732	1.1
Scandinavian	18,310	0.7	12,310	0.4	9,550	0.3	9,167	0.2	7,128	0.2	–	–
Hungarian	23,345	0.9	22,685	0.8	22,150	0.7	24,666	0.6	20,412	0.5	19,627	0.4
Polish	51,210	1.9	47,690	1.6	51,800	1.5	73,999	1.9	79,776	1.9	80,593	1.7
Ukranian	60,705	2.3	50,705	1.7	45,650	1.3	42,566	1.1	38,628	0.9	41,649	0.9
Croatian, Serbian, etc. (Balkan)	–	–	–	–	38,400	1.1	51,833	1.3	67,212	1.6	75,976	1.6
Greek	51,470	2.0	65,025	2.2	62,800	1.8	64,166	1.7	62,712	1.5	63,138	1.4
Italian	271,775	10.3	297,205	10.0	295,500	8.7	309,997	8.0	312,012	7.4	314,804	6.8
Portuguese	43,640	1.7	88,885	3.0	96,650	2.8	124,399	3.2	127,620	3.0	132,784	2.9
Spanish	6,495	0.2	20,060	0.7	–	0.0	33,400	0.9	26,352	0.6	–	–
Jewish	109,865	4.2	109,240	3.7	109,850	3.2	115,299	3.0	98,388	2.3	95,735	2.1
Other European	118,780	4.5	115,730	3.9	98,200	2.9	69,366	1.8	69,696	1.6	117,151	2.5
European (sing.)	916,705	34.9	946,685	31.8	933,600	27.5	1,018,123	26.4	992,736	23.5	1,019,395	21.9

Table 2.1. (concluded)

Ethnic origins	1971* Population	%	1981* Population	%	1986 Population	%	1991 Population	%	1996 Population	%	2001 Population	%
West Asian & Arab	–	–	–	–	29,600	0.9	61,799	1.6	81,504	1.9	124,857	1.7
South Asian	14,545	0.6	69,725	2.3	106,200	3.1	190,031	4.9	280,332	6.6	419,225	9.0
Chinese	26,355	1.0	89,590	3.0	126,750	3.7	222,298	5.8	321,732	7.6	381,559	8.2
Filipino	–	–	–	–	36,850	1.1	66,566	1.7	87,840	2.1	116,844	2.5
Vietnamese	–	–	–	–	–	–	22,033	0.6	35,460	0.8	34,672	0.7
Other East & Southeast Asian	–	–	–	–	42,150	1.2	42,266	1.1	50,112	1.2	65,277	1.4
Other Asian	27,870	1.1	62,555	2.1	–	–	–	–	–	–	–	–
Asian (sing.)	68,770	2.6	221,870	7.5	341,550	10.0	604,994	15.7	856,980	20.2	1,142,434	24.6
African	–	–	–	–	–	–	–	–	68,256	1.6	84,020	1.8
Caribbean	–	–	–	–	–	–	–	–	168,948	4.0	185,092	4.0
African & Carib. (sing.)	27,965	1.1	78,445	2.6	116,750	3.4	178,798	4.6	237,204	5.6	269,112	6.8
Latin, Central & South Am. (sing.)	–	–	–	–	–	–	24,600	0.6	38,556	0.9	46,929	1.0
Other (sing. or mult.)*	20,660	0.8	78,080	2.6	117,750	3.5	17,066	0.4	252,756	6.0	299,621	6.4
Native & Inuit (sing.)	6,935	0.3	11,380	0.4	6,050	0.2	5,867	0.2	5,724	0.1	9,439	0.2
Total	2,628,325	100.0	2,975,495	100.0	3,399,600	100.0	3,861,695	100.0	4,232,880	100.0	4,647,809	100.0

Sources: Statistics Canada 1971 and 1981 census data are as reported by Kalbach (1990, 18); 1986, 1991, 1996, and 2001 census data are based on public use samples.

*In 1971 and 1981 data, the category 'Other' includes Syrian/Lebanese.

Table 2.2. Population of Toronto (CMA) by ethnic origins and race, 1996

Ethnic Origins	White Count	White % Row	White Col.	Chinese Count	Chinese % Row	Chinese Col.	South Asian Count	South Asian Row	South Asian Col.	Black Count	Black Row	Black Col.	Other Visible Minority Count	Other Visible Minority Row	Other Visible Minority Col.	N/A (incl. aboriginal) Count	N/A Row	N/A Col.	Table Total Count	Table Total Col.
Canadian	293,292	94.2	10.2	1,116	0.4	0.3	2,376	0.8	0.7	10,188	3.3	3.7	3,276	1.1	0.8	1,116	0.4	6.7	311,364	7.4
Canadian & Br. or Fr. (& other)[a]	300,456	97.0	10.4	828	0.3	0.2	648	0.2	0.2	3,708	1.2	1.3	2,304	0.7	0.6	1,656	0.5	9.9	309,600	7.3
Canadian and other	64,080	73.7	2.2	3,492	4.0	1.0	3,060	3.5	1.0	9,540	11.0	3.4	5,328	6.1	1.3	1,404	1.6	8.4	86,904	2.1
British	679,824	97.8	23.6	1,080	0.2	0.3	2,016	0.3	0.6	9,648	1.4	3.5	2,124	0.3	0.5	216	0.0	1.3	694,908	16.4
French	33,840	97.6	1.2				72	0.2	0.0	468	1.3	0.2	36	0.1	0.0	252	0.7	1.5	34,668	0.8
British and French	66,168	98.9	2.3	72	0.1	0.0	36	0.1	0.0	360	0.5	0.1	108	0.2	0.2	180	0.3	1.1	66,924	1.6
British & other	234,684	85.2	8.2	5,652	2.1	1.7	6,624	2.4	2.1	16,776	6.1	6.0	9,180	3.3	2.3	2,628	1.0	15.7	275,544	6.5
French & other	21,420	80.8	0.7	180	0.7	0.1	180	0.7	0.1	1,404	5.3	0.5	2,232	8.4	0.6	1,080	4.1	6.4	26,496	0.6
Brit. French & other	37,296	87.9	1.3	648	1.5	0.2	288	0.7	0.1	1,296	3.1	0.5	1,296	3.1	0.3	1,620	3.8	9.7	42,444	1.0
British or French (sing. & mult.)	1,073,232	94.1	37.3	7,632	0.7	2.4	9,216	0.8	2.9	29,952	2.6	10.8	14,976	1.3	3.7	5,976	0.5	35.7	1,140,984	27.0
Dutch	27,504	97.4	1.0	108	0.4	0.0	396	1.4	0.1	36	0.1	0.0	180	0.6	0.0	0			28,224	0.7
German	54,288	99.5	1.9				72	0.1	0.0	108	0.2	0.0	108	0.2	0.0	0			54,576	1.3
Other Western Europe	7,128	100.0	0.2				0			0			0			0			7128	0.2
Hungarian	20,376	99.8	0.7				0			36	0.2	0.0	0			0			20,412	0.5
Polish	79,632	99.8	2.8	36	0.0	0.0	0			36	0	0.0	0			72	0.1	0.4	79,776	1.9
Ukrainian	38,340	99.3	1.3				144	0.4	0.0	108	0.3	0.0	0			36	0.1	0.2	38,628	0.9
Balkan origins	67,176	99.9	2.3				0			36	0.1	0.0	0			0			67,212	1.6
Greek	62,568	99.8	2.2	36	0.1	0.0	36	0.1	0.0	36	0.1	0.0	36	0.1	0.0	0			62,712	1.5
Italian	311,040	99.7	10.8	108	0.0	0.0	108	0	0.0	216	0.1	0.1	396	0.1	0.1	144	0.0	0.9	312,012	7.4
Portuguese	125,496	98.3	4.4	36	0.0	0.0	648	0.5	0.2	324	0.3	0.1	1,116	0.9	0.3	0			127,620	3.0
Spanish	7,704	29.2	0.3				0			180	0.7	0.1	18,468	70.1	4.6	0			26,352	0.6
Jewish	97,812	99.4	3.4	36	0.0	0.0	108	0.1	0.0	108	0.1	0.0	324	0.3	0.1	0			98,388	2.3
Other European	69,408	99.6	2.4	36	0.1	0.0	72	0.1	0.0	72	0.1	0.0	108	0.2	0.0	0			69,696	1.6
European (sing.)	968,472	97.6	33.6	396	0.0	0.1	1,584	0.2	0.5	1,296	0.1	0.5	20,736	2.1	5.2	252	0.0	1.5	992,736	23.5

Table 2.2. (concluded)

Ethnic Origins	White			Chinese			South Asian			Black			Other Vis. Min.			N/A (incl. aboriginal)			Table Total	
	Count	% Row	Col	Count	Row	Col	Count	Row	Col	Count	Row	Col	Count	Row	Col	Count	Row	Col	%	Col
West Asian & Arab	18,252	22.4	0.6	216	0.3	0.1	2,448	3	0.8	216	0.3	0.1	60,372	74.1	15.0	0			81,504	1.9
South Asian	4,032	1.4	0.1	288	0.1	0.1	257,004	91.7	80.7	1,296	0.5	0.5	17,676	6.3	4.4	36	0.0	0.2	280,332	6.6
Chinese	1,440	0.4	0.1	312,948	97.3	92.3	72	0	0.0	108	0	0.0	7,164	2.2	1.8	0			321,732	7.6
Filipino	936	1.1	0.0	36	0	0.0	0			36	0	0.0	86,832	98.9	21.6	0			87,840	2.1
Other East & Southeast Asian	1,368	1.6	0.0	1,944	2.3	0.6	792	0.9	0.2	0			81,468	95.2	20.3	0			85,572	2.0
Asian (sing.)	26,028	3.0	0.9	315,432	36.8	93.0	260,316	30.4	81.7	1,656	0.2	0.6	253,512	29.6	63.1	36	0.0	0.2	856,980	20.2
African	2,592	3.8	0.1	396	0.2	0.1	684	1	0.2	63108	92.5	22.6	1872	2.7	0.5	0			68,256	1.6
Caribbean	7,200	4.3	0.3				4,932	2.9	1.5	134,892	79.8	48.4	21,528	12.7	5.4	0			168,948	4.0
African & Caribbean. (sing.)	9,792	4.1	0.3	396	0.2	0.1	5,616	2.4	1.8	198,000	83.5	71.0	23,400	9.9	5.8	0			237,204	5.6
Latin, C. & S. Am.	6,228	16.2	0.2				0			144	0.4	0.1	32184	83.5	8	0			38,556	0.9
Other single origins	2,628	85.9	0.1	0			0			288	9.4	0.1	144	4.7	0.0	0			3,060	0.1
Other mult. origins	133,308	53.4	4.6	9,720	3.9	2.9	35,676	14.3	11.2	239,04	9.6	8.6	45,684	18.3	11.4	1,404	0.6	8.4	249,696	5.9
Aboriginal origins	756	13.2	0.0	0			0			72	1.3	0.0				4,896	85.5	29.2	5,724	0.1
Total	2,878,272	68	100	339,012	8	100	318,492	7.5	100	278,748	6.6	100	401,580	9.5	100	16,776	0.4	100	4,232,880	100
(Sample data)	(79,952)			(9,417)			(8,847)			(7,743)			(11,155)			(466)			(117,580)	

aMultiple origins including 'Canadian,' plus British, French, or both, and in some cases also in combination with other origins.

Source: 1996 Public Use Microdata file, 2.8% sample; for population estimates, cases weighted by 36.0.

of those of British or French origin – over 95 per cent, although somewhat less for those with multiple origin that included British or French, among whom between 10 and 20 per cent are racial minorities – and virtually all of those of European origins (over 99 per cent for those with most single European origins, an exception being Spanish origin, among whom only 29 per cent were white). These two categories constituted about 50 per cent of Toronto's population. In addition, among the roughly 700,000 Torontonians who described themselves as 'Canadian,' the vast majority – more than 657,000, or 92 per cent – reported themselves as 'white.' Only a few self-described 'Canadians' were racial minorities. About 8 per cent of blacks in Toronto described themselves as 'Canadian' (either solely or in combination with another origin), and over 10 per cent of blacks described themselves as 'British' (either solely or in combination with other origins).

Table 2.2 also clarifies the racial composition of other ethnic groups. The size of certain specific Asian groups seems somewhat underestimated based on the single-origin 'ethnic' data alone. For example, 7.4 per cent of Torontonians described themselves as Chinese in response to the ethnic origin question, but 8.0 per cent of Torontonians described themselves as Chinese in response to the race question. For South Asians, the figures were 6.6 per cent using the ethnic origin question and 7.5 per cent based on the race question. Most of those who described themselves as of Asian ethnic origin included themselves in a non-white racial group; however, the West Asian and Arab group was a significant exception to this: 22.4 per cent described themselves as 'white.'

The population identified by African and Caribbean ethnic origins – 5.6 per cent – was somewhat less than the 6.6 per cent identified as black by the race question. That said, although the two groups were roughly the same size, the overlap was less than in the case of the Chinese or the South Asians. Regarding people of African or Caribbean origin, 83.5 per cent described themselves as black, 4.1 per cent as white, and 2.4 per cent as South Asian; the rest gave various other origins. And regarding those described as black, only 71 per cent gave a single African or Caribbean origin. At least one British origin was mentioned by 10.8 per cent, and 8.4 per cent mentioned at least one Canadian origin. Among the small Latin American group, most gave minority racial origins, but 16.2 per cent described themselves as white.

Most members of Toronto's racial minority communities were immigrants, as Figure 2.1 shows. In each case, between 80 and 100 per cent

Figure 2.1. Percentage immigrant, by ethnic origins, for Toronto (CMA), 1996

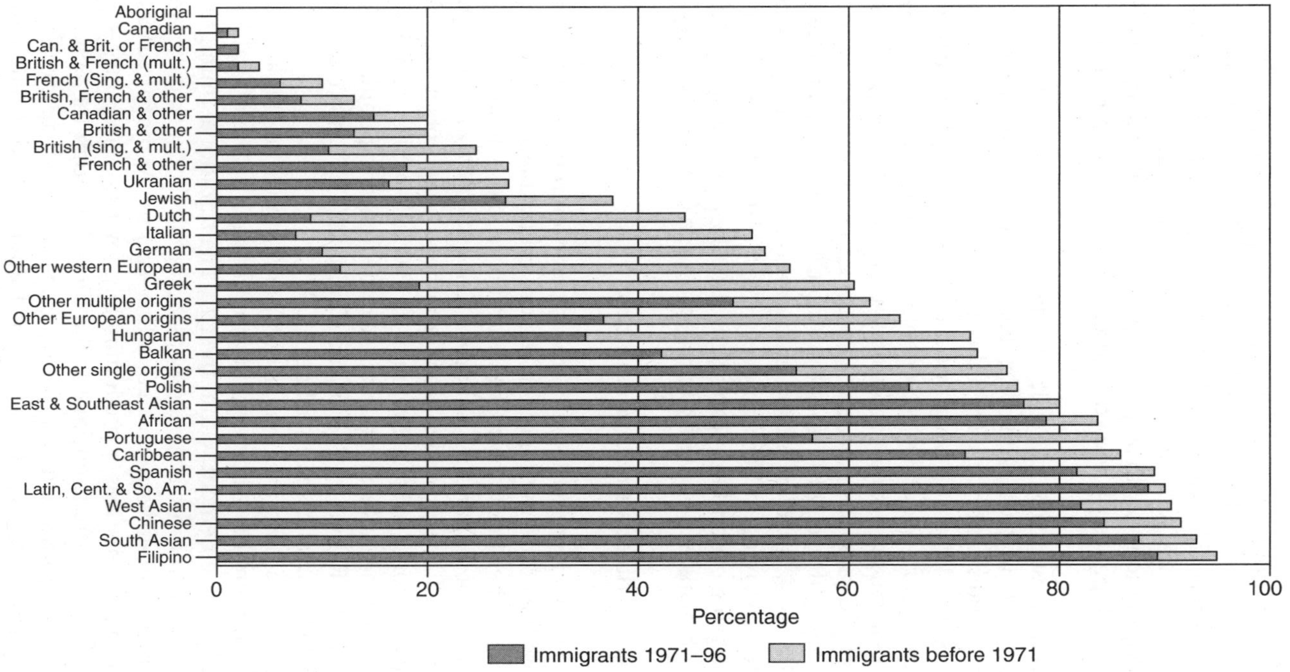

Percentage

■ Immigrants 1971–96   □ Immigrants before 1971

were immigrants. In contrast, most of those of British or French origins, and virtually all of those describing their ethnic origin as 'Canadian,' were born in Canada. Most European ethnic-origin groups fall between those extremes, with fewer immigrants among the Ukrainian and Jewish populations (20 to 30 per cent), more among Italians and Germans (nearly 50 per cent), and still more among Poles and Hungarians (60 to 80 per cent).

Toronto, with a 32 per cent 'visible minority' population in 1996, and 37 per cent in 2001, is likely to become even more racially diverse as immigration continues. The Liberal government, in power since 1993, has repeatedly promised to boost immigration to 1 per cent of population per year – about 300,000 people. Current levels of about two-thirds of 1 per cent are actually reduced somewhat from the numbers reached under the previous Conservative government of Brian Mulroney, but they are still roughly triple the American immigration rate on a per capita basis. Based on current immigration patterns, with about 100,000 persons arriving in Toronto every year, and with over 75 per cent of these being of non-European origin, it can be projected that by 2017, most Torontonians will be of non-European origin (Statistics Canada 2005, 29).

Neighbourhoods and Communities

Immigrants have settled in various neighbourhoods and communities across the entire metropolitan region. Ethnic neighbourhoods are layered together throughout the central core and extend in all directions towards the expanding suburbs. Kalbach (1990) and Bourne (2000, Section 5) have provided demographer's maps of ethnic residential concentrations (see also Breton et al. 1990, 21–31; Ley and Smith 1998). A taste of the cultural landscape can be found in popular articles such as those by Relph (1997, 100) and Caulfield (1997); more encyclopaedic coverage is available in Kashner (1997).

As the Toronto area has grown, and ethnic neighbourhoods have shifted, there have been significant changes in the overall pattern of immigrant settlement within the city. The traditional immigrant reception area in Toronto has been Kensington Market, just to the west of the central business district near Spadina Avenue. At the turn of the twentieth century this was a predominately Jewish community – Toronto's largest single ethnic enclave at the time. Although the Spadina area is still a base for the textile industry, the main Jewish district now runs up Bathurst Street towards the City of Toronto's border, where the largest synagogue in North America is located. In Kensington, the Italians and then the Portuguese and West Indians moved in, creating what is now an even more multiethnic street market; its Anglo-Saxon origins are preserved only in its street names.

Most of the larger ethnic groups have concentrations in several distinct neighbourhoods. Italians settled not only in Kensington but also along the Corso Italia on St Clair Avenue West between Bathurst and Old Weston Road, in the 'Junction Triangle' near Keele and Dundas (named after the junction of two railway lines), and in the district around Lansdowne and Davenport. Some Italians have migrated to Mississauga or north to the Toronto suburb of Woodbridge (which is now 75 per cent Italian).

Toronto also has one of the largest Chinese communities in northeastern North America, and today supports four separate Chinatowns. The original Chinatown has moved several times and now is only a few steps from Kensington. It is still expanding and has attracted Vietnamese immigrants, who have set up their distinctive restaurants and groceries alongside Chinese businesses. Substantial numbers of Hong Kong Chinese have settled in North York, Scarborough, and the northern suburbs of Richmond Hill and Markham; in these places, they have stimulated the development of large shopping malls with restaurants, grocery stores, cinemas, book and music stores, medical clinics, dentists, pharmacies, and other establishments catering to the Chinese community.

Other recent immigrants have settled in one or more downtown areas and in suburban neighbourhoods, where apartment towers provide affordable housing. Koreans are on Bloor Street west of the University of Toronto towards Bathurst. Greeks settled first along the Danforth near Pape and created what is now a lively souvlaki-house strip. Today many live in sections of Scarborough. West Indians are concentrated near St Clair West, in the Jane–Finch corridor in North York, and near Warden Avenue in Scarborough. South Asians have a busy commercial centre of curry houses and other businesses along Gerrard Street, and also in the Tuxedo Court complex at Markham and Highway 401 in Scarborough. Ethiopian and Somali groups have settled in a northwestern suburb (Relph 1997, pp. 54–64).

Specific areas of immigrant settlement reflect the economic levels typical for a particular group (Ley and Smith 1998; Halli and Kazemipur 1998), as well as social distances between racial groups (Fong, in this volume). The implications of this have changed over time as Toronto has changed. Lower-income immigrant groups have always chosen the Kensington area and other downtown communities as settlement areas. But in Toronto, as in many Canadian cities (and different from the American pattern), the oldest traditional middle- or upper-class neighbourhoods have been close to the core, and some of the most affordable housing has been located in high-rise suburbs (Goldberg and Mercer 1986). Hence, these outlying areas also have attracted many immigrant groups. This trend towards the suburbanization of immigrants intensified as older downtown neighbourhoods were gentrified (the classic case in Toronto being 'Cabbagetown,' today known for its beautifully restored Victorian townhouses).

However, over the past thirty years, most population growth has been in the new suburbs beyond North York, Etobicoke, and Scarborough. The City of Toronto population has stayed steady at about two million; meanwhile, the outlying suburban population has grown to comprise about half the current CMA total of nearly five million. These new suburbs, known locally as the '905' suburbs because of their telephone area code, have a distinct identity. The high-end housing in these outlying suburbs has attracted new immigrant settlement (such as the Hong Kong Chinese areas noted above), but much of the population is of traditional ethnic ancestry. The '905' area includes 57.4 per cent of the Toronto population of British ancestry and 63.8 per cent of those the census describes as 'Canadian,' but only 34.7 per cent of Toronto's Jamaicans, 34.5 per cent of its Chinese, 33.4 per cent of its Filipinos, and 26.5 per cent of its Greeks (*Toronto Star*, 22 January 2000: H4). This means that most new immigrant communities are within the City of Toronto. Thus the City of Toronto is where the racial composition of Toronto has changed most rapidly. In the city, the racial-minority population will become the majority much earlier than in the Toronto CMA as a whole, if it has not done so already.

Trends in Intergroup Relations

The city planning critic Jane Jacobs, author of *The Death and Life of Great American Cities* (1961), a former New Yorker but resident in Toronto since the 1960s, was one of the first internationally visible figures to comment positively on the distinctive quality of urban life in Toronto, including its immigrant communities. In *City Limits*, a 1971 production by the National Film Board of Canada devoted to her urban philosophy, she described herself as one among many immigrants to Toronto who found it to be 'a place where you can work, where you can live well, a place where there is still hope.' Although not without problems, Toronto was a place where 'there's still room to solve problems, there's still hope that they can be solved.' In 1997 an international symposium on human ecology celebrated her contribution to Toronto – 'the city that Jane helped build' (Hume 1997, Allen 1997). Her enthusiasm for Toronto continues after decades of change and further immigration (Jacobs 1991, 1993).

Support for this positive view is easy to find. Toronto's cultural diversity flourishes in many ways. CHIN radio station broadcasts in thirty-two different languages; there is also multicultural television alongside the mainstream English offerings (Kashner 1997, 240). Toronto boasts numerous ethnic theatres as well as foreign-language bookshops, newspapers, video outlets, and music stores. There are community-based foreign-language educational programs and community and religious institutions, as well as myriad ethnic restaurants, grocery stores, and so on. The most prominent festival undoubtedly is Caribana, the biggest Carnival parade outside the Caribbean. There is also Caravan, a week-long network of ethnic organizations converted to cabarets and dancehalls, which highlights the traditions and cuisines of many of Toronto's cultural communities.

Educational institutions have incorporated minority groups with surprisingly little conflict. The majority of students at the University of Toronto's three campuses (the downtown St George campus and the outlying Mississauga and Scarborough campuses) are now of Asian and other non-European origins; York University's main North York campus has an even larger non-European majority; and Ryerson University has experienced similar changes; the response has been largely positive and sometimes even enthusiastic.

At the same time, inequality has emerged as an issue for 'visible minorities' and conflicts with racial overtones clearly have increased in Toronto (see Breton et al. 1990; Henry et al. 1995). Racial discrimination in labour markets was demonstrated dramatically in field trials conducted by Henry and Ginzberg (1985; see also Reitz and Breton 1994, 113–23), and may be an important reason why racial-minority workers earn substantially less than those of European origins with the same levels of education and experience. There have been a series of controversies over racial bias in the media and in cultural life – for example, the Royal Ontario Museum's 1989 exhibition 'Into the Heart of Africa' presented artefacts from the colonial period in a way that could be seen as disparaging, and commercial productions of the musicals *Showboat* and *Miss Saigon* drew protests (Tator et al. 1998). Regarding Toronto's black community, police shootings and perceptions of a biased justice system have provoked both violence and government intervention in the form of a commission of inquiry (Task Force on Race Relations and Policing 1992; Lewis 1992). Chinese shopping malls in the suburbs have disturbed some local officials, causing an eruption of controversy. Fears about illegal immigration and bogus refugee claims have generated concerns about an expected negative impact on Toronto (Go 1997). In 1995, for the first time in Ontario, race became an election issue. The Progressive Conservatives under Mike Harris won the election and unceremoniously scrapped the previous New Democratic government's equal job opportunity legislation with the provocatively titled Bill to Repeal Job Quotas and Restore Merit Based Employment Practices in Ontario (Ontario Statutes and Regulations 1995). It also ordered employers to destroy information they had collected as part of internal workforce surveys under the earlier legislation (Lum 1998). In place of employment equity, the government introduced a non-legislative and voluntary Equal Opportunity Plan (Ontario Ministry of Citizenship, Culture and Recreation 1998). Because of tensions surrounding these new racial issues, some have feared that Toronto really may be a racial 'time-bomb,' a place where the true extent of ethnic and racial conflict is now hidden but will eventually burst.

Immigration and refugee settlement issues remain lightning rods for public debate and controversy, and anti-immigrant sentiment is strong according to polls, yet so far Canada has not made it a national priority to limit immigration, as has happened in the United States and Australia. A few years ago, Canada's official opposition party, the Canadian Alliance, tapped into the sentiments of some Canadians with its proposals to limit immigration and curtail social services to immigrants. However, that party's successor, the Conservative Party of Canada – the result of a merger with the more moderate Progressive Conservative Party – has yet to put forward major proposals to reform immigration policies. The government has reacted to public perceptions that Canada is an 'easy' country to enter and a haven for criminals and illegal immigrants with tough new 'law and order' legislation, the Immigration and Refugee Protection Act (Thompson 2001a, 2001b). Still, no public official has expressed the Thatcherite fear of being 'swamped.' In fact, the Liberal government continues to call for *increased* immigration, and in a recent poll, 74 per cent of Canadians mentioned 'our multicultural and multiracial makeup' as 'an important part of what makes us Canadian' (*Maclean's*, December 1999, 34). These sentiments prevail despite unemployment rates that have edged over 10 per cent in recent years, major government spending cuts, and massive reductions in social services (Swimmer 1996).

If intergroup relations in Toronto are relatively calm, why is this? And are there forces of change that may cause a deterioration in intergroup relations in the future?

The Multiculturalism Factor

Official 'multiculturalism' policies are often credited as a key factor in Canada's favourable intergroup relations. Along with gun control and universal health insurance, official multiculturalism seems distinctively Canadian. The Ontario government and municipal governments across greater Toronto proudly proclaim themselves officially multicultural. For Canadians, multiculturalism means a 'live and let live' cultural tolerance, which arguably is very different from American-style multi-culturalism, which entitles minorities to make equity claims. This brand of multiculturalism emerged out of the debate over French-language rights, the status of Quebec, and the political reluctance of the federal Liberals under Trudeau to alienate immigrant voters. The federal government's multiculturalism policy was officially launched in 1971; it was immediately embraced like motherhood by all parties at all levels of government and was later entrenched in Canada's Charter of Rights and Freedoms.

The race issue was not present at the birth of Canadian multi-culturalism, and as with any uninvited guest, there has been an awk-wardness about its arrival. Multicultural programs originally focused on the cultural identities of European minorities. When new groups began talking about equity, access, and discrimination, it became clear that these issues did not quite fall under the rubric of culture. Although some multiculturalism programs have now shifted to include antiracism and antidiscrimination activities, the policy discourse around multi-culturalism has continued to play down the significance of race.

Policies directly addressing race tend to be ambiguous and ineffec-tive. Canada's federal employment-equity legislation, introduced in 1986, is a good example. Visible minorities (a Canadian term reflecting a desire to avoid the word 'race') were included as one of four groups designated for attention (the others being women, Native people, and the disabled). The 1986 law covered only about 5 per cent of the workforce and included no effective monitoring or enforcement mechanisms (Lum 1995). The new employment-equity law, passed in 1995, is stronger because it authorizes the Canadian Human Rights Commission (CHRC) to enforce compliance through on-site employer audits. However, it still covers only 8 per cent of the Canadian workforce and restricts the commission's purview to investigating third-party complaints of systemic discrimination in employment, or to initiating its own complaint if an employer's statistical reports offer reasonable grounds to believe there may be systemic issues affecting the employment opportunities of designated groups, including racial minorities (Lum and Williams 2000). Despite evidence that racial discrimination is no less prevalent in Toronto and other Canadian cities than in American cities (Reitz and Breton 1994), the issue is much further from the public agenda.

Whether or not multiculturalism is the glue binding ethnic and racial groups in Toronto (there is virtually no research about its impact), its persistence both as an ideology and as a government policy probably reflects the relative lack of conflict. As racial issues have grown, some racial minorities have begun to oppose multiculturalism on the grounds that it assigns minorities a marginal status (Bissoondath 1994). Others oppose it because they see it as underpinning identity politics that support the rights of certain minority groups at the expense of either majority rights (Bibby 1990) or the rights of other minority groups (Kay 1998). Still others view multiculturalism as an attempt to maintain the traditional ethnic hierarchy – the 'vertical mosaic' as John Porter (1965) once called it. Multiculturalism, it is argued, socially constructs cultural identities but does little to recognize and remedy inequalities based on race (Bannerji 2000). Criticisms like these have prompted governments to look hard for ways to cut their already small multiculturalism budgets or abandon programs altogether while still being politically correct. For example, as a result of the 1994 Federal Program Review, funds allotted to multiculturalism have been reduced by 28 per cent and reoriented from program to project funding. Also, the question of whether municipal budgets should continue to fund a Multicultural Grants Program has been raised regularly (Peries 1997, 88).

In short, although observers have often credited official multiculturalism with improving intergroup relations, it is questionable whether the policy actually ever had this effect. And today the growth of racial minority populations seems to be changing the role of multiculturalism, making it less a socially cohesive force and more a rallying point for demands for stronger public policies to address issues of equality and human rights.

The Importance of Immigration Selection

Perhaps the positive impact of immigration can be explained by Canada's highly selective screening process. For example, the American economist George Borjas (1990), among others, argues that compared to the United States, Canada has tried to be more skill selective. In 1967, Canada introduced a points-based selection system that numerically assessed independent applicants according to a number of characteristics, including language skills, educational attainment, and occupational expertise. This formally colour-blind policy not only removed discriminatory obstacles to non-European immigration but also opened the immigration doors to people from Asia, Africa, the Caribbean, and Central and South America, many of whom had higher educational levels than past waves of immigrants from southern Europe. In fact, these new immigrants often possessed stronger academic credentials than native-born Canadians, which boosted their employment success. Moreover, the selection criteria have been raised several times, especially in recent years, further enhancing the skills of Canada's immigrants. The implication here – and the lesson for the United States according to Borjas – is that in picking and choosing its immigrants more wisely than its southern neighbour, Canada has succeeded better in forging a racial and ethnic population mix that is more harmonious than in the United States.

The data, however, do not support this line of argument. According to immigration statistics (Duleep and Regets 1992; Reitz 1998, 69–97), Canada is not really more skill selective than the United States. Quite the reverse – that country actually out-competes Canada for highly skilled immigrants from every major source country except Mexico. The reasons for this are not entirely clear; processes of selection and self-selection may be involved.[5] In any case, effective immigration management and screening for the best cannot be trumpeted as the reason why there is less racial tension in Canada than the United States. If immigration selection has had an impact, it is perhaps in the selection of a greater diversity of groups. This has resulted – most likely inadvertently – in an immigration population mix in which no single group is large enough to emerge as a focal point for conflict.

Illegal immigration exists in Toronto but is far less prominent than in many American cities. The relative lack of illegal immigration may be attributed to Canada's isolation from all countries other than the United States. Immigration control remains an issue, but the apparently small size of what Americans call the 'undocumented' population helps support a sense that immigration is successfully managed in the public interest. This undoubtedly contributes to positive perceptions of immigrants and immigration in Canada and in Toronto (Reitz 2004).

Labour Markets and the New Economy: Beyond the 'Global City'

Canada's immigrants in most origin groups (other than Mexicans) may be less skilled than immigrants to the United States, and benefit little from multiculturalism or less discrimination; even so, they have experienced greater employment success. It is possible that the relatively successful integration of immigrants into Toronto's labour market is a factor in Canada's fairly harmonious intergroup relations. In contrast, in the United States, especially in the high-immigration cities, most immigrant-origin groups have significantly lower relative earnings than their counterparts in Canadian cities (Reitz 1998). Sassen's (1988) concept of the 'global city' suggested a link between immigration and inequality in certain cities. According to her, global cities (New York being the prototype) contain super-elites who occupy the command posts of the entire global economy. Their affluence generates a demand for personal services, and these are supplied by new waves of immigrants who are willing to work for low wages. This hypothesis may or may not apply to the United States but it certainly does not hold for Canada. If Canada had a global city it would be Toronto. However, Toronto's high immigration levels can hardly be explained entirely by the elite's demand for personal services. There are too many immigrants and too few super-elites. As well, immigrants in Toronto have not been confined to low-level service jobs. Employment success for Toronto's immigrants has been greater, not only compared to New York's minorities, but also compared to immigrant minorities in some less strategic American cities.

A comparison of the institutional bases of immigrants' employment success in Canada and the United States shows the importance of a range of institutions, including education and labour market structures, in determining overall earnings inequalities (Reitz 1998). Educational institutions are most significant. The earlier and more rapid expansion of postsecondary education in the United States contributed to a large accumulation of educational credentials by the native-born population; this created formidable obstacles for immigrants seeking to compete for jobs. The impact of this native-born education on immigrants in the United States has been magnified by the tendency for the best-educated members of the population to be concentrated in the most dynamic urban centres – in cities that also happen to be most attractive to immigrants. Furthermore, among immigrants it is the *least* educated who have settled in these major immigration cities, probably because of the selective effects of personal networks in immigrant settlement. This had added to the skills gap they face.

Postsecondary education in Canada expanded later than it did in the United States. As a consequence, Canada's immigrants have experienced easier access to middle-class status. Yet the seeds of change are clearly present in this situation. If immigrant employment success in the past was due to lower levels of education of the native-born, the recent rapid expansion of education in Canada will likely create greater obstacles for immigrants to Canada over time.

Trend data on the employment experiences of newly arriving immigrants to Toronto suggest that this is exactly what is happening. Recent immigrant cohorts have been far less successful than those in the past in obtaining jobs, especially well-paying jobs. Figures 2.2 and 2.3 are based on data from men and women aged twenty to sixty-four in Toronto from four successive Canadian censuses: 1981, 1986, 1991, and 1996. Two aspects are considered: employment participation (measured as the percentage with any earnings during the previous year – Figure 2.2), and relative earnings for those who have employment (measured as the ratio of mean earnings for immigrants to mean earnings for the native-born – Figure 2.3). When we compare immigrants who have been settled for roughly the same periods of time – fewer than five years, six to ten years, and so on – we see a very clear downward trend. More recent immigrant cohorts are far less likely to get jobs quickly when they arrive, and the jobs they do get are much less attractive. These trends apply to immigrants in general and also to specific minority groups such as Chinese and blacks (see Tables 2.3 and 2.4). The result has been high rates of poverty in a number of immigrant groups in Toronto. In 1996 the poverty rate for all families of non-European origin in Toronto was 34.3 per cent, more than double the rate for families of European origin (Ornstein, 2000).

Further analysis shows a similar downward employment trend for

Figure 2.2. Percentage of immigrants with earnings, compared to native-born, for men and women 20–64, by time in Canada, Toronto CMA, 1971–96

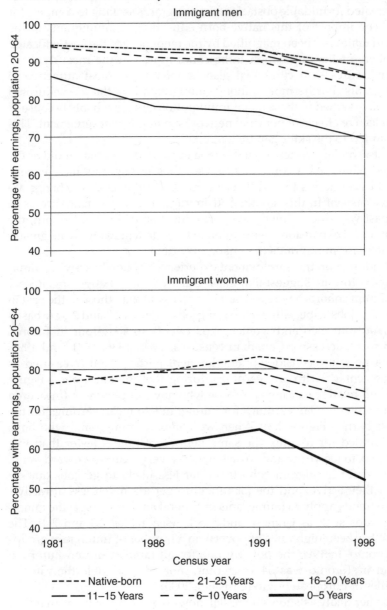

Figure 2.3. Ratios of mean earnings of immigrants to mean earnings
of native-born, for immigrant men and women 20–64, by time in
Canada, Toronto CMA, 1971–96

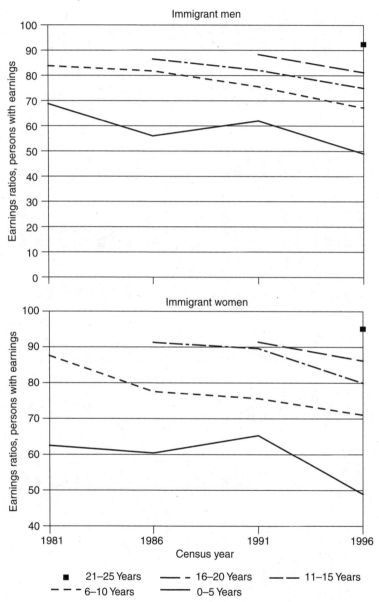

Table 2.3. Percentage of Toronto's immigrants with earnings,[a] for those arriving since 1970 and 20–64, by gender and years in Canada, for the census years 1981–1996 (N = cases)

Origins	Years in Canada	Men				Women			
		1981	1986	1991	1996	1981	1986	1991	1996
Native-born[b]	–	94.3	93.2	92.6	88.7	76.5	79.3	83.1	80.6
	(N)	(9,658)	(11,862)	(18,621)	(17,630)	(10,111)	(12,436)	(19,356)	(18,400)
Immigrants	Total	92.6	89.9	87.8	80.7	71.3	72.8	74.3	66.3
	(N)	(8,381)	(9,470)	(16,559)	(17,598)	(8,483)	(9,664)	(17,339)	(18,941)
Immigrants since 1970	0–5	86.0	78.0	76.4	69.3	64.5	60.7	64.7	51.9
	(N)	(880)	(1051)	(3,425)	(3,799)	(1,055)	(1,089)	(3,601)	(4.537)
	6–10	93.9	91.0	89.8	82.6	80.0	75.4	76.7	68.2
	(N)	(1,572)	(1,114)	(1,588)	(2,985)	(1,692)	(1,190)	(1,752)	(3,112)
	11–15		92.4	91.6	85.4		79.2	79.0	71.8
	(N)		(1,665)	(1,844)	(1,435)		(1,835)	(2,002)	(1,594)
	16–20			92.9	85.6			81.3	74.2
	(N)			(2,916)	(1,714)			(3,022)	(1,884)
	21–25				85.5				75.6
	(N)				(2,562)				(2,723)
White immigrants	0–5	90.4	85.0	82.8	78.4	65.1	59.5	68.3	56.2
	(N)	(270)	(302)	(766)	(663)	(307)	(309)	(775)	(767)
	6–10	95.6	94.1	93.6	87.0	74.0	75.2	78.9	74.1
	(N)	(542)	(322)	(439)	(648)	(599)	(358)	(460)	(659)
	11–15		603	541	378		632	554	397
	(N)		(604)	(541)	(378)		(633)	(554)	(397)
	16–20			94.6	87.3			78.0	73.6
	(N)			(1,147)	(463)			(1,118)	(531)
	20–25				86.1				71.1
	(N)				(932)				(984)

Table 2.3. (continued)

Origins	Years in Canada	Men 1981	Men 1986	Men 1991	Men 1996	Women 1981	Women 1986	Women 1991	Women 1996
Black Immigrants	0–5	82.8	78.4	78.4	70.8	77.9	73.6	73.4	52.5
	(N)	(64)	(89)	(296)	(391)	(86)	(72)	(335)	(476)
	6–10	91.4	93.3	90.4	77.1	86.4	86.4	83.3	68.8
	(N)	(162)	(105)	(135)	(310)	(154)	(147)	(210)	(320)
	11–15		92.5	87.6	85.0		86.2	80.8	72.0
	(N)		(200)	(202)	(140)		(276)	(281)	(193)
	16–20			93.3	84.6			82.0	70.0
	(N)			(357)	(209)			(505)	(233)
	21–25				82.4				78.1
	(N)				(290)				(438)
Chinese immigrants	0–5	85.2	69.4	75.0	56.9	58.2	56.7	64.6	45.6
	(N)	(128)	(183)	(673)	(837)	(182)	(238)	(777)	(1,045)
	6–10	90.6	83.7	83.5	79.5	81.1	74.9	71.5	69.1
	(N)	(170)	(208)	(291)	(595)	(196)	(179)	(354)	(661)
	11–15		90.6	87.7	76.2		81	79.2	70.3
	(N)		(170)	(325)	(257)	(195)	(336)	(337)	
	16–20			89.5	82.9			80.7	74.5
	(N)			(295)	(293)			(306)	(333)
	21–25				87.4				79.8
	(N)				(277)				(257)

Table 2.3. (concluded)

Origins	Years in Canada	Men				Women			
		1981	1986	1991	1996	1981	1986	1991	1996
So. Asian immigrants	0–5		76.2	75.6	70.4		62.7	58.8	46.6
	(N)		(168)	(578)	(801)		(636)	(532)	(874)
	6–10		92.3	93.3	84.0		70.1	73.3	62.7
	(N)		(130)	(240)	(494)		(135)	(225)	(475)
	11–15		92.7	94.3	92.2		81.5	72.4	64.2
	(N)		(261)	(230)	(204)		(260)	(246)	(187)
	16–20			92.8	86.7			83.3	71.7
	(N)			(443)	(195)			(401)	(240)
	21–25				83.2				74.6
	(N)				(411)				(378)

[a] The percentage having received any earnings during the previous year from wages, salaries, or self-employment.
[b] Percentages for native-born whites do not vary by more than 0.5 per cent.
Source: Statistics Canada, Census of Canada, Public Use Microdata Files for Individuals.

Table 2.4. Relative earnings[a] of Toronto's immigrants, among those with earnings,[b] for those arriving since 1970 and 20–64, by gender and years in Canada, for the census years 1981–1996 (N = cases)

Origins	Years in Canada	Men 1981	Men 1986	Men 1991	Men 1996	Women 1981	Women 1986	Women 1991	Women 1996
Mean native-born Born Earnings	–	$20,361	$28,439	$39,045	$41,225	$10,911	$16,656	$24,848	$28,164
	(N)	(9,103)	(11,058)	(17,242)	(15,629)	(7,739)	(9,859)	(16,091)	(14,837)
Mean immigrant earnings		$19,207	$27,052	$34,936	$34,002	$10,342	$15,373	$22,073	$23,400
	(N)	(7,757)	(8,514)	(14,531)	(14,206)	(6,051)	(7,032)	(12,883)	(12,536)
Immigrants since 1970	0–5	.688	.560	.620	.490	.625	.604	.653	.490
	(N)	(757)	(820)	(2,621)	(2,366)	(681)	(661)	(2,329)	(2,349)
	6–10	.838	.818	.756	.672	.876	.776	.756	.711
	(N)	(1,476)	(1,014)	(1,431)	(2,456)	(1,354)	(897)	(1,344)	(2,122)
	11–15		.865	.821	.750		.913	.896	.800
	(N)		(1,539)	(1,691)	(1,225)		(1,453)	(1,585)	(1,145)
	16–20			.883	.812			.914	.862
	(N)			(2,713)	(1,468)			(2,460)	(1,398)
	21–25				.924				.951
	(N)				(2,190)				(2,059)
White	0–5	.886	.792	.621	.678	.686	.747	.620	.544
	(N)	(244)	(256)	(634)	(520)	(200)	(184)	(529)	(431)
	6–10	.945	.955	.880	.761	.844	.845	.883	.728
	(N)	(518)	(303)	(411)	(564)	(443)	(267)	(363)	(488)
	11–15		.930	.910	.880		.885	.906	.863
	(N)		(566)	(507)	(327)		(460)	(442)	(309)
	16–20			.910	.943			.914	.900
	(N)			(1,085)	(404)			(872)	(390)
	21–25				.933				.921

Table 2.4. (continued)

Origins	Years in Canada	Men				Women			
		1981	1986	1991	1996	1981	1986	1991	1996
	(N)				(802)				(698)
Black	0–5	.576	.398	.494	.422	.566	.554	.590	.495
	(N)	(53)	(69)	(232)	(277)	(67)	(53)	(246)	(250)
	6–10	.679	.587	.568	.547	.926	.774	.664	.626
	(N)	(148)	(98)	(122)	(239)	(133)	(127)	(175)	(220)
	11–15		.683	.667	.651		.820	.756	.694
	(N)		(185)	(177)	(119)		(238)	(227)	(139)
	16–20			.712	.677			.867	.810
	(N)			(333)	(176)			(414)	(163)
	21–25				.762				.833
	(N)				(239)				(342)
Chinese	0–5	.56	.541	.639	.488	.68	.552	.772	.492
	(N)	(109)	(127)	(505)	(476)	(106)	(135)	(502)	(476)
	6–10	.83	.660	.674	.685	.102	.816	.685	.803
	(N)	(154)	(174)	(243)	(473)	(159)	(134)	(253)	(457)
	11–15		.991	.760	.665		1.18	.902	.764
	(N)		(154)	(285)	(195)		(158)	(266)	(237)
	16–20			1.01	.820			1.06	.933
	(N)			(264)	(243)			(247)	(248)
	21–25				1.03				1.23

Table 2.4. (concluded)

Origins	Years in Canada	Men				Women			
		1981	1986	1991	1996	1981	1986	1991	1996
South Asian	(N)				(242)				(205)
	0–5		.512	.531	.411		.550	.616	.423
	(N)		(128)	(437)	(564)		(84)	(313)	(407)
	6–10		.775	.725	.676		.740	.668	.670
	(N)		(120)	(224)	(415)		(94)	(165)	(476)
	11–15		.892	.788	.733		.910	.879	.783
	(N)		(242)	(217)	(188)		(212)	(178)	(120)
	16–20			.902	.851			.931	.890
	(N)			(411)	(169)			(334)	(172)
	21–25				.956				.980
	(N)				(342)				(282)

[a] Relative earnings is the ratio of mean earnings for an immigrant group to mean earnings of the native-born workforce (reported in unadjusted dollars).
[b] See Table 2.3.

Source: Statistics Canada, Census of Canada, Public Use Microdata Files for Individuals.

immigrants across Canada and that these trends are continuing (Statistics Canada 2003, 12; Frenette and Morrisette 2003; Galarneau and Morrissette 2004). It also suggests that these trends have arisen from the increasing importance of education in labour markets, and also from the emergence of a 'knowledge economy' (Reitz 2001). The more recent immigrants have faced more stringent selection standards and have higher levels of education; however, the educational levels of the native-born population have risen even more rapidly. Although immigrants are still better educated than the native-born, their advantage is less salient now than in the past. Furthermore, in the increasingly credentialist environment, immigrants' foreign credentials seem to have decreasing value. For most Canadians, earnings returns to education have been rising; for immigrants, they are falling. And finally, earnings inequalities are rising, and the gap between the best-paid and least-paid workers is widening; as a consequence, the implications of losing out in the job competition are becoming more negative.

In short, fundamental changes in education and the labour market are undercutting some of the major advantages that in the past contributed to employment success for immigrants. The success of immigration to Canada today is measured largely in terms of the employment success of immigrants and (it follows) their contribution to the Canadian economy. Immigrants with higher earnings pay more taxes, use fewer social services, buy more goods, start more businesses, and create more jobs. Conversely, immigrants with lower earnings may encounter more difficulties in many areas of life. Also, they are perceived as accessing more social support services. The social consequences of these trends are likely to become manifest, perhaps in increasing intergroup tension and conflict.

The Changing Fabric of Urban Life

Some of the reasons for Toronto's ethnoracial dynamics may lie in the broader social or cultural framework, and this too is changing in many respects. Canadian cities have less poverty and crime of all kinds. According to S.M. Lipset (1989), Canada's emphasis on social programs and a social safety net constitutes a key social and cultural difference between Canada and the United States. However, because of growing concerns over government finance and taxation, government across Canada have weakened their commitments to social programs, including in Toronto. Unemployment insurance benefits have been reduced.

Health care funding has been cut, and in 1996 the Ontario Conservative government established an independent Health Services Restructuring Commission with the power to make radical changes to the province's health system – changes that included amalgamating and closing hospitals (Ontario Health Services Restructuring Commission 1997). University tuition levels have increased dramatically, with students now expected to pay a larger share of their education costs. These reductions do not target immigrants; they may, however, affect the ease with which immigrants become integrated into the community (Lum et al. 2001). For example, up until now the children of immigrants have pursued advanced education in large numbers; tuition increases and the impact of lower earnings by immigrants may well change this.

Settlement programs specifically for immigrants have been scaled back. In Toronto, many community-based agencies offering immigrant services such as language training, job placement, skills training, counselling, and community education (represented by a coalition group, the Ontario Council of Agencies Serving Immigrants – OCASI) rely on funding from a variety of sources – primarily the federal government but also provincial and municipal governments, the United Way, and donations and grants from foundations and corporations. Between 1996 and 1998, funding for Ontario's immigrant settlement programs was reduced from $6.1 million to $3.9 million. Programs and services such as antiracism grants, Ontario Welcome Houses, the Multilingual Access to Social Assistance Program, and Citizenship Development grants were eliminated (Peries 1997, 87–9; Richmond 1996). Another Ontario government initiative has reduced benefits for sponsored immigrants on the assumption that sponsors provide a minimum of support (whether or not they actually have done so).

There are other possible forces. Jane Jacobs's enthusiasm for Toronto arose from her admiration for downtown neighbourhoods and human-scale streetscapes. According to her (1993, xi), neighbourhoods in the central cores of Canadian cities have been preserved for several reasons, including the weaker commitment to urban renewal in the 1950s and 1960s and the much smaller federal highway program. In the United States, she contends, the larger-scale urban renewal and federally sponsored expressway construction devastated communities in many city centres. She also contends that in the United States, the creation of racial ghettos and white flight to the suburbs were in part a result of 'block-busting' tactics by developers and the real estate industry, the purpose of which was to create property-value panics. Prejudice and discrimination were also present in Toronto, but 'these evils were not exacerbated and intensified' by a development industry working in concert with banks and local authorities.

If such differences matter, they may be declining in significance. Fong (1994, 1996) suggests that patterns of residential concentration for new immigrant groups do not differ substantially between Canadian and American cities. In any case, Toronto's distinctive urban landscape applies primarily to neighbourhoods in the old city of Toronto – neighbourhoods that now comprise less than 20 per cent of the city's population. Today's vast and expanding suburban tracts are much harder to distinguish from American models. Only now are researchers beginning to examine how such changes are affecting the social reception of immigrants in Toronto, and opportunities for immigrants to launch businesses or create viable communities (see Michelson, in this volume). Antipathy between the suburban '905' and central-city '416' areas is sometimes linked to the relative sizes of their racial minority immigrant populations. This urban–suburban polarization related to race, if it exists, would be a relatively new feature of life in Toronto.

In the realm of politics, the amalgamation of municipal governments in the Toronto area has increased the sizes of constituencies; this has the potential to reduce the clout of immigrant groups during local elections (see Siemiatychi and Isin 1998; Siemiatychi and Saloojee 2000). Amalgamation also eliminated the various race relations committees, which had provided a forum for expressing issues arising in the community, and which had tried to maintain positive race relations.

Conclusions

Intergroup relations arising from immigration in Toronto may well be more positive than in comparable situations elsewhere, although systematic comparative evidence is lacking. Yet the evidence that prejudice and discrimination are substantially less is quite weak. Perhaps multicultural policies have helped. This discussion has pointed to a number of other institutional forces, including education, labour markets, community life, and local government, that perhaps also had an impact in Toronto.

Many institutional features that may have helped foster effective immigrant integration in the past are now changing rapidly. Most significantly, rising levels of education and increased labour market disparities linked to the 'new economy' have greatly reduced the employment success of immigrants. Reduced support for multiculturalism, American-style suburbanization, and rapid changes in community-based local government also may be having an impact on race relations in Toronto. Canadian cities continue to be distinctive in many ways, but they are clearly also changing in many ways, partly in response to outside forces such as the North American Free Trade Agreement. All these changes raise questions about the future of race relations in Toronto. Will they be as positive as in the past?

NOTES

This paper is revised and enlarged from an earlier paper (Reitz and Lum 1997). The research was supported in part by a grant from the Social Sciences and Humanities Research Council. The authors wish to thank Michelle Maenck for her excellent research assistance.

1 In 2003, of 221,352 immigrants arriving in Canada, 97,476, or 44.0 per cent, named Toronto as their city of intended destination (Citizenship and Immigration Canada 2004, 38).
2 The census question asked about each person in the household in 1991, 1996, and 2001 was 'To which ethnic or cultural group(s) did this person's ancestors belong?' Examples were listed (including French, English, German, Scottish, Canadian, and many others, including non-European and aboriginal origins). Respondents were invited to 'specify as many groups as applicable.' The census questions asked in 1971, 1981, and 1986 varied somewhat in wording, the most important difference being that 'Canadian' (or other North American) responses were excluded.
3 The following question was asked about each person in the household: 'Is this person ...' with the following response options provided: White, Chinese, South Asian, Black, Arab/West Asian, Filipino, South East Asian, Latin-American, Japanese, Korean, and other.' Although the word 'race' does not appear in the question, the Microdata File codebook describes the resulting data as a 'visible minority indicator.' The response options are similar to those used in the U.S. census question on race.
4 Multiculturalism has been viewed negatively as reflecting a weak national identity – for example, by the American historian Arthur Schlesinger Jr. (1992, 13). Supposedly this leaves Canada vulnerable to breakup along French-English lines.
5 Self-selection might favour more highly skilled immigrants in the United

States because of that country's superior market position, or because of labour market structures as discussed by Borjas (1990). Skilled immigrants represent a greater proportion of total immigration in Canada than in the United States, but partly for this reason the criteria of selection in Canada must be somewhat less demanding. The skill levels of immigrants entering under family reunification would to some extent reflect the skill levels of those entering under the skill-selective streams.

REFERENCES

Allen, Max. 1997. *Ideas That Matter: The Worlds of Jane Jacobs*. Owen Sound, ON: Ginger Press.

Bannerji, Himani. 2000. *The Dark Side of the Nation: Essays on Multiculturalism, Nationalism and Gender*. Toronto: Canadian Scholars' Press.

Bibby, Reginald. 1990. *Mosaic Madness: The Poverty and Potential of Life in Canada*. Toronto: Stoddart.

Bissoondath, Neil. 1994. *Selling Illusions: The Cult of Multiculturalism in Canada*. Toronto: Penguin.

Bourne, Larry S. 2000. *People and Places: A Portrait of the Evolving Character of the Greater Toronto Area* (Report to the Neptis Foundation). Toronto: Department of Geography/Program in Planning, January.

Borjas, George. 1990. *Friends or Strangers: The Impact of Immigrants on the United States Economy*. New York: Basic Books.

Breton, Raymond, Wsevolod W. Isajiw, Warren E. Kalbach, and Jeffrey G. Reitz. 1990. *Ethnic Identity and Equality: Varieties of Experience in a Canadian City*. Toronto: University of Toronto Press.

Caulfield, Jon. 1997. 'Walking and Looking in Inner Toronto: Elements of the City's Fabric.' *Footnotes* 25(2) 1, 7.

Citizenship and Immigration Canada. 2004. *Facts and Figures 2003, Immigration Overview*. Ottawa: Citizenship and Immigration Canada.

Conniff, Richard. 1966. 'Toronto.' *National Geographic* (June): 121.

Duleep, Harriet, and Mark C. Regets. 1992. 'Some Evidence on the Effects of Admissions Criteria on Immigrant Assimilation.' Pp. 410–39 in Barry Chiswick, ed., *Immigration, Language and Ethnicity: Canada and the United States*. Washington, DC: AEI Press.

Fong, Eric. 1994. 'Residential Proximity among Racial Groups in American and Canadian Neighborhoods.' *Urban Affairs Quarterly* 30(2): 285–97.

– 1996. 'A Comparative Perspective of Racial Residential Segrega-tion: American and Canadian Experiences.' *Sociological Quarterly* 37(2): 501–28.

Frenette, M., and R. Morrissette. 2003. Will They Ever Converge? Earnings
    of Immigrants and Canadian-born.' Ottawa: Statistics Canada, Cat. No.
    11F0019MIE2003215.
Galarneau, D., and R. Morrissette. 2004. 'Immigrants: Settling For Less?
    Perspectives on Labour and Income 5(6) (June): 5–16.
Go, Avvy. 1997. 'Xenophobia, Politics and Sound Bites: Immigrants, Refugees
    and Public Perception.' Pp. 58–65 in Patrick Hunter, ed., *Toronto: Who's
    Listening? The Impact of Immigration and Refugee Settlement on Toronto.*
    Toronto: Report of the Advisory Committee On Immigration and Refugee
    Issues in Metropolitan Toronto.
Goldberg, Michael A., and John Mercer. 1986. *The Myth of the North American
    City: Continentalism Challenged.* Vancouver: UBC Press.
Halli, S.S., and A. Kazemipur. 1998. 'Plight of Immigrants: The Spatial Con-
    centration of Poverty in Canada.' *Canadian Journal of Regional Science* 20(1,2):
    11–28.
Henry, Frances, and Effie Ginsberg. 1985. *Who Gets the Work? A Test of Racial
    Discrimination in Employment.* Toronto: Urban Alliance on Race Relations
    and Social Planning Council of Metropolitan Toronto.
Henry, Frances, Carol Tator, Winston Mattis, and Rim Rees. 1995. *The Colour of
    Democracy: Racism in Canadian Society.* Toronto: Harcourt Brace Canada.
Hume, Christopher. 1997. 'The City That Jane Helped Build.' *The Toronto Star*,
    12 October, F1, 5.
Jacobs, Jane. 1993. Foreword to John Sewell, *The Shape of the City: Toronto
    Struggles with Modern Planning.* Toronto: University of Toronto Press.
– 1991. 'Putting Toronto's Best Self Forward.' *Places* 7(2): 50–3.
– 1961. *The Death and Life of Great American Cities.* New York: Random
    House.
Kalbach, Warren E. 1990. 'Ethnic Residential Segregation and Its Significance
    for the Individual in an Urban Setting.' Pp. 92–134 in Breton et al., *Ethnic
    Identity and Equality.*
Kashner, Robert. 1997. *Ethnic Toronto: A Complete Guide to the Many Faces and
    Cultures of Toronto.* Toronto: Passport Books.
Kazemipur, A., and S.S. Halli. 2001. 'Immigrants and New Poverty: The Case
    of Canada.' *International Migration Review* 35(4): 1129–56.
Kay, Jonathan. 1998. 'Explaining the Modern Backlash against Multi-
    culturalism.' *Policy Options* (May): 30–4.
Lewis, Stephen. 1992. *Report to the Office of the Premier* [on race relations].
    Toronto: Government of Ontario.
Ley, David, and Heather Smith. 1998. 'Immigration and Poverty in Canadian
    Cities, 1971–1991.' *Canadian Journal of Regional Science* 20(1/2): 29–48.

Lipset, Seymour Martin. 1989. *Continental Divide: The Values and Institutions of the United States and Canada*. Toronto: C.D. Howe Institute.

Lum, Janet M. 1998. 'Backward Steps in Equity: Health System Reform's Impact on Women and Racial Minorities in Ontario.' *National Women's Studies Association Journal: Special Issue Affirmative Action Edition* 10(3): 101–14.

– 1995. 'The Federal Employment Equity Act: Goals vs. Implementation.' *Canadian Public Administration* (Spring): 45–76.

Lum, Janet M., and Paul A. Williams. 1995. 'Out of Sync with a "Shrinking State"? Making Sense of The Employment Equity Act (1995).' Pp. 194–211 in M. Burke, C. Mooers and J. Shields, eds., *Restructuring and Resistance: Canadian Public Policy in an Era of Global Capitalism*. Halifax: Fernwood.

Lum, Janet M., Paul A. Williams, Joseph H. Springer, and Raisa B. Deber. 2001. 'From Medicare to Home and Community: Overtaking the Limits of Publicly Funded Health and Social Care: Implications for Chinese and Caribbean Seniors In Toronto.' Paper prepared for presentation at the Congress of the Social Sciences and Humanities: Annual Meeting of the Canadian Political Science Association, 23–30 May.

Municipality of Metropolitan Toronto. 1993. *Towards a Metropolitan Anti-Racism Policy And Implementation Strategy*. Toronto: Chief Administrative Officer's Department, Municipality of Metropolitan Toronto.

Ontario Health Services Restructuring Commission. 1997. *Metropolitan Toronto Health Services Restructuring Report*. March.

Ontario Ministry of Citizenship, Culture and Recreation. 1998. *Equal Opportunity in Ontario*. Toronto: Queen's Printer.

Ontario Statutes and Regulations. 1995. *Bill 8: Job Quotas Repeal Act*. Toronto: Queen's Printer.

Ornstein, Michael. 2000. *Ethno-Racial Inequality in Metropolitan Toronto: Analysis of the 1996 Census*. Toronto: Institute for Social Research, York University. March.

Peries, Sharmini. 1997. 'Funding of Settlement Services.' Pp. 87–9 in Patrick Hunter, ed., *Toronto: Who's Listening? The Impact of Immigration and Refugee Settlement on Toronto*. Report of the Advisory Committee on Immigration and Refugee Issues in Metropolitan Toronto.

Porter, John. 1965. *The Vertical Mosaic: An Analysis of Social Class and Power in Canada*. Toronto: University of Toronto Press.

Precourt, Geoffrey, and Anne Faircloth. 1996. 'Best Cities: Where the Living Is Easy.' *Fortune* 134(9) (11 November): 126–49.

Relph, Edward. 1997 (revised and updated). *The Toronto Guide: The City, Metro, The Region*. Toronto: University of Toronto Centre for Urban and Community Studies. Prepared for the Association of American Geographers.

Reitz, Jeffrey G. 2004. 'Canada: Immigration and Nation-Building in the Transition to a Knowledge Economy.' Pp. 97–133 in *Controlling Immigration: A Global Perspective*, 2nd ed., ed. Wayne A. Cornelius, Philip L. Martin, James F. Hollifield, and Takeyuki Tsuda. Stanford, CA: Stanford University Press.

– 2001. 'Immigrant Success in the Knowledge Economy: Institutional Change and the Immigrant Experience in Canada, 1970–1995.' *Journal of Social Issues* 57(3): 577–611.

– 1998. *Warmth of the Welcome: The Social Causes of Economic Success for Immigrants in Different Nations and Cities*. Boulder, CO: Westview.

– 1988. 'Less Racial Discrimination in Canada, or Simply Less Racial Conflict? Implications of Comparisons with Britain.' *Canadian Public Policy/Analyse de Politiques* 14(4): 424–41.

Reitz, Jeffrey G., and Raymond Breton. 1994. *The Illusion of Difference: Realities of Ethnicity in the United States and Canada*. Toronto: C.D. Howe Institute.

Reitz, Jeffrey G., and Janet M. Lum. 'Immigration and Toronto's "Stylish New Personality,"' *Footnotes* 25(3): 1, 8.

Richmond, Ted. 1996. 'Effects of Cutback on Immigrant Service Agencies.' Toronto: City of Toronto Public Health Department.

Sassen, Saskia. 1988. *The Mobility of Labor and Capital: A Study in International Investment and Labor Flow*. Cambridge: Cambridge University Press.

Schlesinger, Arthur M., jr. 1992. *The Disuniting of America: Reflections on a Multicultural Society*. New York: W.W. Norton.

– 1991. *The Global City: New York, London, Tokyo*. Princeton, NJ: Princeton University Press.

Siemiatychi, M., and E. Isin. 1998. 'Immigration, Diversity and Urban Citizenship in Toronto.' *Canadian Journal of Regional Science* 20(1/2): 73–102.

Siemiatychi, M., and A. Saloogee. 2000. 'Ethno-racial Political Representation In Toronto: Patterns and Problems.' Paper prepared for presentation at the 5th International Metropolis Conference, Vancouver, November.

Simon, R.J., and J.P. Lynch. 1999. 'A Comparative Assessment of Public Opinion toward Immigrants and Immigration Policy.' *International Migration Review* 33(2): 455–67.

Statistic Canada. 2003. 'Earnings of Canadians: Making a Living in the New Economy.' Cat. no. 96F0030XIE2001013. Ottawa: Minister of Industry.

– 2005. 'Population Projections of Visible Minority Groups, Canada, Provinces and Regions, 2001–2017.' Cat. no. 91-541-XIE. Ottawa: Minister of Industry.

Swimmer, Gene. ed. 1996. *How Ottawa Spends 1996–97: Life under the Knife*. Ottawa: Carleton University Press.

Task Force on Race Relations and Policing. 1992. *The Report of the Race Relations and Policing Task Force*. Toronto: Office of the Solicitor General, Government of Ontario.

Tator, Carol, Frances Henry, and Winston Mattis. 1998. *Challenging Racism in the Arts: Case Studies of Controversy and Conflict*. Toronto: University of Toronto Press.

Thompson, Allan. 2000a. 'Immigration Bill Tough on Criminals.' *Toronto Star*, 14 June.

– 2001b. 'Immigration bill called "un-Canadian": Diminishes the Rights of Thousands of People, Lawyers Say.' *Toronto Star*, 16 March.

Troper, Harold. 2003. 'Becoming an Immigrant City: A History of Immigration into Toronto since the Second World War.' Pp. 19–62 in *The World in a City*, ed. Paul Anisef and Michael Lamphier. Toronto: University of Toronto Press.

3 Residential Segregation of Visible Minority Groups in Toronto

ERIC FONG

Racial and ethnic residential integration has been viewed as an indicator of group relations in any society. It is a basic form of association that provides the mechanisms and occasions for intergroup interaction. Intergroup contact in neighbourhoods is unique because it is informal and not competitive (White 1987; Park 1967). Thus it fosters intergroup friendships and corrects misunderstandings among groups (Sigelman et al. 1996; Jackman and Crane 1986).

Racial and ethnic residential segregation is perceived as a barrier that minority groups must overcome in order to achieve full integration with the larger society (Massey and Mullan 1984). Massey and Mullan contend that assimilation cannot occur in a vacuum. Most interactions occur in a physical environment. Thus the residential integration of minority groups facilitates other types of assimilation, such as labour force participation (Massey and Shibuya 1995) and educational achievement (Wilson 1987; Kasarda 1989).

In explaining residential segregation patterns, Park suggested that 'physical and sentimental distances reinforce each other, and the influences of local distribution of the population participate with the influences of class and race in the evolution of the social organization' (1967:10). Later work delineated three main complementary, albeit sometimes competing, explanations for residential segregation patterns.

The first explanation is that racial and ethnic residential segregation is a reflection of group desirability (Massey and Denton 1993; Clark 1986; Farley et al. 1978). The hypothesis is that every group has neighbourhood preferences in terms of racial and ethnic composition. The racial preferences in the neighbourhood reflect the social distance of various groups (Fong 1997a). A group not welcomed in the neighbour-hood is seen as having a greater social distance from other groups.

The racial and ethnic preferences of a neighbourhood affect the residential mobility of minority groups in two ways. First, institutionalized discrimination in the housing market arises to minimize the chances of the unwanted group moving into certain neighbourhoods (Massey and Denton 1993). Through a variety of discriminatory mechanisms, entry by the undesirable group is blocked by local residents. Sometimes the unwanted group must pay higher prices than other groups to move into the same neighbourhoods (Fong 1997b; Massey and Fong 1990). Moreover, some groups go to any lengths to avoid living in the same neighbourhoods as undesirable groups, even if it means paying to move away (Clark 1991; Schelling 1971). Thus when members of an unwelcome group do move into a neighbourhood, rapid residential turnover often follows. Studies have suggested that minority groups are more likely to be treated as undesirable. It has been shown that in the United States and Canada, blacks pay higher prices to move into certain neighbourhoods (Fong 1997; Massey and Fong 1990). 'White flight' from American urban neighbourhoods because of an increase in black residents has been well documented (Massey and Denton 1993; Farley et al. 1978).

The second explanation for residential patterns was offered by Burgess (1967) in his classic study of the growth of Chicago. Burgess linked residential patterns to the integration processes of immigrants. He elegantly demonstrated how residence in neighbourhoods changes and evolves according to the integration process. He observed that recently arrived immigrants usually cluster in areas next to the central business district, mainly because of lower housing costs. As they stay longer and become socially mobile, they move out of these areas and into better-quality neighbourhoods.

Studies of ethnic communities provide explanations for the residential segregation pattern described by Burgess. When immigrants first settle in a new country, they stay close to their compatriots in order to ease the adjustment process (Portes and Sensenbrenner 1993; Piore 1979). Strong ethnic networks can provide financial, social, and emotional support. As immigrants stay in the country longer, they establish their own networks. At the same time, their attachment to their ethnic group may decrease. At that point they feel less need to stay in the established ethnic community and have more motivation to move out (Alba et al. 1997).

The third explanation for racial and ethnic residential segregation patterns suggests that these patterns reflect differences in the socio-economic resources of groups (Massey 1981; Clark 1986). Because residential locations are associated with a variety of resources, such as schools, housing, services, and job opportunities, they differentiate the life chances of the groups. Thus once families improve their socio-economic situation, they seek neighbourhoods with better qualities. Yet in any society, for various sociohistorical reasons, different groups have different socio-economic resources. Groups with fewer socio-economic resources are less competitive in the housing market. Thus when other groups move into neighbourhoods with better qualities, they are left behind. They are less able to move into and share the more desirable neighbourhoods with the other groups (Fong 1997b).

Given that the residential segregation patterns of racial and ethnic groups reflect various aspects of race and ethnic relations, I will discuss the residential segregation of visible minority groups in Toronto. I will focus on visible minority groups because their populations have been growing rapidly as Toronto has become increasingly diversified racially and ethnically. There is extensive literature on racial residential patterns, yet there have been only a few analyses of the racial residential patterns of visible minorities in Toronto, and all of these have been descriptive in nature.

Residential Segregation in Toronto

As Toronto increased its population size and its racial and ethnic diversity at in the beginning of the twentieth century, its segregation levels also rose (Herberg 1989). These levels have become relatively high compared to other Canadian cities. For instance, using the 1981 census data, Balakrishnan and Selvanathan (1990) have documented that Toronto has the second-highest mean segregation scores for all major racial and ethnic groups among the major Canadian census metropolitan areas (CMAs).

Research has also found that segregation levels among racial and ethnic groups in Toronto vary substantially. Until recently, most studies focused on the segregation patterns of European groups before 1980. Visible minorities represented a small proportion of the population, and information about their segregation patterns was limited. Recent studies are beginning to include visible minority groups such as Asians and blacks (Balakrishnan 1976, 1982; Balakrishnan and Selvanathan

1990; Fong 1996, 1997a, 1997b). The results in general show that both these groups experience higher levels of residential segregation from the Charter groups than do other European groups. South Asians in particular usually experience high levels of segregation, similar to those of blacks.

Most studies that explain the differences in residential segregation patterns do not focus on Toronto but explore general patterns of major Canadian cities. Thus, Balakrishnan (1982) posited the importance of social distance among groups. He compared the segregation levels of groups in various Canadian cities and identified persistent residential segregation patterns among groups that corresponded closely to their social distance. Since visible minority groups are at the bottom of the social hierarchy and the Charter groups are at the top, their residential segregation levels are high. In recent studies using the 1991 census (Fong 1997b) found that blacks and South and Southeast Asians have lower levels of spatial contact with the Charter groups, controlling for socio-economic and demographic variables. Similarly, Fong and and Gulia (1997, 1999) found that these two groups must pay higher prices than whites to live in neighbourhoods with similar amenities. Fong and his colleagues suggested some possible effects of social distance among groups on the attainment of neighbourhood qualities. However, these studies did not directly or explicitly explore how social distance affects the segregation patterns of visible minority groups.

Another account of the residential segregation patterns of minority groups focused on levels of social integration, which usually are measured by nativity or the length of time since immigration. Fong (1997b) showed that the proportion of immigrants in a group substantially affects the group's spatial contact with Charter groups. Even among minority groups, members who have been in the country for a longer time usually encounter lower levels of segregation from other groups. However, a detailed multivariate study by Fong and Wilkes (1999) showed that among blacks, the effects of length of time in the country on the improvement of neighbourhood qualities become insignificant when other factors are controlled. In addition, Kalbach (1990) obtained mixed results when he compared the segregation levels of major ethnic groups across generations. He found a gradual decline in segregation levels for successive generations of older European immigrant groups (that is, the Charter groups, northern Europeans, and southern Europeans). However, this general pattern of decline did not apply to recent European immigrants (such as southern and eastern Europeans) or to visible minority groups. Taken as a whole, the empirical evidence suggests that the effects of social integration may apply more to Charter groups and older immigrant groups than to others.

Studies in the United States have identified the importance of a group's socio-economic resources in determining its residential segregation level; however, the impact is not as significant for residential patterns in major Canadian cities (Fong 1996). An early study by Darroch and Marston (1972), based on the 1961 census, showed that the education, occupations, and income of groups explained only very small proportions of residential segregation among groups. In a series of studies based on unique data from the 1986 and 1991 censuses, Fong and his colleagues developed causal models to disentangle the residential segregation patterns of major racial and ethnic groups (Fong and Gulia 1994, 1997, 1999; Fong 1996). They found repeatedly that the effects of socio-economic resources on residential patterns in Canadian cities are insignificant for all groups, including visible minority groups. However, studies by Balakrishnan (1982) and Balakrishnan and Selvanathan (1990) offered a different picture. They discovered a consistent effect of socio-economic resources on residential segregation patterns between 1961 and 1981. Comparing the dissimilarity indexes of census tracts with different socio-economic status, they found segregation levels to be lower in tracts with higher socio-economic status.

It is in this context of mixed research findings and scant information about the residential segregation of visible minority groups in Toronto that I examine the patterns and test the effects of social distance, social integration, and social mobility on the residential segregation patterns of these groups.

Data and Methods

Data for this study were obtained from specially requested tables of the 1996 Canadian census (Statistics Canada 1998). These tables provide detailed socio-economic and demographic information about major racial and ethnic groups. The central purpose of this paper is to compare the residential patterns of these groups. To do so, I have used the census tract as the unit of analysis. Tracts are small areas with an average of four thousand residents. They are drawn to maximize socio-economic homogeneity and are the closest approximation to 'neighbourhoods.'

The major racial and ethnic groups included in the study are British, French, northern European, western European, eastern European, southern European, East and Southeast Asian, South Asian, and black. Among all these groups, special attention will be given to visible minority groups, including East and Southeast Asians, South Asians, and blacks. Asians are treated as two separate groups because of their different social and cultural backgrounds. For all groups except British and French, I use broad categories (such as East and Southeast Asians) rather than specific ethnic groups (such as Koreans) because using broad geographic locations minimizes the likelihood of suppression due to confidentiality. Statistics Canada requires the suppression of all information about groups in a geographic unit if their number is smaller than fifty. I am confident about using the broader geographic designations because past studies have shown that the housing experiences of specific ethnic groups from the same geographic locations are similar (Balakrishnan 1982; Balakrishnan and Selvanathan 1990).

To measure the level of residential segregation, I used the index of dissimilarity, which measures the uneven distribution of two groups. Despite some reviews that have identified limitations of the index, it has been widely used over the past several decades (Pielou 1977; Zoloth 1976). One major advantage is that the index is easy to interpret (White 1986). In addition, the dissimilarity index allows the results obtained from this study to be directly compared with the results obtained from past studies using the same index.

The index is calculated as follows:

$$D = \frac{1}{2} \sum_{i=1}^{n} \left| \frac{X_i}{X} - \frac{Y_i}{Y} \right|$$

where X_i and Y_i are the populations of group X and Y in tract i. X and Y are the total populations of group X and Y in the city. The value of the index indicates the percentage of a group that would have to relocate to achieve the same percentage as its distribution in the city. The index ranges from 0 to 100. Total segregation is reflected in the maximum value (that is, 100); a completely unsegregated situation yields a value of 0.

Results

Table 3.1 presents the dissimilarity index for major racial and ethnic groups in Toronto. Although these statistics represent the residential segregation patterns of visible minorities in the city, our discussion

Table 3.1. Residential segregation of major racial and ethnic groups in Toronto, 1996

	British	French	Northern Europeans	Western Europeans	Eastern Europeans	Southern Europeans	East & Southeast Asians	South Asians	Blacks
British		13.1	33.3	16.6	38.3	47.8	52.5	55.7	52.2
French			35.2	20.9	37.5	46.2	50.0	53.8	50.0
Northern Europeans				35.0	47.0	56.4	54.9	61.7	59.1
Western Europeans					38.7	47.0	53.0	56.5	53.5
Eastern Europeans						45.0	49.9	54.7	52.1
Southern Europeans							48.6	48.7	45.0
East & Southeast Asians								41.8	43.4
South Asians									30.4

Source: 1996 Canadian Census, specially requested table.

focuses on the residential patterns of these groups. The table reveals two interesting findings. First, there are pronounced residential segregation levels between visible minority groups and the Charter groups and northern Europeans and western Europeans. The lowest segregation level between visible minority groups and any of these groups is 50 (French vs blacks; French vs East and Southeast Asians); the highest is 62. Second, the results also show that the segregation levels of eastern and southern Europeans from Asians and blacks are all above 45 – slightly lower than those of the Charter groups and northern and western Europeans. Although the periods of arrival of these groups (eastern Europeans, southern Europeans, Asians, and blacks) were close, they have still experienced high levels of residential segregation along racial lines.

Although our study is about the residential segregation of visible minority groups, I would like to point out a few important patterns among European groups that provide a context for understanding the patterns of visible minority groups. Segregation levels among the Charter groups and northern and western Europeans are low, ranging from 13 to 35. In addition, there are moderate levels of residential segregation of the Charter groups and northern and western Europeans from eastern and southern Europeans. Among these groups, the lowest value of the segregation index is 37.5 (eastern Europeans vs French), and the highest reaches 56.4 (southern vs northern Europeans). The results suggest that northern and western Europeans share similar residential patterns but also that their residential patterns are different from those of southern and eastern Europeans.

It is reasonable to suspect that these patterns indicate the effects of the groups' social integration. Asians and blacks are the most recently arrived groups, followed by southern and eastern Europeans. The average years of arrival among members of the Charter groups and northern and western Europeans were earlier than for any other group. The results closely correspond to length of time in Canada: for Asians and blacks, segregation levels are high with the earlier groups, moderate with southern and eastern Europeans. However, one can argue against this hypothesis about the effects of social integration on residential segregation patterns because the close arrival periods of southern and eastern Europeans vis-à-vis Asians and blacks should not result in their high levels of segregation from one another. The patterns may equally well reflect the socio-economic resources of groups. The relatively lower socio-economic resources of blacks and Asians may affect their ability to move into neighbourhoods with the Charter groups and northern and western Europeans. The patterns may also reflect a stable hierarchy of social distance among groups. According to past studies, visible minorities (Asians and blacks) are at the bottom of the social hierarchy, followed by southern and eastern Europeans (Pineo 1977). The Charter groups and northern and western Europeans are at the top.

The Prevalence of Residential Segregation among Visible Minorities

The first table documents consistently higher levels of residential segregation of visible minority groups (Asians and blacks) from the Charter groups and other European groups. To further assess the prevalence of residential segregation among visible minority groups in Toronto, I report the proportion of visible minorities living in neighbourhoods with different concentration levels (more than 30, 50 and 70 per cent) of non-visible minority groups. To simplify the presentation I have combined the Charter groups and all European groups into one category labelled 'whites.' I have then created two subcategories: 'old European immigrant groups' are the two Charter groups and northern and western Europeans, whereas 'new European immigrant groups' include southern and eastern Europeans. These two categories reflect the results of Table 3.1: the two Charter groups and northern and western Europeans share similar residential patterns that are uniquely different from those of eastern and southern Europeans. The last two columns in the table show the percentage of visible minorities living in old and new European immigrant neighbourhoods. I define neighbourhoods as old European immigrant neighbourhoods when the concentration of old immigrant groups in the tract is more than half their percentage in the city. The same criterion was used to define new European immigrant neighbourhoods.

The second to fourth columns in Table 3.2 give the average percentages of the three visible minority groups in neighbourhoods with different percentages of whites. The results show a very clear picture. As the percentage of whites living in neighbourhoods rises, the percentages of visible minorities drastically shrink. For example, in neighbourhoods where whites are more than 30 per cent, the average percentage of South Asians is 6 per cent. The percentage drops to 1 per cent in neighbourhoods where whites are more than 70 per cent – a reduction of 75 per cent. Similarly, the presence of blacks decreases from 5 per cent in neighbourhoods with more than 30 per cent white population to

Table 3.2. Distribution of visible minority groups in neighbourhoods by percentages of white in Toronto, 1996

	Average	White > 30%	White > 50%	White > 70%	Old European immigrant groups	New European immigrant groups
East & Southeast Asians	11.7	8.8	5.9	3.0	10.8	13.6
South Asians	6.8	5.5	3.1	1.4	5.6	8.6
Blacks	5.9	5.1	3.3	1.3	4.9	7.9

Source: 1996 Canadian Census, specially requested table.

1 per cent in neighbourhoods with more than 70 per cent white population. Given the difficulties visible minorities have in gaining access to
predominantly white neighbourhoods, it is not surprising to find other
research in Canada which shows that visible minorities must pay high
prices to live in neighbourhoods with higher proportions of whites
(Fong 1997a).

The last two columns break the white population into old and new
European immigrant groups. The results show that lower percentages
of Asians and blacks live in neighbourhoods with predominantly old
European immigrant groups than in neighbourhoods with new European immigrant groups. When we fold these findings into the results
reported in Table 3.1, we see that even when visible minority groups
share neighbourhoods with whites, a smaller proportion of them live in
neighbourhoods with the old European immigrant groups that have
been in Canada for a longer time and that are socially and culturally
established. This segregation between old immigrant groups and visible minority groups in the city suggests that it may be difficult for visible
minority groups to achieve full participation in the larger society and to
share neighbourhoods with the more established groups in Canada.

Distribution of Visible Minorities in Toronto

Our analyses so far only show the levels of residential segregation; they
do not reveal the geographic distribution or the locations where the
racial and ethnic groups reside. This information is important because
it provides a glimpse of the desirability and accessibility of the locations
where groups reside. In the following discussion I present two series of
maps. The first shows the distribution of groups in the city of Toronto
and neighbouring suburbs. The second displays the distribution of
groups in the Toronto CMA designated by Statistics Canada. The area
covered is much larger since it includes the outer suburbs of Toronto. To
facilitate this discussion, I have classified census tracts into three types:
a particular group's population in the tract is either 4 per cent above its
city distribution, or 0 to 4 per cent above its city distribution, or below
its city distribution. These classifications can be interpreted as high,
moderate, and low concentrations of a group in the tract.

Figure 3.1 shows the distribution of East and Southeast Asians in the
city of Toronto and neighbouring suburbs. Most East and Southeast
Asians live in middle-class suburbs such as Markham and Scarborough
or near the downtown area of Toronto. Those living in the middle-class

Figure 3.1. Distribution of East and Southeast Asians in City of Toronto and
neighbouring suburbs, 1996

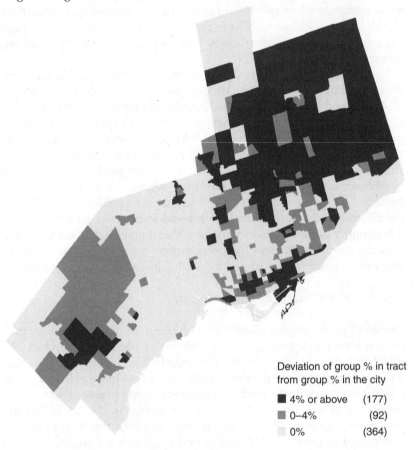

Deviation of group % in tract
from group % in the city

■ 4% or above   (177)
▨ 0–4%   (92)
▢ 0%   (364)

Source: 1996 Census, specially requested table.

suburbs may represent recent immigrants from Hong Kong, Taiwan,
and Korea who have financial resources. East and Southeast Asians are
highly concentrated in a few locations. About 177 of the 633 census
tracts have a proportion of East and Southeast Asians that is 4 per cent
or more than their city proportion. The number of such tracts is much
higher for other groups. Most South Asians, as shown in figure 3.2, live
in middle-class suburbs such as Mississauga; however, a closer look
suggests that most of them live in relatively poorer areas of these

Figure 3.2. Distribution of South Asians in city of Toronto and neighbouring suburbs, 1996

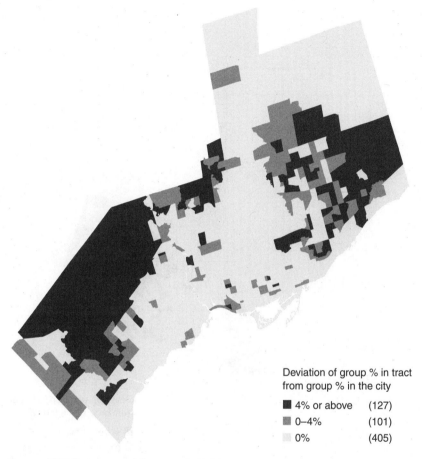

Deviation of group % in tract
from group % in the city

■ 4% or above   (127)
■ 0–4%   (101)
  0%   (405)

Source: 1996 Census, specially requested table.

suburbs, such as southern Scarborough. This suggests that their socio-economic resources may be limited. Figures 3.3 and 3.4 show clearly that both Asian groups are underrepresented in the outer suburbs.

Figures 3.5 and 3.6 show the distribution of blacks. Figure 3.5 shows that blacks are scattered in diverse areas of Toronto. These areas are always associated with poorer amenities, echoing Fong and Shibuya's earlier finding (2000) that poor blacks are highly segregated in Canadian cities. These maps also reveal that blacks are underrepresented in

Figure 3.3. Distribution of East and Southeast Asians in Toronto Metropolitan Area, 1996

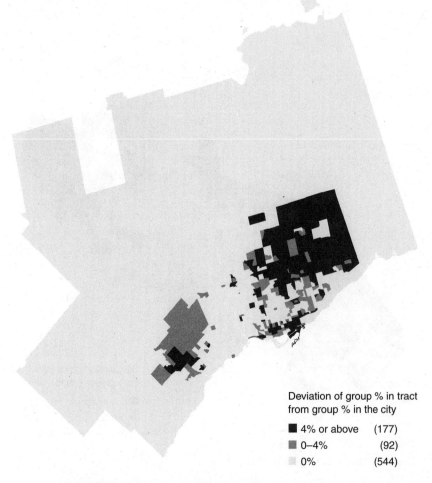

Deviation of group % in tract
from group % in the city

■ 4% or above   (177)
▨ 0–4%   (92)
▢ 0%   (544)

Source: 1996 Census, specially requested table.

more affluent suburbs such as North York and Richmond Hill. Figure 3.6 shows that blacks, like other visible minorities, are underrepresented in the outer suburbs.

In sum, these maps present a diverse geographic distribution of visible minority groups in Toronto. East and Southeast Asians are highly concentrated in middle-class communities and the downtown area; South Asians are living in poor pockets of suburbs; blacks are scattered

Figure 3.4. Distribution of South Asians in Toronto CMA, 1996

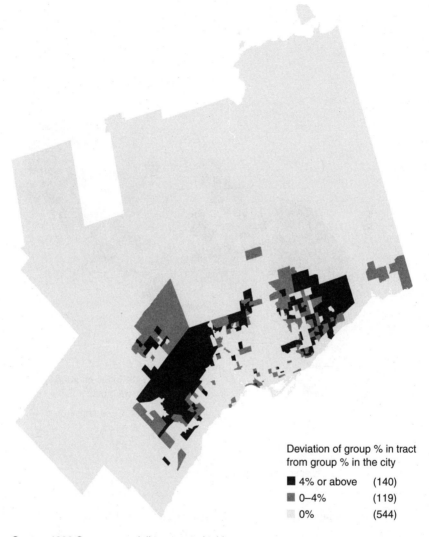

Deviation of group % in tract
from group % in the city

■ 4% or above   (140)
■ 0–4%   (119)
  0%   (544)

Source: 1996 Census, specially requested table.

in poor neighbourhoods in different parts of the city. Clearly, visible
minority groups are not living in the outer suburbs. All of this suggests
significant variations in the residential patterns of visible minority
groups. To thoroughly examine the residential patterns of groups, I
now turn to a multivariate causal analysis.

Figure 3.5. Distribution of blacks in City of Toronto and neighbouring suburbs, 1996

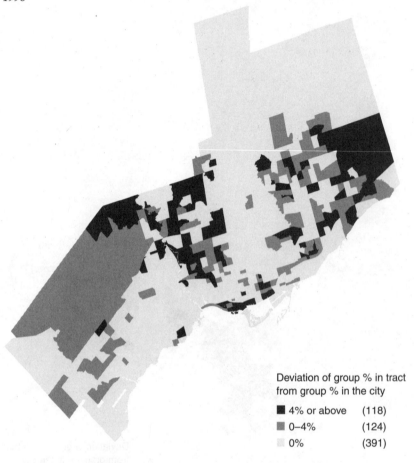

Deviation of group % in tract
from group % in the city

■ 4% or above   (118)
■ 0–4%   (124)
  0%   (391)

Source: 1996 Census, specially requested table.

The Relative Importance of Social Distance, Social Integration, and Social Mobility

Past analyses have suggested the possible effects of social integration, social distance, and social mobility on the residential patterns of visible minority groups in Toronto. However, the relative importance of these factors has yet to be determined. In this section I develop causal models to compare their relevance.

Figure 3.6. Distribution of blacks in Toronto CMA, 1996

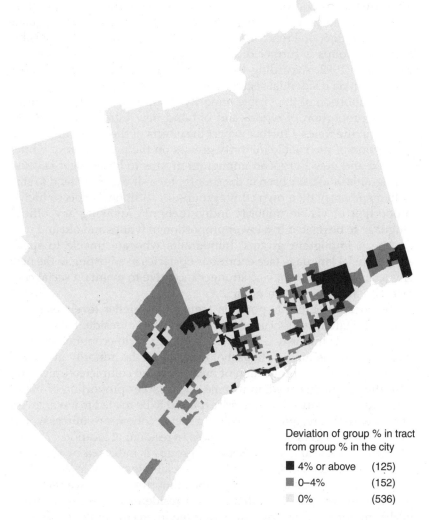

Deviation of group % in tract
from group % in the city

■ 4% or above   (125)
■ 0–4%   (152)
  0%   (536)

Source: 1996 Census, specially requested table.

I compare the effects of the three possible factors on the residential segregation levels of visible minority groups. The dependent variables are the proportion of whites, older European immigrant groups, and new European immigrant groups. I have included three sets of independent variables in order to capture the possible effects of social integration, social mobility, and social distance. The first set of variables is intended to measure the social integration of visible minority groups. They are the proportion of minority groups in the tract who are immigrants and the proportion who do not know either official language (that is, English or French). The immigrant population of the visible minority groups is further differentiated into the proportion who arrived after 1992. According to the discussion of the effects of social integration on residential segregation, one would expect a larger immigrant proportion of the visible minority group to be associated with a smaller proportion of whites and old and new European immigrant groups in the tracts. I further expect the effects of the recent immigrant proportion of the visible minority groups on the proportion of whites and old and new European immigrant groups to be stronger because immigrants who have been in the country for a short period tend to stay with members of their own ethnic groups. In addition, I expect a higher proportion of visible minority individuals not knowing any official language to be related to a lower proportion of whites and old and new European immigrant groups. Immigrants who are unable to speak either official language face enormous obstacles in adjusting to the new environment, so they have a stronger incentive to maintain social contact with their ethnic community.

The social mobility hypothesis argues that higher levels of socio-economic status are associated with lower levels of residential segregation for visible minority groups. In this study, socio-economic status is measured by the median household income of the minority groups in the tract and by the proportion of members who completed university education. A higher median income and a larger proportion of members with university education are expected to be related to lower levels of residential segregation. More group socio-economic resources would imply that members have more choices in residential location.

Finally, the social distance between groups is indicated by the intercept of the model. Once we control for social integration levels and for the socio-economic status of the visible minority groups, we can interpret the intercept as the initial level of residential segregation of the visible minority group. By comparing the intercepts of the models for different groups, we will be able to see the relative distance of each visible minority group with whites, older European immigrant groups, and newer European immigrant groups.

In Table 3.3 I present the results of a set of regression equations that estimate the effects of the three proposed factors (social integration, socio-economic status, and social distance) on the proportion of whites,

Table 3.3. Estimated coefficients for selective variables on proportion of whites, old European immigrant groups, and newer European immigrant groups in Toronto neighbourhoods, 1996

	Proportion of whites	Proportion of old European immigrant groups	Proportion of new European groups
East and Southeast Asians			
Median education	0.121*	0.255**	−0.147**
Median income	0.002	0.027	0.001
Prop. not knowing English/French	−0.173**	−0.190**	0.024
Prop. immigrants	−0.318**	−0.433**	0.123*
Prop. recent immigrants (arrived after 1992)	−0.259**	−0.145**	−0.111*
Intercept	0.736**	0.561**	0.160**
R²	0.214	0.314	0.022
N	733	733	733
South Asians			
Median education	0.097**	0.175**	−0.078*
Median income	−0.003	−0.001	−0.000
Prop. not knowing English/French	−0.039	−0.177*	-0.177*
Prop. immigrants	−0.111**	−0.086*	−0.025
Prop. recent immigrants (arrived after 1992)	−0.154**	−0.138**	-0.016**
Intercept	0.586**	0.346**	0.306**
R²	0.059	0.114	0.019
N	733	733	733
Blacks			
Median education	0.138**	0.178**	−0.036
Median income	−0.008**	0.002	−0.040
Prop. not knowing English/French	−0.755*	−0.953**	0.198
Prop. immigrants	−0.116**	−0.172**	0.056
Prop. recent immigrants (arrived after 1992)	0.004	−0.244**	0.248**
Intercept	0.572**	0.399**	−0.173**
R²	0.043	0.135	0.065
N	733	733	733

Note: p** < 0.05; p*< 0.1
Source: 1996 Canadian Census, specially requested table.

the proportion of old European immigrant groups, and the proportion of newer European immigrant groups in the neighbourhoods. I ran separate models for each visible minority group. The results can be used to compare the possibly different effects of social integration, socio-economic status, and social distance on the residential patterns of visible minority groups.

The first column delineates the results of the models for the proportion of whites. There is strong and significant support of the social integration hypothesis for East and Southeast Asians. For those two groups, all three variables intended to capture the effects of social integration (proportion of group members not knowing any official language, proportion of immigrants, and proportion of recent immigrants) are negatively related to the proportion of whites. For the two other groups – South Asians and blacks – not all three variables are related to the proportion of whites. However, the effects of any of the social integration variables that are related to the proportion of whites are markedly strong. Although the literature suggests that income and education should be positively related to the proportion of whites in the neighbourhood, results show that for all three visible minority groups, only education is significant (moderately) to the proportion of whites in the neighbourhood.

Since the intercept of the model can be interpreted as the beginning segregation level of the visible minority group, the comparison of intercepts among models identifies the relative social distance of the three visible minority groups from whites. The results of this analysis correspond to the relative social distances of the three visible minority groups documented in other studies: both South Asians and blacks have distinctively disadvantaged beginning levels compared to East and Southeast Asians.

In columns 2 and 3, I further compare the effects of social integration, socio-economic status, and social distance at the spatial contact level with old and newer European immigrant groups. The comparison shows the relative importance of the three proposed factors on residential patterns for visible minority groups with whites who arrived in different time periods.

In general, the results in column 2 reflect a consistently strong effect of social integration and a moderate effect of socio-economic resources on the spatial contact between older immigrant groups and visible minorities. All visible minority groups with higher levels of education, lower proportions of members not knowing any official language, lower proportions of immigrants, and lower proportions of recent immigrants have increased levels of spatial contact with older European immigrant groups. A closer look suggests that most of the effects of socio-economic variables on the proportion of old European immigrant groups are consistently stronger when compared with the previous models. When the intercepts of all three visible minority groups are compared, the results show a similar picture: both South Asians and blacks are at more disadvantaged beginning levels of spatial contact with older European immigrant groups than are East and Southeast Asians.

Column 3 shows a different picture. The level of social integration is not always related to the proportion of new European immigrant groups in the neighbourhoods. A higher proportion of immigrants and a higher proportion of recent immigrants – if the effects are statistically significant – are not always related to lower proportions of new European immigrant groups. Similar patterns are also found with the socio-economic variables. Even when socio-economic variables are related to the proportion of newer European immigrant groups, they are not in the expected direction.

Taken together, the results show a clear picture. Groups with higher socio-economic status and integration levels are associated with higher proportions of whites in the neighbourhoods. In other words, the socio-economic and social integration levels of a visible minority group explain its residential patterns. Some visible minority groups face disadvantaged beginning positions in improving their residential integration with whites; this corresponds to their social distance from whites in society. However, when the analysis further compares the old and newer European immigrant groups, the results reveal that these relationships only apply to the older groups. The findings regarding spatial contact between new European immigrant groups and visible minority groups give another picture: Socio-economic status is not necessarily related to the proportion of new European immigrants, and a higher proportion of immigrants in the visible minority group is related to a higher proportion of newer European immigrant groups in the neighbourhoods.

Conclusion

This chapter documented the residential segregation levels of visible minority groups, the fastest-growing and newest immigrant groups in Toronto. Based on the 1996 census data, results show that the residential segregation levels of visible minority groups are higher with the older European immigrant groups than with recent European immigrant groups. The extent of segregation in the city between the old immigrant groups and visible minority groups suggests that it may be difficult for visible minority groups to achieve full participation in the larger society and to share neighbourhoods with the more established groups in Canada. The results also suggest significant variations in the geographic distribution of the visible minority groups. East and Southeast Asians are highly concentrated in middle-class communities and the down-town area; South Asians are living in poor pockets of suburbs; blacks are scattered in different parts of the city where poor neighbourhoods are usually found. Visible minority groups clearly are not living in the outer suburbs. The information suggests substantial differences in the residential patterns of visible minority groups.

To disentangle the factors affecting the residential segregation levels of visible minority groups, I examined their social integration levels, socio-economic status, and social distance from other groups. The data indicate that all three processes are operating. First, the effects of social integration on the residential segregation of visible minority groups are strong and consistent. The results suggest that as visible minority groups – especially old European groups – stay in the country longer, their residential segregation levels from European groups decline. However, this optimistic picture is blurred by another major finding in the study – the social distances among groups also play a significant role in the residential patterns of visible minority groups. South Asians and blacks at the bottom of the social hierarchy are in a more disadvantaged position in the beginning process of residential integration. Finally, the results show that socio-economic resources affect the residential segre-gation levels of visible minority groups. However, this effect is more applicable in relation to old European immigrant groups than to new European immigrant groups.

The data form a complex picture. On the one hand, as visible minor-ity groups stay in the country longer, their residential segregation levels from European groups decline. On the other hand, the spatial integra-tion processes for some visible minority groups are hampered by their social distance from European groups. The evidence suggests that the spatial integration processes of visible minority groups do not rely solely on their ability to integrate and their socio-economic achieve-ments, but rather depend on other factors – such as social distance from other groups – that are beyond their control.

NOTE

The research was supported by a grant from the Social Sciences and Humanities Research Council of Canada.

REFERENCES

Alba, Richard D., John R. Logan, and Kyle Crowder. 1997. 'White Ethnic Neighborhoods and Assimilation: The Greater New York Region, 1980–1990.' *Social Forces* 75: 883–912.
Balakrishnan, T.R. 1982. 'Changing Patterns of Ethnic Residential Segregation in the Metropolitan Areas of Canada.' *Canadian Review of Sociology and Anthropology* 19:92–110.
– 1976. 'Ethnic Residential Segregation in the Metropolitan Areas of Canada.' *Canadian Journal of Sociology* 1:481–98.
Balakrishnan, T.R., and K. Selvanathan. 1990. 'Ethnic Residential Segregation in Metropolitan Canada.' Pp. 393–413 in *Ethnic Demography*, ed. Shiver S. Halli, Frank Trovato, and Leo Driedger. Ottawa: Carlton University Press.
Burgess, Ernest W. 1967. 'The Growth of the City: An Introduction to a Research Project.' Pp. 47–62 in *The City*, ed. Robert E. Park, Ernest W. Burgess, and Roderick D. McKenzie. Chicago IL: University of Chicago Press.
Clark, William A.V. 1991. 'Residential Preferences and Neighborhood Racial Segregation: A Test of the Schelling Segregation Model.' *Demography* 28:1–20.
– 1986. 'Residential Segregation in American Cities: A Review and Interpretation.' *Population Research and Policy Review* 5:95–127.
Darroch, Gordon A., and Wilfred G. Marston. 1971. 'The Social Class Basis of Ethnic Residential Segregation: The Canadian Case.' *American Journal of Sociology* 77:491–510.
Farley, Reynolds, Howard Schuman, Suzanne Bianchi, Diane Colasanto, and Shirley Hatchett. 1978. 'Chocolate City, Vanilla Suburbs: Will the Trend toward Racially Separate Communities Continue?' *Social Science Research* 7:319–44.
Fong, Eric. 1997a. 'A Systemic Approach to Racial Residential Patterns.' *Social Science Research* 26:465–86.
– 1997b. 'Residential Proximity with the Charter Groups in Canada.' *Canadian Studies in Population* 24(2):103–24.
– 1996. 'A Comparative Perspective of Racial Residential Segregation: American and Canadian Experiences.' *Sociological Quarterly* 37:501–28.

Fong, Eric, and Milena Gulia. 1999. 'Differences in Neighborhood Qualities among Major Racial/Ethnic Groups in Canada.' *Sociological Inquiry* 69(4):575–98.

– 1997. 'The Effects of Group Characteristics and City Contexts on Neighborhood Qualities of Racial and Ethnic Groups.' *Canadian Studies in Population* 24:45–66.

– 1994. 'Residential Proximity among Racial Groups in American and Canadian Neighborhoods.' *Urban Affairs Quarterly* 30:285–97.

Fong, Eric, and Kumiko Shibuya. 2000. 'Spatial Separation of the Poor in Canadian Cities.' *Demography* 37(4):449–59

Fong, Eric, and Rima Wilkes. 1999. 'An Examination of Spatial Assimilation Model.' *International Migration Review* 33:594–620.

Herberg, Edward N. 1989. *Ethnic Groups in Canada: Adaptations and Transitions*. Scarborough, ON: Nelson Canada.

Jackman, Mary R. and Marie Crane. 1986. "Some of my best friends are black ...": Interracial Friendship and Whites' Racial Attitudes.' *Public Opinion Quarterly* 50:459–86.

Kalbach, Warren E. 1990. 'Ethnic Residential Segregation and Its Significance for the Individual in an Urban Setting.' Pp. 92–134 in *Ethnic Identity and Inequality*, ed. Raymond Breton, Wsevolod W. Isajiew, Warren E. Kalbach, and Jeffrey G. Reitz. Toronto: University of Toronto Press.

Kasarda, John D. 1989. 'Urban Industrial Transition and the Underclass.' *American Academy of Political and Social Science* 501:26–47.

Massey, Douglas S. 1981. 'Social Class and Ethnic Segregation.' *American Sociological Review* 46:641–50.

Massey, Douglas S., and Nancy A. Denton. 1993. *American Apartheid: Segregation and the Making of the Underclass*. Cambridge, MA: Harvard University Press.

Massey, Douglas S., and Eric Fong. 1990. 'Segregation and Neighborhood Quality: Blacks, Hispanics, and Asians in the San Francisco Metropolitan Area.' *Social Forces* 69:55–75.

Massey, Douglas S., and Brendan P. Mullan. 1984. 'Processes of Hispanic and Black Spatial Assimilation.' *American Journal of Sociology* 89:836–71.

Massey, Douglas S. and Kumiko Shibuya. 1995. 'Unraveling the Tangle of Pathology: The Effect of Spatially Concentrated Joblessness on the Well-Being of African Americans.' *Social Science Research* 24:352–66.

Park, Robert E. 1967. 'The City: Suggestions for the Investigation of Human Behavior in the Urban Environment.' Pp. 1–46 in *The City*, ed. Robert E. Park, Ernest W. Burgess, and Roderick D. McKenzie. Chicago: University of Chicago Press.

Pielou, E.C. 1997. *Mathematical Ecology*. New York: Wiley.

Pineo, Peter C. 1977. 'The Social Standing of Ethnic and Racial Groupings.' *Canadian Review of Sociology and Anthropology* 14:147–57.

Piore, Michael. 1979. *Birds of Passage: Migrant Labor and Industrial Societies*. New York: Cambridge University Press.

Portes, Alejandro, and Julia Sensenbrenner. 1993. 'Embeddedness and Immigration: Notes on the Social Determinants of Economic Action.' *American Journal of Sociology* 98:1320–50.

Sigleman, Lee, Timothy Bledsoe, Susan Welch, and Michael W. Combs. 1996.'Making Contact? Black–White Social Interaction in an Urban Setting.' *American Journal of Sociology* 101:1306–32.

Schelling, T. 1971. 'Dynamic Models of Segregation.' *Journal of Mathematical Sociology* 1:143–86.

Statistics Canada. 1998. *1996 Census Custom Data – Job E00352*. Toronto: Statistics Canada.

White, Michael. 1987. *American Neighborhoods and Residential Differentiation*. New York: Russell Sage Foundation.

– 1986. 'Segregation and Diversity Measures in Population Distribution.' *Population Index* 52:198–221.

Wilson, William Julius. 1987. *The Truly Disadvantaged*. Chicago: University of Chicago Press.

Zoloth, B.S. 1976. 'Alternative Measures of School Segregation.' *Land Economics* 52:278–98.

4 Metropolitan Government and the Social Ecology of Minority Residential Distribution: The Experience of Metropolitan Toronto

WILLIAM MICHELSON

The postwar suburbanization of Toronto sheds light on how the particular implementation of a two-tiered metropolitan government had a surprising impact on minority residential distributions, which now differ greatly from those in other countries and in different circumstances. This example of social ecological dynamics, in which many factors interacted, suggests that to explain minority residential patterns we must understand the unique combination of circumstances in individual cities.

Toronto is interesting, first, for the extent of its recent immigration. 'The United Nations has designated Toronto as the world's "most ethnically-diverse city"'(Tourism Toronto 1997). It has evolved to the point where no ethnic group constitutes a majority; in 1991 nearly three-quarters of the residents of the Toronto Census Metropolitan Area (CMA) identified themselves as having a single or dual ethnic origin among almost eighty origins other than simple British or Canadian ethnicity (calculated from Statistics Canada 1994).

Toronto is interesting in quite another way. This city has been the object of intensive experimentation in municipal government, including what was widely regarded as a successful implementation of metropolitan government when it was in force.

In the postwar years, largely under the structure of this metropolitan governance structure, rapid suburbanization and population growth occurred, as a result of both immigration and in-migration. What happened with patterns of minority residential distribution in these circumstances? To what extent can one attribute these growth and settlement patterns to the presence of metropolitan government? Surely Toronto's unique metropolitan government and its implications for attracting and accommodating immigrants in particular locations served as the context for immigration of an unprecedented nature and amount, above and beyond the traditionally potent locational factors of social integration, socio-economic status, and social distance from other groups (see Fong in chapter 3).

This is not a simple matter of cause and effect, nor is it a claim that a form of government unilaterally brought about a particular form of minority population distribution in a deterministic way. I view this analysis as a form of social ecology in that the relationships among Toronto's attributes are complex and interactive and require consideration of a number of additional factors if we are to understand them. This chapter describes the patterns of minority residential distribution during an era of large-scale immigration and widespread suburbanization, and also explores how these patterns emerged in the way that they did in this time and place.

Do Municipal Boundaries Matter?

Is it plausible to examine minority residential distribution with respect to formal aspects of municipal structure such as the nature and extent of urban boundaries? With the expansion of communication and transportation technology in recent decades, sociologists are beginning to view specific municipalities in a region as anachronisms. However, Weiher (1991) has published a corrective to the notion that local areas are declining in significance. His research, which focused on small municipalities in suburban St Louis, examined the extent to which local municipalities maintain and reinforce unique images and packages of activities that attract distinct populations. Boundaries serve to contain qualities and processes: 'Indeed, because of the certainty with which these units are defined, and the interaction that such precise boundaries encourage between geography, political power and publicly provided services, economic activity, and the social characteristics of residents, political boundaries are quite instrumental in creating place identity' (60).

Do boundaries of even larger metropolitan or regional areas represent meaningful entities? Many observers doubt it. This empirical question was put to the test in a study in and around Toronto (Michelson 1997; Popenoe & Michelson 2002).[1] A telephone survey was conducted of 904 randomly selected households in the Municipality of Metropolitan Toronto (commonly referred to as 'Metro') and two contiguous

Figure 4.1. Perceived impacts of municipality, ethnicity, and religion on outcomes (percentage respondents choosing 'some' or 'a lot' of impact) (n = 904)

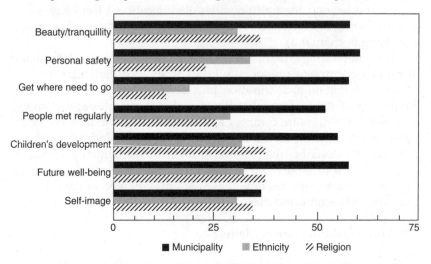

regional municipalities, Durham and York. In comparing their own regional municipality to those nearby, the respondents declared that their own areas were unique. Moreover, they stated very strongly that their regional municipality made a difference in their daily lives, both in general and with respect to specific aspects of their lives. The differences people attributed to their regional municipality were considerably greater than those they attributed to some crucial social characteristics of the sort protected by law: religion and race/ethnicity. Figure 4.1 plots the percentage of respondents who attributed 'some' or 'a lot of' impact on selected aspects of everyday life to municipal place of residence, religion, and national/ethnic origin. Much more impact was accorded to municipal place of residence than to the others on six of seven aspects: beauty or tranquillity, personal safety, get where you need to go, kind of people met on a regular basis, children's development, and future well-being. And in each of these cases a plurality said that municipal place of residence had 'a lot' of impact. In most of the breakdowns having to do with religion and national/ethnic origin, an absolute majority felt that these personal characteristics had 'no impact at all' on these aspects of life.

Part of the reason why respondents felt that metropolitan and regional municipalities are salient may lie in the leverage each offers to control factors that bear on quality of life. More respondents said they had the most control over decisions at the level of the metropolitan/ regional municipality; fewer than half picked the provincial and federal levels combined.

Thus even places as large as regional municipalities are viewed as tangible, mutable, and meaningful entities that strongly affect people's everyday lives. And boundaries help define the nature and potential impacts of these places.

'Metro' and the Growth of Toronto

A short review of Toronto's growth and suburbanization is required if we are to understand how the boundaries and subsequent policies and processes of this realization of metropolitan government fit into and become a dynamic part of the setting for the residential distribution of minorities.

Toronto more than tripled its population in forty years – from 1951 to 1991 – from somewhat over one million to nearly four million, based on the 1991 CMA boundaries. At the start of this period, however, most Torontonians – 706,613 – lived in the central city, the City of Toronto (which then included several municipalities that were later annexed). Another 187,496 people lived in contiguous, fully settled municipalities referred to locally as inner boroughs. What the Dominion Bureau of Statistics (later named Statistics Canada) then called the CMA had a much larger ring of so-called outer boroughs, with great amounts of undeveloped land (much of it farmland) and a relatively small population of 223,361 (calculated from Dominion Bureau of Statistics 1953). The even larger 'outer ring,' which has since been added over the years to the 1951 CMA, then housed only 144,391 people (calculated from Nader 1976: 203).

When the Municipality of Metropolitan Toronto was formed in 1953, it was assigned the 1951 CMA boundaries as its outer limits. This was logical for its purpose, as it included almost all the population of the area around Toronto and also fulfilled the criteria reflecting daily interdependence.

The proportions of the respective areas changed dramatically over the ensuing forty years, as did the total population. The population of the City of Toronto declined by about 10 per cent over this period, to 627,785. The inner boroughs increased by about 50 per cent but still represented a modest percentage of the total. The outer boroughs grew by nearly 600 per cent, to 1,386,045 in 1991, much of this *before* 1971. However, by 1991, the outer ring of the CMA had the largest single share of population, 1,607,965 (or 41 per cent), amounting to a gain of 1100 per cent (calculated from Statistics Canada 1994; see also Ley and Bourne 1993, 8), the greatest part *after* 1971. As 792,000 immigrants arrived in Toronto during the 1990s, the disproportionate growth of the outer ring increased (Statistics Canada 2003, 28).

What this means for minority residential distribution cannot safely be assumed from experiences elsewhere (cf. Phillips 1996). That is, it is not appropriate to assume that Toronto followed the pattern of accommodating newly arriving immigrants in the central city, at the same time that the existing population there deserted the central city for the suburbs. Population growth, the existence and dynamics of Metro, and the need to house great numbers of immigrants representing a wide range of ethnic minorities together placed Toronto's suburbanization in a unique context.

The Dynamics of Metro Toronto

What kind of imprint did Metro Toronto put on the territory within its boundaries?

The creation of the Municipality of Metropolitan Toronto (aka Metro) in 1953 followed nearly a decade of advocacy in planning circles, much political debate, and a report of the Ontario Municipal Board (1953). It was a formal response to the need to deal with housing and accompanying urban infrastructure that accompanied the end of the Second World War, the baby boom, and the expansion of immigration. Other cities advocated metropolitan government as a way of coping with the financial, social, and infrastructural problems of the *central city*; in contrast, Toronto's metropolitan government was a response to the developmental problems of the *suburbs*.

Metro Toronto was established as part of *two-tiered* municipal government. A division of labour between functions that required metropolitan coordination and/or redistribution, on the one hand, and local control, needs, and lifestyle, on the other, was struck between the metropolitan level and local municipalities that either already existed or were amalgamations of existing municipalities. The Metro government was given specific departments; for some functions it was directed by an (indirectly) elected council, for others by boards or commissions with appointed members. Among the functions dealt with by Metro departments were water, sewage disposal, roads, health and welfare, parks, and assessment. At the Metro level, boards and commissions dealt with public transportation, educational facilities, public housing, and planning (cf. Rose 1972, 25–6; Frisken et al. 1997, 33).

Uniform assessment practices and the creation of a Metro budget based on levies from the constituent municipalities proportionate to their assessment levels made possible a metropolitan tax base on the basis of which redistribution among subareas could take place. According to Frisken and colleagues (1997, 35), 'the redistribution of property tax revenues ... has had important consequences for Metro. Not only has it helped prevent the appearance of wide inter-municipal disparities in the quality of services funded in this way, but it has also allowed the governments of Metro's poorer municipalities ... to provide a higher standard of local services than they would have been able to provide otherwise.'

This approach worked particularly well when it came to creating physical infrastructure. As Kaplan (1967, 251) put it: 'Of those metropolitan problems cited by Ontario officials as the reasons for Metro's creation, the problems requiring public construction were quickly met to the satisfaction of almost all relevant actors.' Roads and bridges were built, water lines were extended, and sewers were connected. The metropolitan area was connected and opened up for more complete development.

Furthermore, some of the specific boards and commissions made decisions with far-reaching consequences to development within Metro Toronto.

First, a Metropolitan Toronto Planning Board (MTPB) was established, with the power to review all subdivision approvals carried out by lower-level planning boards within its territory. A unique feature of this was that the MTPB was given jurisdiction over an area one-third larger than Metro Toronto, one that included thirteen surrounding municipalities, mainly to the north. These consisted mostly of undeveloped farmland (Rose 1972). During its first years, the MTPB rejected more than half the applications for development. Particularly concerned about the amount of water available and limits to the amount of sewage that would wend its way southward into Lake Ontario, the MTPB effectively restricted large-scale development to the area within the boundaries of Metro. To all intents and purposes, the outlying areas became a greenbelt during the years in which the MTPB enjoyed this extraterritorial jurisdiction. Kaplan (1982, 725 and 727) described the situation: 'MTPB had to stop profit-hungry, unscrupulous land developers from leaping about the suburbs, picking choice sites, and, in the process, producing low-density sprawl or scattered pockets of development, both of which were extraordinarily expensive to provide with proper municipal services ... The implementation of this "orderly suburban development" policy was one of metro's most important successes.'

The MTPB had the power to stop development north of the Metro line until 1971, when regional municipalities with their own planning powers were created outside the Metro borders. According to the Ontario Economic Council (1973, 87), reviewing the original Metro system: 'The efficacy of the resultant planning controls is perhaps illustrated most dramatically at Bathurst Street and Steeles Avenue, where twenty-storey apartments on the south side of Steeles tower over green farmland on the north side.'

Sewell (1994) illustrates the impact of this change in policy as follows: 'In 1971, it was estimated that by 1990 the Town of Markham, on the outskirts of Toronto, would have a population of 20,000. However, in 1974 it was decided to offer Markham substantial sewage capacity ... by 1985, Markham's population exceeded 100,000' (29). (By 2001, Markham's population had reached 207,940; see Statistics Canada 2003, 61.)

Second, a consolidated Toronto Transit Commission built (and constantly extended) two subway lines – north/south and east/west – as well as bus and streetcar routes from subway stations along nearly all major thoroughfares. The subway lines were oriented to shuttle riders to the downtown core and back; the bus and streetcar lines fanned out into the residential areas. Transfers between all vehicles were free, and after 1972 a single, flat-rate fare could take riders anywhere within Metro. (Still later, passes for unlimited travel within Metro were introduced.)

However, people living outside the Metro borders had very limited access to the comprehensive services of the TTC. Again, the borders of Metro were given increased impact by the kinds of decisions being made in implementing a Metro function.[2]

Third, with the support of a metropolitan tax base, new schools were built throughout the newly settling areas of Metro, as needed. Health and welfare facilities, although not as prominent as school buildings, followed the same pattern. These buildings and services added to the habitability of the entire area within Metro, although they were not as visible a commitment as physical infrastructure. Apropos the emphasis in chapter 2 on access to various institutions by immigrant groups, many basic institutions were built and distributed quite evenly throughout Metro.

Fourth, the The Metropolitan Toronto Housing Authority (MTHA) provided social housing throughout the Metro area. Buildings and projects were well distributed throughout the constituent municipalities within the Metro boundaries (cf. Frisken et al. 1997, 39–42).

At least until 1971, Metro's policies had the effect of focusing intensive residential and commercial development within Metro territory. This made Metro land a relatively scarce and expensive commodity. According to the Ontario Economic Council (1973, 88): 'By shutting off further growth in the smaller fringe communities, the Province has turned off the last safety valve for land prices in the Metro Toronto area.'

As single-family houses reached the limits of affordability, in view of land costs per unit, the focus within Metro increasingly turned to the construction of high-rise apartments in the outer boroughs of Metro. At first, most of these were rental accommodation; condominium buildings came much later. Given the presence also of social housing complexes, the housing available in these outer boroughs represented a great mixture of housing types and costs. Metro's suburban areas represented a much more concentrated but varied form of housing – with extensive infrastructure of all kinds – than was at the time common in the suburban areas of most American cities.

What, if anything, does this mean for minority residential distribution? Did the rapid but concentrated development of suburbia mean that polarization occurred, with a majority group flooding the suburbs and the 'ethnics,' be they new or old, increasingly isolated in the central city? Are there major differences – possibly between visible minorities and others – among ethnic groups in their centralization or suburbanization? Among visible minorities, are there locational differences of the sort found in the United States between black and, for example, Chinese settlement patterns? How are minority residential patterns affected by the emerging absence of a majority group? In the next section I turn to the suburbanization of minorities throughout the history of the Metro system.

Minorities and Suburbanization in Metro Toronto

In this section I recalculate published data at the municipality level from the 1951, 1971, and 1991 Canadian censuses (Dominion Bureau of

Statistics 1953; Statistics Canada 1974, 1994), reducing and simplifying the data presented in light of frequent alterations in definitions and categories prompted by historical trends and publication decisions by Statistics Canada. The data from these censuses have been chosen to reflect the situation prior to the establishment of Metro, the period in its midlife before the end of extraterritorial planning controls, and a final full census in the Metro regime – a forty-year span, overall. I analyse residential distribution at these three census checkpoints and then look at decentralization trends more specifically.

1951

In 1951 the Toronto CMA had the same boundaries as Metro was given at its inception two years later. For analytic purposes, I will differentiate between the City of Toronto (the central city), the (settled) inner boroughs (the areas that evolved into East York and York), and the outer boroughs (eventually, Etobicoke, North York, and Scarborough).

As Table 4.1 indicates, most of the CMA's population (63 per cent) lived in the City of Toronto, with the rest divided nearly evenly between the inner and outer boroughs. This was true for each of the categories of 'origin or cultural group' (Dominion Bureau of Statistics 1953); all were concentrated in the central city. Some, however, were more concentrated there than others. Among the Asian category, 85 per cent were centralized, as were 81 per cent of Ukrainians, compared to 'only' 60 per cent of the British. These differences are statistically significant on the basis of chi-square (p < .001). It is absolutely clear that all the groups were centralized but had some presence in both the inner and outer boroughs.

Table 4.2 shows that in each concentric ring, the overwhelming majority of the population was of British origin (69 to 80 per cent), with the remaining population divided in each case into many small-percentage clusters. There were more people of non-British origin in the central city, but this was more or less in proportion to the population of the municipality.

1971

The 1951 census reflected immigration from northern and western Europe to Toronto (and to Canada more generally). The 1971 census reflected the emergence of a strong wave of immigration from southern

Table 4.1. Breakdown of ethnic groups by location of residence, 1951 (%)

Origin or cultural group	City of Toronto	Inner boroughs	Outer boroughs	Totals
British	60	18	22	100 (812,498)
French	70	12	18	100 (31,853)
Italian	67	19	14	100 (27,962)
Jewish	78	16	6	100 (59,448)
Polish	78	10	12	100 (26,998)
Ukrainian	81	7	12	100 (29,262)
Asian	85	8	7	100 (9,786)
Other	66	14	20	100 (119,663)

Source: Calculated from Dominion Bureau of Statistics, 1953.

Table 4.2. Ethnic breakdown of residential locations, 1951 (%)

Origin or cultural group	City of Toronto	Inner boroughs	Outer boroughs
British	69	78	80
French	3	2	3
Italian	3	3	2
Jewish	7	5	2
Polish	3	1	1
Ukrainian	3	1	1
Asian	1	*	*
Others	11	9	11
Totals	100 (706,613)	99 (187,496)	100 (223,361)

*Under 1 per cent, rounded down.
Source: Calculated from Dominion Bureau of Statistics, 1953.

Europe (Balakrishnan and Hou 1995). The numbers of Metro residents with Italian ethnicity increased nearly tenfold during these two decades, from 27,962 to 271,755. Table 4.3 includes the outer ring (that is, outside the Metro border); this became part of the CMA as its population increased from 144,391 to 542,110. The City of Toronto held a much smaller percentage of the CMA's population – less than one-third, a huge shift in twenty years – even though its absolute population had actually increased. Even ignoring the ring outside Metro, the City of Toronto's population by 1971 had fallen to only a little more than one-third of the Metro total.

The suburbanization of the ethnic groups was uniformly high during these years. Even if we ignore the population of the inner suburbs, as neither purely central city nor suburb, the majority of every ethnic

86   William Michelson

Table 4.3. Breakdown of ethnic groups by location of residence, 1971 (in percent)

Origin or cultural group	City of Toronto	Inner boroughs	Outer boroughs	Outer ring	Totals
British	22	9	44	26	101 (1,495,295)
French	29	8	41	22	100 (91,975)
Italian	33	18	41	8	100 (271,755)
Polish	44	7	34	15	100 (51,185)
Ukrainian	37	9	39	15	100 (60,755)
Other N. Eur.	21	10	43	26	100 (208,045)
Asian	47	9	36	8	100 (71,030)
Others	39	8	42	11	100 (378,085)

Source: Calculated from Statistics Canada, 1974.

Table 4.4. Ethnic breakdown of residential locations, 1971 (%)

Origin or cultural group	City of Toronto	Inner boroughs	Outer boroughs	Outer ring
British	46	51	59	71
French	4	3	3	4
Italian	13	19	10	4
Polish	3	1	2	1
Ukrainian	3	2	2	2
Other N. Eur.	6	9	8	10
Asian	5	2	2	1
Others	21	13	14	7
Totals	101 (713,130)	100 (251,920)	100 (1,120,965)	100 (542,000)

Source: Calculated from Statistics Canada, 1974.

group now lived in suburbs. The outer boroughs surpassed the central city in this regard for all but two of the groups, and the outer ring held many of them as well. It should be noted that the outer ring was settled more heavily by people with northern European origins than by others.

Table 4.4 shows that the pattern of ethnic heterogeneity in each ring was continuing in 1971, but with the diminution of the British-origin majority in every ring. The British were not going away (other than by changes in census definitions). However, they were being joined by increasing numbers of people from less traditional sources of immigration. The Italian influx shows up very clearly in Table 4.4. Between 1951 and 1971, the City of Toronto lost a majority group, even though those with British origins still represented a large plurality.

Table 4.5. Breakdown of ethnic groups by location of residence, 1991 (%)

Ethnic origin	City of Toronto	Inner boroughs	Outer boroughs	Outer ring	Totals	
British	14	6	32	48	100	(747,250)
Canadian	11	5	32	52	100	(266,420)
French	19	6	30	45	100	(52,085)
Italian	9	7	40	44	100	(311,215)
Chinese	23	4	47	26	100	(231,820)
East Indian	7	5	43	45	100	(141,415)
Black	11	7	53	30	101	(125,610)
Other origins	20	8	39	33	100	(1048,070)
Multiple origins	18	5	30	47	100	(939,225)

Source: Calculated from Statistics Canada, 1994.

1991

Over the next twenty years, as noted in chapters 2 and 3, additional waves of immigration from the Caribbean and from Asia (most prominently from Hong Kong and China, but also from India and Pakistan and to a lesser extent from Korea and Vietnam) began to land in Toronto in great numbers. According to Balakrishnan and Hou (1995), more than half the immigrants to Canada in the 1980s were visible minorities (see also Sewell 1994, 29). This added to the number of ethnic groups reflected in the census. During this period, the tilt of the population to the outer boroughs and, even more so, to the outer ring was carried even further. By 1991 the City of Toronto contained only one-sixth of the CMA's population – and only just over one-quarter of the Metro population.

The general suburbanization of the population, without more than a small decline in the central-city population, was common to *all* the ethnic categories. As seen in table 4.5, the overwhelming majority in all ethnic categories were residing beyond the inner boroughs. They differed, however, in the extent to which they settled beyond the Metro boundaries. A significantly smaller percentage of the Chinese and black populations (the latter only now formally recognized in decennial census publications) lived in the outer rings in 1991. But this difference must be placed in context: nearly half of 'East Indians' – also a large visible minority – lived in the outer rings, and more affluent, recent Chinese immigrants have chosen to do so increasingly since 1991. By 2001, 55.5 per cent of the people of suburban Markham were visible

Table 4.6. Ethnic breakdown of residential locations, 1991 (%)

Ethnic origin	City of Toronto	Inner boroughs	Outer boroughs	Outer ring
British	17	18	17	22
Canadian	5	5	6	9
French	2	1	1	1
Italian	5	10	9	8
Chinese	8	4	8	4
East Indian	1	3	4	4
Black	2	4	5	2
Other origins	34	33	29	22
Multiple origins	26	21	20	27
Totals	100 (627,785)	99 (241,315)	99 (1,386,045)	99 (1,607,965)

Source: Calculated from Statistics Canada, 1994.

minorities, mainly of Chinese heritage (Statistics Canada 2003, 60). In any case, more than one-quarter of the people in each category of ethnicity lived in the outer ring in 1991.

Table 4.6 shows that although people of British origin still hold a plurality in each ring compared to other single categories of ethnicity, this has declined to under 20 per cent in all but the outer ring, where it is nonetheless only 22 per cent. In every ring, the rest of the population once again is divided up into many minorities.[3] Yet many of these minorities represent critical masses in the rings where they live, given their large absolute numbers. For example, people of Italian origin represent 10 per cent of residents in the inner boroughs and 9 per cent in the outer boroughs – not far from the percentage of British origin; Chinese make up 8 per cent of the population in both the central city and the outer boroughs. In contrast, the Black population is 83 per cent suburbanized but makes up only between 2 and 5 per cent of the population of the individual rings.

Decentralization

Figures 4.2 and 4.3 summarize the suburbanization of the specific ethnic groups for which data were published for the 1951, 1971, and 1991 censuses (plus the category of black population in 1991). (Sources: Dominion Bureau of Statistics 1953; Statistics Canada 1974, 1994.) There are many ways to measure the distribution of racial and ethnic groups in cities. Most commonly used are measures of segregation and concentration (cf. James and Taeuber 1985; Lieberson 1962; Davies and Murdie

Figure 4.2. Index of decentralization for selected ethnicities in 1951, 1971, and 1991*

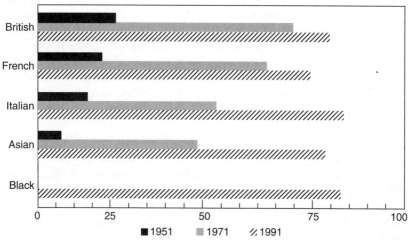

*Including the outer ring in 1971 and 1991.

Figure 4.3. Index of decentralization for selected ethnicities in 1951, 1971, and 1991*

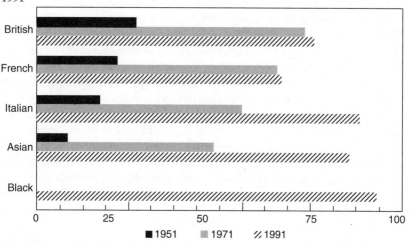

*Excluding the outer ring at all times.

1993; Massey and Denton 1988). For the question of suburbanization, however, the literature holds a relatively simple measure – of central-ization, that is, the percentage of a group whose members reside in the central city. Massey and Denton (1988) note that this measure is impre-cise in metropolitan areas that contain inner suburbs, which might be considered part of the central city except for historical borders. For this reason I turn in the opposite direction and use an index of decentraliza-tion: the percentage of group members who live outside the central city and the inner suburbs. In the case of Toronto, this means those living in the outer boroughs and outer ring.

Figure 4.2 includes the outer ring only after its inclusion in 1971, with the effect that the geographic area is not constant at the three check-points, although the functional entity being measured remains similar. What is evident from this figure is that regardless of their original degree of decentralization, all the groups changed in their degree of decentralization by a large amount between 1951 and 1971. The original settlement groups, the British and French, decentralized somewhat more, but the Italians and Asians also did so to nearly the same extent. Indeed, in Figure 4.3, which restricts its view for each decade to the borders of Metro – within which so much development was concen-trated by administrative fiat – it seems that the percentage of decentrali-zation taking place within the outer boroughs – which were 'opened up' as a consequence of Metro – was almost exactly the same for all the groups (between 31 and 37 per cent).

However, between 1971 and 1991, when there was far less immigra-tion of people of British and French origins relative to others, the major gains in decentralization were made by these others. What we see is a suburban localization of immigrant groups in aggregate as their mem-bers arrived in Toronto, not simply the mobility of individuals outward. By the end of these years, the decentralization values for all the groups measured fell within a narrow range, between 75 and 83 per cent for the CMA. There may be important qualitative differences in the settlement histories and lifestyles of different ethnic groups in Toronto, as noted in chapter 3, but these have not been an impediment to the decentralization of these groups towards suburban areas to roughly the same degree.

Segregation and Concentration

Although the focus of this chapter is on suburbanization, some mention of the actual texture of settlement by the many ethnic groups might supplement the preceding distributional information.

Toronto has always had residential and commercial ethnic areas, and this has continued in the suburbs. Insofar as there are no pronounced invidious differences marking the different group turfs, it has not been considered an ongoing problem. The choice to render institutional completeness through residential proximity differs from segregation engineered and enforced by outside parties. Indeed, the City of Toronto planners have thought it desirable to garnish and reinforce homogeneous local areas through street signs, which are written in Chinese or Greek or which designate areas such as 'Little Italy' or 'Portugal Village' or 'The Annex' or 'Fashion District.'

One cannot generalize about all the many ethnic groups. By and large, though, even the existence of an area bearing 'Corso Italia' street signs does not mean that those of Italian origin are concentrated in a single ghettolike area. As the preceding data show, many areas in both the central city and the suburbs have residents with Italian heritage, and there is no pressure from outside making it difficult for these people to live elsewhere. There are arguably five Chinatowns – three in the central city, one in an outer borough, and another in the outer ring. Many analyses of segregation and concentration in Toronto over the years have confirmed the absence of large, involuntary ghettos.

In 1951, when most of the Metro population, including minorities, lived in the central city, indices of dissimilarity were not especially high (where 0 represents total integration and 1.0 complete segregation). When matched against the residential distribution of the dominant British origin group, the French had an index of .20, Poles .521, Ukrainians .512, Italians .346, and Jews, the highest, .63. As of 1971, with much more suburbanization, indices for the first three of these groups declined appreciably, whereas they increased to .569 and .74 for Italians and Jews, respectively, each of which had thriving community institutions. Chinese and blacks had indices of .532 and .508 respectively (Kalbach 1990, 94). In 1991 – much later in the suburbanization process – the index values were substantially unchanged. The Jewish population index of dissimilarity was .787; for Chinese .573, for Italians, .562, and for blacks .517 (Balakrishnan and Hou 1995, 24).

Citing data gathered by Balakrishnan and Selvanatham from the 1981 census, Driedger (1991, 138) indicated that the mean segregation index for Toronto was .433 when based on all possible pairs and .331 when based on each group with the rest of the population.

Balakrishnan and Hou (1995, 12 and 14) have presented Gini measures of concentration calculated from 1991 census data, to indicate the extent to which residential clustering occurs in large concentrations.

They have found a high correlation of .9 between the indices of dissimilarity and those of concentration. Thus, the Jewish population, which shows the highest index of dissimilarity at .787, also has a very high Gini index of concentration, at .901. Also, 50 per cent of the Jewish population is found in just 3.1 census tracts in Toronto, and 90 per cent within 14.5 of the more than 600 tracts. In contrast, the Chinese population has a Gini of .532, with 50 per cent of Chinese in 9.6 tracts, and 90 per cent in 44.4 tracts. The black population has a Gini of .557, with 50 per cent in 12.9 tracts and 90 per cent in 46.3 tracts.

Fong's research on racial residential patterns in the United States and Canada suggests that 'all groups consistently live in neighborhoods with higher proportions of their own group'; yet his data on Asians and blacks also show that the greatest portion of these same neighbourhoods in Canada consist of whites (1997, Tables 1 and 2). These findings, and others indicating high levels of education and non-problematic mean incomes among black and Asian populations that have immigrated in recent years, suggest that the invidious differences among these groups found in American cities have not arisen in Canada (Fong 1996). Indeed, in Canadian cities the consistently most isolated (and deprived) group has been Native Canadians (Driedger 1991).

In short, the minority residential distribution in Toronto, as it has extended to the suburbs, has resembled a quilt but largely not one involving a high degree of segregation or concentration – certainly not centralization. Figure 4.4 (reproduced electronically from Statistics Canada 2002) shows that the percentage of visible minorities in Toronto CMA census tracts is highly variable, although these people are found more commonly in the outer boroughs and outer ring areas. Indeed, the most segregated and concentrated group in Toronto is a relatively affluent one, whose institutions are reinforced and partly made possible by propinquity.

Social Ecology

The objective of this chapter was not just to show the pattern of immigrant settlement accompanying the suburbanization of Toronto and the establishment of a metropolitan government, but to gain some understanding of its dynamics. In that regard, the materials I have presented suggest that although the boundaries accompanying metropolitan government are a necessary factor if we are to understand trends in residential settlement, they are part of a complex, interactive system of

Figure 4.4. Toronto CMA, visible minorities by 2001 census tract

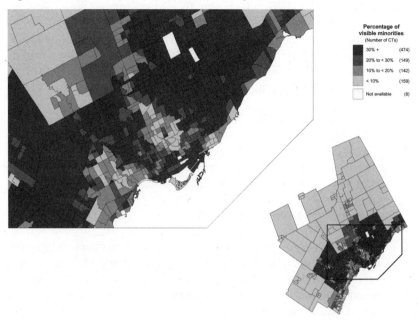

Source: 2001 Census of Canada. Produced by the Geography Division, Statistics Canada, 2002.

factors. The impact of boundaries is a function of what is put inside them through policies and practices. The goals, plans, and infrastructures that emerged from the departments, boards, and commissions of Metro were instrumental to the opening up of great numbers of housing units, which took a great variety of forms and prices inside Metro boundaries within a relative handful of years. Moreover, research suggests that the professional, apolitical actions of many of the principal actors in the initial bureaucracy of Metro (its chairman and many of the department heads) constituted another vital ingredient in this social ecology (Kaplan 1967).

Furthermore, not all the factors were at the Metro level. It has been argued that Metro would not have succeeded without a modicum of cooperation from the lower-level municipalities within Metro. However, it was the provincial government that exercised its absolute power over municipalities to research, legislate, and implement Metro, against the will of existing local political leaders. Also, the provincial level maintained the tenacious subdivision controls that found their way into the actions of the MTPB, which was fixated on intensifying development within the borders of Metro (Ontario Economic Council 1973). The federal government has no direct jurisdiction over municipal affairs in Canada; however, it has jurisdiction over immigration, and in the postwar years it turned on the immigration taps and then redirected the resulting flows as conditions changed at the national and global levels.

Thus, understanding the dynamics that link metropolitan government and immigrant residential distribution requires a much more inclusive social ecology, in terms of both factors and scale. Multiple factors must be considered if we are to understand the locational dynamics of immigrant and ethnic groups in a given area.

Final Perspectives from Current Events

The thrust of this paper is underscored by continuing events relating to Toronto and the Province of Ontario. One feature of the Metro structure was that it involved periodic reviews and was open to structural changes as deemed desirable. The review of Metro (Greater Toronto Area Task Force 1996), commissioned by the NDP government, which lost power in an election in June 1995, highlighted the fact that more people in the Greater Toronto Area (GTA) – an area somewhat larger than the CMA – now live in the outer ring than within Metro borders. This task force recommended assigning a GTA level of government responsibility for some of the most crucial functions done best at the greatest level of scale. This recommendation was an updating of the original intentions of Metro, corrected to reflect the current geographic distribution of population. Also parallel to the original Metro legislation was a recommendation to retain the lower-level municipalities as responsive local governments. But, staying with the notion of two-tiered local government, the *existing* Metro government would be abolished.

The Progressive Conservative government, elected on a neoconservative 'common sense revolution' platform, refused to accept these recommendations or, subsequently, even those of several of its own appointed ad hoc committees. Instead it eventually declared and implemented its own legislation, developed without apparent research or rationale other than a combination of positive and negative political payback.

The new legislation dictated the following: (1) the abolition of all the constituent lower-tier municipalities within Metro; (2) the amalgamation of these municipalities into a single City of Toronto, with an entirely different governmental structure than existed before; and (3) the shelving of integration and redistribution involving the outer ring to subsequent legislation in the future. Metro Toronto ceased to exist on 1 January 1998, and there are only faint prospects of a structure with the same objectives being established to meet current realities.

The subsequent legislation covering the larger GTA region resulted in the formation of a regional 'services board.' The only function given it at the outset was responsibility (but no longer financing) for the suburb-to-CBD commuter trains and buses that had been originated by a previous Government of Ontario (hence the name of GO Transit). The services board was given the conflict-laden job of determining how to apportion the costs between the new City of Toronto and the outer-ring municipalities. This board no longer functions.

At the same time, in separate legislation, the provincial government has almost totally restructured the provincial–municipal division of fiscal responsibilities and control, thus placing a potentially greater economic burden on municipalities that wish to retain accustomed levels of services while relieving them of local fiscal control over education (but only half the cost). The new City of Toronto has been saddled with disproportionate demands for revenue generation, even though it is increasingly less affluent than the fast-growing outer ring (cf. Frisken et al. 1997). The full slate of legislation – created at a time in history when many people have sufficient knowledge and experience to understand its invidious implications – raises the familiar spectre of an increasing bifurcation between a disadvantaged urban core (within the former borders of Metro) and an affluent outer ring. And, as the most recent data indicate (cf. figure 4.4), it makes suburban location increasingly attractive for newly arriving immigrants with sufficient financial means.

If the main message of this paper is that municipal borders matter and that actual outcomes also reflect the motives, substance, and structure of policies, current events support this message just as clearly as the experience of the late Metro Toronto.

NOTES

An earlier draft of this chapter was commissioned by the Harvard Civil

Rights Project for presentation to the conference on Suburban Racial Change,
Harvard Civil Rights Project, and the Taubman Center on State and Local
Government, Harvard University, Cambridge, Massachusetts, 28 March 1998.
I am grateful to my colleagues, L.S. Bourne, Eric Fong, David Hulchanski,
John Miron, and Richard Stren, for a generosity of thoughts and materials for
this paper. Joseph Moosman sent me a useful file from the Web. Joel Lau and
Boxu Yang provided informed interpretation. And, not least, Jennifer Redman
contributed some helpful sources as part of her work with this university's
Research Opportunity Program. I am solely responsible, however, for the
direction and specific content of this paper.

1 I conducted this study in part-fulfilment of a contract with Cassels Brock &
   Blackwell, Barristers and Solicitors. I am grateful to Environics Ltd. for
   collecting the data.
2 Although there have been marginal improvements in transit services across
   the traditional boundaries in recent years, the implementation of an integrated regional transportation system remains an elusive goal.
3 Note that in 1991, Statistics Canada allowed people to classify themselves as
   of Canadian origin, but relatively few did. More chose this option in the
   2001 Census.

REFERENCES

Balakrishnan, T.R., and Feng Hou. 1995. 'The Changing Patterns of Spatial
   Concentration and Residential Segregation of Ethnic Groups in Canada's
   Major Metropolitan Areas, 1981–1991.' London, ON: Population Studies
   Centre, University of Western Ontario, Discussion Paper no. 95–2.
Davies, W.K.D., and R.A. Murdie. 1993. 'Measuring the Social Ecology of
   Cities.' Pp. 52–75 in *The Changing Social Geography of Canadian Cities*, ed. L.S.
   Bourne and D.F. Ley. Montreal: McGill-Queen's University Press.
Dominion Bureau of Statistics, 1953. *Ninth Census of Canada: Population and
   Housing Characteristics by Census Tracts, Toronto.* Bulletin: CT-6, 1953. Ottawa:
   Queen's Printer.
Driedger, Leo. 1991. *The Urban Factor: Sociology of Canadian Cities.* New York:
   Oxford University Press.
Fong, Eric. 1997. 'A Systemic Approach to Racial Residential Patterns.' *Social
   Science Research* 26:465–86.
– 1996. 'A Comparative Perspective on Racial Residential Segregation: Ameri-
   can and Canadian Experiences.' *Sociological Quarterly* 37:199–206.

Frisken, Frances, L.S. Bourne, Gunter Gad and Robert A. Murdie. 1997. 'Governance and Social Well-Being in the Toronto Area: Past Achievements and Future Challenges.' Toronto: Centre for Urban and Community Studies, University of Toronto, Research Paper no. 193.

Goldberg, Michael, and John Mercer. 1986. *The Myth of the North American City: Continentalism Challenged*. Vancouver: UBC Press.

Goldenberg, H. Carl. 1965. *Report of the Royal Commission on Metropolitan Toronto*. Toronto: Province of Ontario.

Greater Toronto Area Task Force, 1996. *Greater Toronto*. Toronto: Queen's Printer.

Hulchanski, David, 1993. 'Barriers to Equal Access in the Housing Market.' Toronto: Centre for Urban and Community Studies, University of Toronto, Research Paper no. 187.

James, David, and Karl E. Taeuber. 1985. 'Measures of Segregation.' Pp. 1–32 in *Sociological Methodology 1985*, ed. Nancy B.Tuma. San Francisco: Jossey-Bass.

Kalbach, Warren. 1990. 'Ethnic Residential Segregation and Its Significance for the Individual in an Urban Setting.' Pp. 92–134 in *Ethnic Identity and Equality*, ed. Raymond Breton, W.W. Isajiw, Warren Kalbach and J.G. Reitz. Toronto: University of Toronto Press.

Kaplan, Harold. 1982. *Reform, Planning, and City Politics*. Toronto: University of Toronto Press.

– 1967. *Urban Political Systems: A Functional Analysis of Metro Toronto*. New York: Columbia University Press.

Ley, D.F., and L.S. Bourne. 1993. 'Introduction: The Social Context and Diversity of Urban Canada.' Pp. 3–30 in *The Changing Social Geography of Canadian Cities*, ed. L.S. Bourne and D.F. Ley. Montreal: McGill-Queen's University Press.

Lieberson, Stanley. 1962. 'Suburbs and Ethnic Residential Patterns.' *American Journal of Sociology* 67:673–81.

Massey, Douglas, and Nancy Denton. 1988. 'The Dimensions of Residential Segregation.' *Social Forces* 67:281–315.

Michelson, William. 1997. 'Municipal Boundaries and Prospective LULU Impacts.' *Research in Community Sociology* 7:117–40.

Nader, George. 1976. *Cities of Canada*. Vol. 2. *Profiles of Fifteen Metropolitan Centres*. Toronto: Macmillan of Canada.

Ontario Economic Council. 1973. *Subject to Approval: A Review of Municipal Planning in Ontario*. Toronto: Ontario Economic Council.

Ontario Municipal Board. 1953. *Municipality of Metropolitan Toronto, 1953*. Toronto: Province of Ontario.

Phillips, E. Barbara. 1996. *City Lights: Urban-Suburban Life in the Global Society,*

2nd ed. New York: Oxford University Press.

Popenoe, David, and William Michelson. 2002. 'Macroenvironments and People: Cities, Suburbs, and Metropolitan Areas.' Pp. 137–65 in *Handbook of Environmental Sociology*, ed. Riley Dunlap and William Michelson. Westport, CT: Greenwood Press.

Rose, Albert. 1972. *Governing Metropolitan Toronto: A Social and Political Analysis*. Berkeley: University of California Press.

Sewell, John. 1994. *Houses and Homes: Housing for Canadians*. Toronto: James Lorimer.

Statistics Canada. 2003. *Canada's Ethnocultural Portrait: The Changing Mosaic*. Ottawa: Statistics Canada.

– 2002. *2001 Census of Canada*. Ottawa: Statistics Canada, Geography Division.

– 1994. *Profile of Census Tracts in Toronto, Part B*. 95–354. Ottawa: Statistics Canada.

– 1974. *Population and Housing Characteristics by Census Tracts: Toronto*. 95–751 (CT-21B). Ottawa: Ministry of Industry, Trade and Commerce.

Tourism Toronto. 1997. 'About Toronto,' www.tourism-toronto.com/ho_abou.html.

Weiher, Gregory R. 1991. *The Fractured Metropolis: Political Fragmentation and Metropolitan Segregation*. Albany, NY: SUNY Press.

5 Immigration and the Environment: Polemics, Analysis, and Public Policy

JOHN VEUGELERS

Research on international migration is broadening its focus to better capture the range and complexity of immigration's effects, even those which are difficult to quantify (Kanjanapan and Rosenzweig 1995, 3). How immigration affects the natural environment of industrialized countries has received little attention, however, for environmental degradation tends to be treated as a cause rather than a consequence when studied in connection with the movement of people. Understanding how the environment affects migration is important: millions of people are displaced for environmental reasons each year, with heightened social conflict one result among others (Homer-Dixon 1994). But migration also affects the environment, and not just in the developing world (Ghimire 1994).[1]

This chapter treats variation in the condition of the natural environment as a consequence rather than a cause of migration. On the whole, the environmental impact of a given level of population will be greater for developed countries than for developing countries; yet population control does not necessarily generate environmental benefits at the local level. In examining a city of high immigration, Toronto, I argue that we must distinguish between dimensions of environmental quality in reckoning the effects of population. A highly restrictive immigration policy therefore offers an unattractive and unrealistic means of achieving environmental protection. If developed countries are concerned about the environmental effects of immigration, they should adopt cleaner lifestyles and technologies. The purpose of this chapter is not so much to offer new information as to argue that our vision of immigration has been too narrow. The environmental impacts of population growth are significant, so they must be considered in assessing the consequences of immigration for host societies.

Ideological Motives and Policy Discussion

Concern about the environmental effects of immigration has been used to disguise racism, nativism, and right-wing extremism. Partisans of a 'Green fascism' in contemporary Europe have claimed that ecology belongs to a Romantic celebration of nature (Olsen 1999). As a French neo-fascist group puts it: 'Ecology was originally a nationalist topic ... before being picked up by the extreme left. The nationalist state is concerned with the environment and will introduce very strict regulations in this area, unlike the liberals on all sides who have passively put up with several oil-slicks as well as the destruction of the French forest so that property developers can profit' (quoted in Griffin 1995, 362).

Right-wing extremists in Europe say that environmental degradation is like crime, drugs, and unemployment: another unwanted consequence of immigration (Griffin 1995; Davies 2000, 206). Arguing in favour of the separation of peoples, leaders of the far right claim that the fight for racial purity includes 'protecting nature and its diversity' (Olsen 1999, 4). Right-wing extremists have infiltrated environmental groups and have formed similar organizations of their own (Durand 1996, 214; Laqueur 1996, 123–4). In Canada, Australia, and the United States, similarly, some who have lobbied against immigration on environmental grounds are most likely racist propagandists (Fincher 1994, 499; SPLC 2001b).

Racists may be drawn to environmentalism for tactical reasons. Merging a stance that is progressive (environmentalism) with another that is conservative or reactionary (anti-immigrant nativism) may be a ploy, a means of attracting support or confusing the opposition by confounding familiar distinctions between left and right.[2] Right-wing extremists may also seek to weaken their opponents by driving a wedge between environmentalists and those who defend the rights of racial minorities. And by taking a position on environmental protection, nativists gain credibility by addressing issues – such as air pollution, excessive noise, and poor urban planning – that have been ignored or mishandled by the established political parties (Sainteny 1999).

Still, immigration's effects on the environment have become an issue in public debate. In 1998 the 550,000 members of the largest environmental group in the United States, the Sierra Club, were asked to vote on Alternative A. By adopting this resolution the group would have replaced its neutral stance on immigration with a call for severe restrictions. Supporters of Alternative A argued that the United States – which contains only 4 per cent of the world's population but consumes 25 per cent of its resources – should fight environmental degradation by limiting population growth due to immigration. Although defeated by a 60-to-40 margin, the immigration initiative of the Sierra Club stirred up controversy across the country (Goldin 1998; Knickerbocker 1998; Pope 1998). During the 1990s, anti-immigration activists won three of fifteen seats on the Sierra Club's board of governors. In a failed bid to gain control of the organization in 2004, an anti-immigration faction (Sierrans for U.S. Population Stabilization) sponsored five more candidates in general elections to the board (McCarthy 2004, A1, A2; SPLC 2004a, 55–8; SPLC 2004b). Environmental concerns have also been raised by other groups – such as Negative Population Growth, the Alliance for Stabilizing America's Population, and the Federation for American Immigration Reform – that are seeking population control through tight limits on immigration to the United States.[3]

Joining this debate have been civil rights groups such as the Southern Poverty Law Center (2001a, 12), which cites the Cato Institute in asserting that 'since 1965, when the current high levels of immigration began, there is no evidence that the environment has worsened overall,' and the National Wildlife Federation (2000), which cites Paul Ehrlich in countering that population multiplies the environmental impacts of affluence and harmful technology. Even public intellectuals like Witold Rybczynski (2001, 69) have pointed out that the chief cause of urban sprawl in the United States has been immigration. A few articles by academics address the issue. For example, Abernethy (1996, 142) writes that 'a conservation ethic in America should start with the goal of maintaining this country at as small a population size as possible. This goal is incompatible with a relatively open door immigration policy.'

The link between immigration and the environment is now a subject of public discussion in Australia as well. In 1971 a paper by a leading member of the Australian Conservation Foundation asserted that policymakers ought to consider the environmental impacts of population growth: 'We already know enough (more than we did when we embarked on our current immigration policy in 1945) to justify an immediate reduction in the migrant intake' (Warhurst 1993, 199). A study from the early 1980s concluded: 'The Australian population doubled in the thirty years since World War Two. Given Australia's physical geography, its aridity, and the resource-extraction and post-industrial economies which it is likely to have, doubling from 14.6 million to 29 million or so will take much longer to achieve, perhaps fifty to sixty years. To accelerate growth and development, an intensified immigration programme would be necessary. At this time, the necessity for acceleration has not been demonstrated' (Burnley 1982, 134–5). A 1992 report by the National Population Council emphasized the environmental impacts of urban population growth. Meanwhile, environmentalists, anti-immigration activists, and the Australian Democrats – a political party that favours zero population growth – also have argued over immigration policy (Smith 1991; Buetow 1994, 309–10; Jupp 1995, 219–22).

Although tainted by prejudice, the argument that immigrants exacerbate environmental pressures seemed to be winning support by the 1990s (Hugo 1996, 122).[4] At the start of that decade, Australia's Minister for Immigration and Ethnic Affairs was accused of silencing 'any voices in the population debate unless they legitimate the current government's "free trade" and "internationalisation agenda"' (Mercer 1995, 26). But as power shifted from Labor to a Liberal–National coalition, government entered the debate. In 2000 the Minister for Immigration and Multicultural Affairs attributed much of the country's environmental stress to export-oriented economic activities rather than to the size of its population. Adding that population reduction is a 'non-solution' to environmental degradation, he contended that the critical issue is really the location of population. Over the coming decades, many inland areas will become depopulated while most cities and the eastern seaboard will continue to grow. Singling out Sydney, a city facing 'serious environmental challenges' that receives 40 per cent of all overseas migrants and whose population is expected to increase by up to 45 per cent by 2050, the minister said his government was working to encourage migrants to settle elsewhere in the country. But he added that until Australia's population stabilizes, pressure on urban environments 'might also be eased by improvements in their management, the introduction of better technology such as low emission vehicles, better infrastructure and changes in consumption patterns' (Minister for Immigration and Multicultural Affairs 2000).

The immigration–environment linkage has received less attention in Canada. During the 1980s the Conservation Council of Ontario (CCO) warned that environmental protection was becoming inadequate and that population growth would make problems worse. The council claimed that new members of the society, 'whether materializing through natural increase or net immigration, generally accept our ideology of progress through exploitive growth and development ... slight differences in annual net immigration rates can have numerical and environmental implications when influenced by slight changes in distribution patterns' (Barrett et al. 1987, 263, 266). In a CCO report prepared for Employment and Immigration Canada in 1991, the authors stated that they 'know of no case where a positive relationship has been demonstrated between numbers of humans and the health of nature,' and recommended that Canada 'undertake a major study of the environmental impact of any present pro-immigration and pro-natalist policies, and also of some alternative demographic policies' (Regier and Bales 1991, 36–7).

But the government of Canada has danced around this issue. Since 1995, all departments of the federal government have been required to table a Sustainable Development Strategy, a plan for integrating sustainable development into policies, programs, and operations. In its first strategy report, Citizen and Immigration Canada (1997) said: 'While there is a link between population and environmental degradation, there is little agreement on the nature of the link, except that it is more a function of socio-political, institutional and economic factors rather than population growth per se.' Avoiding policy and programs, the department has focused instead on making its operations more environmentally friendly.[5]

A subsequent audit concluded that departments like Citizenship and Immigration Canada were committed to the status quo rather than sustainable development: in consultations on immigration levels with provincial and territorial governments, environmental considerations 'did not figure prominently' (Citizenship and Immigration Canada 2001b). In its next Sustainable Development Strategy, Citizenship and Immigration Canada (2001b) announced that it must 'improve its understanding of how sustainable development can be factored into decision-making processes.' But the department also said it did not control the process that has led to 71 per cent of the country's immigrants being concentrated in just three cities: Toronto, Vancouver, and Montreal. Although it had no reason to believe there are significant differences in behaviour towards the environment between the native-born and immigrants, again the department pointed out that this behaviour lies outside its control. The report also noted little progress in developing information on the environmental impacts of the department's policies.[6] Immigration is thus an area of Canadian policy in which environmental issues are being discussed, but without leading to substantial change.

Motivations that are suspect – racism, nativism, right-wing extremism – undoubtedly stand behind much of the concern about immigration's impact on the environment. Nonetheless, the issue is gaining salience. And although the policy implications are not as straightforward as the anti-immigrant lobby argues, there are good reasons for believing that immigration to developed countries adds to environmental stress.

Population, Development, and the Environment

Population growth in the industrialized world is worrying because it places inordinate stress on the environment. The industrialized countries consume 75 per cent of the world's energy, 79 per cent of all commercial fuels, and 85 per cent of all wood products. They also generate nearly three-quarters of carbon dioxide emissions, which in turn generate half the greenhouse gases on our planet. All things being equal, a small increase in the population of an industrialized country will thus have disproportionate environmental effects.[7] In 1990, a developing country like Bangladesh had 118 million people and a net fertility rate of 4.4; the United States, an industrialized country with 261 million people, had a net fertility rate of 2.1. Yet in one year a Bangladeshi consumed the commercial energy equivalent of only three barrels of oil, whereas an American consumed fifty-five barrels. As a result, population growth in Bangladesh pushed up energy consumption by an estimated 8.7 million barrels of oil per year, compared with 110 million barrels for the United States (UNFPA 1991, 14). Moreover, four-fifths of the world's 445 million cars are concentrated in the more developed regions, which have fewer than five people per car; in the developing world, the corresponding figures are 15 people per car in South America, 52 in Asia, and 75 in Africa (Sherbinin and Kalish 1994, 2). Assuming the number of cars per person stayed constant, a 2 per cent drop in the population of industrialized countries (a decline of 23 million people) would eliminate more than seven million cars; in the developing world, a 2 per cent drop in population (a decline of 89 million people) would eliminate fewer than two million cars. In the words of a UN report: 'Lifestyles in the developed economies of North America, Europe and Asia are responsible ultimately for a large share of environmental degradation carried out elsewhere. Their population growth, averaging 0.8 per cent per year or less, is allied with an exceptional technological and consumerist capacity to exploit resources and generate enormous quantities of waste' (UNFPA 1991, 14). Relatively small changes in the population of the industrialized countries thus have relatively large effects on the environment.

Most population growth in the industrialized countries comes from natural increase. Fertility is already very low, however – the average birth rate is 12 per thousand, compared with 28 per thousand in the developing world – and further decline is not expected (Lutz 1994, Table 1). Fertility thus holds little potential as an instrument for checking or reversing population growth in the industrialized world.

Immigration offers greater potential, at least in countries where it is an important component of population growth. About 40 per cent of the increase in Australia's population between 1947 and 1986 resulted from immigration, with another 20 per cent due to natural increase among the country's postwar immigrants (Moore 1990, 15). In the United States, similarly, immigration accounted for nearly 30 per cent of net population growth during the 1980s and now contributes about 20 per cent of gross addition to the population (Warren 1994, 3). In Canada, 38 per cent of population growth between 1951 and 1981 was due to immigration and births to immigrants. Without this contribution, Canada would have grown from 14.0 million to 20.4 million people; instead, it grew to 24.3 million (Beaujot 1991, 115). Between 1971 and the early 1980s, natural increase was responsible for 71 per cent of growth in Canada's population. With immigration now the major factor, natural increase was responsible for only 41 per cent of the population increase in 1999–2000 (Weber 2000).[8] These three settler societies have attracted a major share of the world's immigrants since 1945, yet many European countries and even Japan are now important destinations as well.

To date, humanity has disconfirmed Malthus's belief that development and population growth are irreconcilable. But population growth remains a concern, for it multiplies the environmental stress of our lifestyles and technologies (UNFPA 1999). From an environmental point of view, population control is needed around the globe: in the developing countries because they contain four-fifths of the world's population, in the industrialized countries because the environmental strain per capita is so high.[9] As fertility is already low and laws limiting the number of children a woman may bear are unlikely, the most obvious instrument for population control in industrialized settler countries is immigration policy.

Environmental Effects Are Not Obvious

Environmental quality is not simply a function of population. It depends on technology and lifestyle, and it varies along multiple dimensions, including (1) biodiversity, (2) air quality, (3) soil quality, (4) and
water quality. Although the assumption that these dimensions are interdependent is a defining feature of the ecological paradigm, treating
them separately permits a more precise understanding of the environmental effects of migration. For despite the postulate of interdependence, these dimensions respond to change in different ways. A decline
in biodiversity might be difficult to reverse, for example, whereas measures might be taken that quickly improve the quality of air.

For a given locality, moreover, the main causes and effects of environmental degradation may be local or non-local, or both. Sources of air
pollution are local (e.g., from motor vehicles or coal-powered energy
plants) as well as non-local (e.g., from motor traffic in other cities or
distant smokestack industries). Similarly, when treatment facilities are
inadequate, a city's sewage pollutes not only adjacent waterways but
also those downstream. The spatial distribution of these cause-and-
effect relationships explains why ecosystems are based on geographic
rather than political units.

In sum, population effects vary by type of environmental degradation and by the geographic distribution of causes and effects. As is often
the case, generalities of this kind are better understood by examining
them in light of specific circumstances; indeed, unless generalities are
so examined they remain unproven. In this chapter the interactions
among population, type of degradation, and location of cause and
effect will be explored by considering a city of high immigration, Toronto.

The Case of Toronto

In terms of climate, watershed, landform, and soil type, the Greater
Toronto Bioregion belongs to an ecosystem that extends into southern
and eastern Ontario as well as the United States. Although human
settlement of the area likely began about 11,000 years ago, the natural
environment hardly changed until the European migrations of the late
eighteenth and early nineteenth centuries. After the Second World War
the population of Toronto increased dramatically, and today the city –
which covers only 1 per cent of Ontario – contains 42 per cent of the
province's 12.1 million people. As Michelson points out in chapter 4 of
this volume, important causes of the city's growth have been the baby

boom, the arrival of migrants from other parts of Canada, and the expansion of immigration. Between 1981 and 1991, Toronto received 39 per cent of all immigration to Canada; by 2001, it was receiving 50 per cent of the intake. Immigration now contributes an estimated 50 per cent to the growth of Toronto, which has become the home for more immigrants than any other metropolitan area in the country (Badets 1993; Citizenship and Immigration Canada 2001a and 2002, 7).

Although it does not single out immigration, the Royal Commission on the Future of the Toronto Waterfront has observed that the 'single greatest challenge facing the Greater Toronto region is probably the number of people who live here, and the expected high rate of population growth' (RCFTW 1992, 23).[10] The commission's report provides an empirical basis for exploring how population change in Toronto is affecting the natural environment. In particular, the findings from this report suggest that the interaction between local population growth and four dimensions of environmental quality – biodiversity and the quality of air, soil, and water – is neither simple nor uniform.

Biodiversity

The diversity of plant and animal life in Toronto today bears little relation to the precolonial past.[11] Major losses resulted from European migration, with wetlands and natural cover disappearing during the nineteenth and twentieth centuries. Settlement, farming, and industrial activity led to the degradation and destruction of wildlife habitats as wetlands were filled in, rivers were dammed, and the shoreline of Lake Ontario was altered. Foreign species were introduced, while chemical contamination affected bird and marine species (RCFTW 1990, 27–45).

The Toronto region still exhibits some biodiversity and even isolated signs of renewal (ibid. 1990, 44–6; Barrett and Kidd 1991, 53–63). Nonetheless, wildlife, green space, water sources, and prime agricultural land have been lost through urban growth. The prospects for protecting biodiversity through limits on population growth are good, but a pristine condition could not be recovered even with a decline in immigrant settlement in Toronto.

Air Quality

Toronto's air contains high concentrations of lead, carbon monoxide, sulphur dioxide, nitrogen oxides, and nitrogen dioxide. Air quality affects both soil and water quality through the transport and deposit of pollutants. The effects are so harsh that in some Toronto areas the lifespan of newly planted trees is no more than ten years. The sources of the toxic substances in the city's air are both non-local and local. Toronto is affected by atmospheric patterns as far away as Hudson Bay and New Brunswick in Canada, and the Dakotas and central Georgia in the United States. American sources are responsible for up to half the smog in the Toronto bioregion, and distant sources seem largely responsible for organic compounds in the air. Locally, industry, energy plants, and motor vehicles are responsible for most emissions, with strains on transportation facilities making the problem worse because congestion on roads and highways is leading to longer and more frequent delays in traffic (RCFTW 1990, 24, 39–41; Barrett and Kidd 1991, 69; City of Toronto 1998, 4).[12]

Reducing immigration settlement in the Toronto area would protect air quality because recent gains from increased control over the main sources of air pollution – motor vehicles, power plants, some industries – have been offset by problems with traffic congestion and more motor vehicles (City of Toronto 1998, 26). However, checks on growth through immigration would leave untouched the remote sources of air pollution. Toronto belongs to an airshed that extends for hundreds of miles around, so those who live in the city and its environs have only partial control over the quality of the air they breathe. Furthermore, change in population growth would have little effect on air pollution caused by local industries. Finally, the thinning of the ozone layer is a global phenomenon that will continue to affect Torontonians even if their city stops growing.

Soil Quality

Less than half the land in the Greater Toronto Bioregion is agricultural or rural, and losses are continuing through development. Adding to this loss is the extraction of sand and gravel for road and building construction. Contamination of soil and groundwater by organic compounds and heavy metals is another problem, especially in port and industrial areas. Landfill and atmospheric deposits account for some of this contamination, but much is a legacy of industry. Municipal services have also contributed to the degeneration of soil quality. Soil at incinerator sites has high toxin levels, while snow dumped from city streets leaves trace metals and high levels of sodium and chloride. The region also has hundreds of abandoned landfill sites. Unregulated until the 1970s, they produce an unknown amount of soil and groundwater contamination. Finally, the area's four million residents produce 4.5 million tonnes of waste annually, of which 40 per cent comes from homes, the rest from institutions, industries and other businesses. Some garbage is recycled, but the rest goes into landfill sites (RCFTW 1990, 24–30; Barrett and Kidd 1991, 74–8).

A decline in immigration settlement would not remove the soil and groundwater contamination that already exits. Nor would it reduce pollution from industries that produce for nonlocal markets. If more immigration adds to urban sprawl, however, snow removal from new roads will worsen the contamination of soil and groundwater. Low-density construction will continue to eat away at rural lands; and as it faces a shortage of local landfill sites, Toronto will increasingly export soil contamination by shipping garbage to other regions.

Water Quality

The Greater Toronto Region sits on the north shore of Lake Ontario and is crossed by rivers and creeks. Water quality off the Toronto waterfront is poor. Concentrations of phosphorus exceed standards set by the provincial government, and nutrients have left some waters in a eutrophic state. Bathing beaches are sometimes closed due to high levels of bacteria, and water and water sediment in Toronto's harbour contain concentrations of heavy metals and other toxic substances (Barrett and Kidd 1991, 79–83).

Apart from industry, transportation, lake filling, and dumping, major sources of contaminants and nutrients are the storm and combined sewers that flow directly into Lake Ontario. Toronto's Main Sewage Treatment Plant channels organic chemicals from hundreds of industries and some 400,000 residences, and a development boom has probably sent additional contaminants and nutrients into the lake (ibid., 79–83). Urban run-off, raw sewage, and industrial waste still flow into the region's rivers. Continued development due to immigration will add more storm water, construction silt, and harmful substances such as herbicides, pesticides, fertilizers, road salt, and polluted snow (RCFTW 1992, 236–8).

As with air quality, water quality in the Toronto section of Lake Ontario is affected by pollution elsewhere, especially in the upstream Great Lakes that straddle the Canada–U.S. border. Revisions and amendments to the Great Lakes Water Quality Agreement signed by Canada and the United States recognize that restoring the waters shared by these two countries cannot be achieved in isolation from other changes in the ecosystem of the Great Lakes Basin. Local sources still have important effects on water quality in the Toronto region, however. Appropriate changes in lifestyle and technology have been shown to reduce water pollution caused by the area's residents and industries. The Don River is actually cleaner than it was half a century ago, for example (RCFTW 1990, 20; Barrett and Kidd 1991, 69).

Reduced immigration settlement in the Toronto region would leave remote sources of water contamination untouched. It would not lessen the impact of local industries that produce mainly for non-local markets, and it would not solve problems stemming from construction, road salting, garbage disposal, improper water treatment, and the use of fertilizers or pesticides. Nonetheless, reduced immigration settlement would moderate the impact of these problems that affect water quality.

Conclusion

This study shares some of the limitations of the inquiry carried out by the Royal Commission on the Future of the Toronto Waterfront. Although the commission's mandate included an investigation of the environment in the Greater Toronto Bioregion, the focus was on the city and its waterfront. Scrutiny of environmental quality outside the downtown area was thinner, and some of the commission's findings may be outdated because the inquiry was conducted from 1988 to 1991 (RCFTW 1992, 1). The commission's report does not provide the data needed to assess the environmental effects of immigration net of other relevant factors, such as industrial production and population losses due to outmigration.

Moreover, an environmental audit cannot be truly comprehensive unless global as well as local exchanges are addressed. Many non-local causes of environmental problems in the Toronto region were recognized by the commission; however, non-local effects were difficult to assess. Much of the garbage produced by Torontonians is disposed of outside the city, while hazardous waste is treated and disposed of in southwestern Ontario, Quebec, and the United States (RCFTW 1990, 31). Some energy is generated locally, but the city imports more energy than it produces. Hence, 'to a large degree, the environmental costs of

energy production are borne elsewhere' (ibid., 29). The audit is otherwise silent on the global consequences of the region's lifestyle and
technology, and on how the environmental impacts of these might be
multiplied by population growth.[13]

Apart from limitations stemming from the commission's report,
longer-term processes – such as the environmental effects of European
migration before the waves of postwar migration from other parts of
the world – also deserve attention. Consider as well that immigrants
tend to adopt not only the lifestyle and technologies of the country they
settle in, but also its fertility patterns. If fertility among immigrants and
their descendants is lower than in the country of origin, population's
multiplier effect on environmental degradation will be reduced, at least
at the global level. Finally, the sources of migration to Toronto are
domestic as well as foreign. According to the most recent census data
available, 34 per cent of the 514,825 migrants five years and over living
in Toronto in 1996 had moved there from within Canada (Statistics
Canada 2000a). This component of the city's population increase will
remain significant.

In examining the possible impact of immigration, it is also important
not to exaggerate the effect of population size. Alberta has about one-
quarter the population of Ontario, for example, yet emits more greenhouse gases than any other Canadian province due to its oil sands
projects and heavy reliance on coal to generate electricity (Mittelstaedt
2001). Furthermore, the environmental effects of population are a function of density as well as size, with urban sprawl encouraging people to
drive instead of walking, cycling, or taking public transit (City of Toronto
1998, 15). As Michelson shows in chapter 4 of this volume, immigrants
and their children contributed heavily to the postwar growth of Toronto's
suburbs. Thanks to the regulatory powers exercised by the Metropolitan Toronto Planning Board, until 1971 urban sprawl was contained
somewhat (as were associated problems such as the disposal of sewage
and the encroachment onto farmlands of real-estate developments). In
this respect, Toronto has done relatively well: at nine feet of road per
inhabitant, it is much denser than the densest American city, Chicago,
which has 16.5 feet per inhabitant (Rybczynski 2001, 69).

Nonetheless, this chapter has shown that the multiplier effect of
population varies for different aspects of environmental quality. Much
of the biodiversity that has been lost from the Greater Toronto Bioregion
cannot be recovered.[14] Reduced immigration settlement in the Toronto
region would lead to an improvement in air quality because it would

affect the volume of traffic on roads, but so would emission controls, regulations limiting automobile traffic, and greater use of mass transit. Reduced immigration settlement would not affect other major causes of local pollution – namely, industry and non-local sources of emissions. Local sources are chiefly responsible for soil loss and contamination, but these are only partly affected by population (primarily through urban growth and the disposal of waste). Other important sources of soil contamination – industry, transportation, groundfill – remain much less sensitive to the size of the local population. Most affected by population – hence by change in immigration settlement – is water quality, in part because treatment facilities have not kept pace with urban growth.

Thus we cannot entirely dismiss the arguments put forth by those who tie immigration to environmental degradation. Although the racism and intolerance that often motivate such arguments are reprehensible, clearly some types of environmental degradation have been accelerated by immigration settlement in Toronto. By raising population levels, migration has exacerbated the harmful effects of the lifestyles and technologies found in Canada. But this study also suggests that controls on population growth through a restrictionist immigration policy would not address problems such as loss of biodiversity and the pollution created by export-producing industries.

It seems doubtful that reductions in levels of immigration to Canada will be used as an instrument for curtailing environmental degradation. Instead of worrying about how many immigrants come to Canada, officials at all levels of government are concerned that 94 per cent of immigrants settle in metropolitan areas, primarily Toronto, Montreal, and Vancouver. The main problem is the strain this places on municipal budgets. In response, the federal government is working to encourage the settlement of immigrants (including refugees) in other regions of Canada (Dunfield 2003). Whether this policy will yield environmental benefits by slowing population growth in the country's biggest cities remains to be seen. Certainly, the premise of the new Official Plan of the City of Toronto (2002) is that the city will continue to be one of the fastest-growing in North America.[15]

The Canadian government will probably avoid a restrictionist policy because it would threaten family reunification and the country's commitment to accept refugees. Of the 229,091 people who immigrated to Canada in 2002, 28 per cent were admitted under the family category while another 11 per cent were refugees (Citizenship and Immigration Canada 2003, 5). Clearly, denying entry to people in these categories on environmental grounds would be politically difficult. Whichever party has held power during the postwar era, government has always been a booster of immigration (Veugelers 2000). No party would risk antagonizing voters or interest-group members – many of them either immigrants or the children of immigrants – by imposing severe restrictions on the number of people allowed into this country.[16]

Countries like Canada therefore face some hard choices if they truly care about protecting the environment. Environmental degradation through population growth seems inevitable, yet population control is not a political option. Canada does not have an official policy on population, and federal politicians will continue to vaunt the benefits of immigration. Big cities are thus faced with the inevitability of continued growth; meanwhile, the society joined by our newcomers remains more or less irresponsible when it comes to urban sprawl, water treatment, mass transit, wasteful consumption, and so forth. There are many ways in which immigration brings benefits to the receiving countries of the developed world. But Canada also faces a predicament: how to benefit from continued immigration without increasing the burden on our natural environment. Changes in lifestyle and technology remain the only alternatives, yet experience suggests that action on these fronts will come slowly, if at all.

NOTES

Fellowship support from the Social Sciences and humanities Research Council of Canada is gratefully acknowledged, as are helpful suggestions from Eric Fong, Gary Freeman, Randy Hart, Jane O'Hare, Beth Savan, and the anonymous reviewers.

1 Forms of environmental degradation attributed to population movements between developing countries include deforestation, soil erosion, water depletion, loss of biodiversity, and air and water pollution (Lonergan 1995; Lohrmann 1996, 337; UNHCR 1998, 6). In 1995 the UN High Commissioner for Refugees established a system to monitor and assess environmental damage in the field (UNHCR 2000).
2 In Vancouver the differences between left and right were blurred in the debate surrounding the construction boom of the 1980s. Many older neighbourhoods underwent rapid change, prompting concerns over urban growth and the loss of green space. Among those building and buying

large new homes in established neighbourhoods were immigrants from Hong Kong, who became scapegoats in a battle to preserve the cityscape (Li 1994).

3 See www.npg.org (Negative Population Growth); www.balance.org (Alliance for Stabilizing America's Population); and www.fair.us (the Federation for American Immigration Reform, an organization with financial and personal ties to racist groups such as the Pioneer Fund; SPLC 2001b, 16–17).

4 Articles in *People and Place,* an Australian journal of academic research and policy debate, include a study which found that 'immigrants to Australia do adopt Australian consumption patterns over time so that their greenhouse gas emissions rise from the levels in their countries of origin' and concludes that 'a high immigration policy would result in Australia's energy-related emissions being 16 per cent higher than they would be with zero net immigration' (Hamilton and Turton 1999, 55, 61).

5 Recommendations from this strategy report include the following: phasing out the department's less fuel-efficient vehicles; encouraging the 'four Rs' (reduce, reuse, recycle, recover) among departmental employees; reviewing contracts with suppliers in light of possible environmental considerations; and developing material on sustainable development and environmental responsibility for newcomers to Canada (Citizenship and Immigration Canada 1997).

6 The department mentions that citizens who participated in consultations in Nunavut and the Northwest Territories 'indicated a preference for the federal government to focus on improving opportunities and conditions for northerners rather than attracting immigrants to the North. They also indicated that, where immigration does take place, the government's emphasis should be on attracting people who are environmentally conscious and who share northerners' high regard and concern for the land' (Citizenship and Immigration Canada 2001b).

7 Differences between countries are great. A person in Italy has the environmental impact of three people who live in the United States; one Bangladeshi has the impact of 140 Americans, whereas a Haitian has the impact of 280 Americans (National Wildlife Federation 2000). The annual level of CO_2 emissions per capita is 21.7 metric tons for the United States, but 11.6 for Germany; levels for two lesser developed countries are 1.3 metric tons for India, but 0.8 for Nigeria (National Wildlife Federation 2003).

8 In calculating population growth, immigration's gross contribution is offset by losses through emigration. For Canada, the impact of emigration

(particularly to the United States) is significant. Between 1 July 1999 and 30 June 2000, the ratio of emigrants to immigrants was 1 to 3.3 (Statistics Canada 2000b).

9 According to the UNFPA (2000), 'the greatest environmental threat comes from both the wealthiest billion people, who consume the most and generate the most waste, and from the poorest billion, who may damage their meager resource base in the daily struggle to avoid starvation.'

10 The commission does not advocate checks or reductions in the population of the Greater Toronto Region. Instead it recommends an increase in the residential population of the downtown area because new housing there consumes less land than in the suburbs (where housing densities are much lower). By reducing travel to the downtown core, a denser city would reduce automobile emissions (RCFTW 1992, 320).

11 Before Europeans came, 'most large North American mammals, including mammoths, saber-toothed tigers, and camels' had already disappeared. Some experts say the main cause was climate change; others blame the extinction of these animal species on overhunting after humans migrated from Asia (Jencks 2001, 57).

12 Motor vehicles are responsible for 93 per cent of the city's carbon monoxide emissions (City of Toronto 1998, 4).

13 In assessing the environmental effects of international migration from a global perspective, three outcomes are possible: (1) the net effect is neutral, because of minimal differences in lifestyle and technology between the sending and receiving societies; (2) the net effect is positive, because the lifestyle and technology of the sending society are more harmful to the environment than those of the receiving society; (3) the net effect is negative, because the lifestyle and technology of the sending society are less harmful than those of the receiving society.

14 Immigration can also promote biodiversity through initiatives such as Where Edges Meet, a community project for creating gardens of native plants. Launched in 1998, this project has included 'the most densely populated and arguably the most multicultural neighbourhood in Canada' (Evergreen Foundation 2001).

15 Toronto's older neighbourhoods have a housing density of ten households per acre; the suburbs, by contrast, have four households per acre. The number of cars is growing more rapidly than the number of inhabitants and is expected to increase from 2.4 million in 1998 to 3.5 million by 2010 (City of Toronto 1998, 15, 26). According to the Official Plan (City of Toronto 2002), urban expansion will threaten the Oak Ridges Moraine; increase air pollution caused by congested traffic; and encroach on farm-

land at the rate of over 3,000 hectares per year. The plan addresses these problems by encouraging higher housing densities in some parts of the city.

16 A restrictionist policy cannot be implemented unless the state enjoys a strong capacity to regulate immigration flows. Only a few high-immigration, industrialized countries have exercised significant control over the entry of foreigners: Australia, Canada, and probably the United Kingdom (Rees 1993, 106; Freeman 1994). Geography, political will, and enforcement seem to be the key factors: Australia and Great Britain are insular, whereas Canada is remote from major sources of international migration (Birrell 1994, 116). Japan is insular, too, but has not stemmed illegal immigration from countries such as Iran, Bangladesh, Thailand, Malaysia, South Korea, and the Philippines (Morita and Sassen 1994, 154). The United States shares a long border with Mexico, the source of perhaps 80 percent of its illegal immigration, and lies near several Caribbean countries that have suffered from civil turmoil and political repression (SOPEMI 1994, 104). Illegal migration to Western Europe has also been high, although the lifting of border controls between the Schengen countries was matched by stricter controls over entry from the non-Schengen countries (Baldwin-Edwards and Schain 1994).

REFERENCES

Abernethy, Virginia. 1996. 'Environmental and Ethical Aspects of International Migration.' *International Migration Review* 30(1):132–50.

Badets, Jane. 1993. 'Canada's Immigrants: Recent Trends.' *Canadian Social Trends* 29:8–11.

Barrett, Michael, Simon Miles, Henry Regier and Chris Winter. 1987. 'Potential Environmental Impacts of Changes in Population Size, Age and Geographic Distribution.' *Canadian Studies in Population* 14(2):261–77.

Barrett, Suzanne, and Joanna Kidd. 1991. *Pathways: Towards an Ecosystem Approach.* Royal Commission on the Future of the Toronto Waterfront. Ottawa: Minister of Supply and Services Canada.

Baldwin-Edward, Martin and Martin A. Schain, eds. 1994. *The Politics of Immigration in Western Europe.* London: Frank Cass.

Beaujot, Roderic. 1991. *Population Change in Canada: The Challenges of Policy Adaptation.* Toronto: McClelland & Stewart.

Birrell, Robert. 1994. 'Immigration Control in Australia.' *Annals of the American Academy of Political and Social Science* 534:106–17.

Buetow, Stephen A. 1994. 'International Migration: Some Consequences for Urban Areas in Australia and New Zealand.' *International Migration* 32(2):307–28.

Burnley, Ian H. 1982. *Population, Society and Environment in Australia: A Spatial and Temporal View*. Melbourne, Australia: Shillington House.

Citizenship and Immigration Canada. 2003. *Facts and Figures 2002: Immigration Overview*. Ottawa: Minister of Public Works and Government Services Canada.

– 2002. *Facts and Figures 2001: Immigration Overview*. Ottawa: Minister of Public Works and Government Services Canada.

– 2001a. *Facts and Figures 2000: Immigration Overview*. Ottawa: Minister of Public Works and Government Services Canada.

– 2001b. 'Sustainable Development Strategy 2001–2003.' www.cic.gc.ca (5 October 2001).

– 1997. 'Sustainable Development Strategy (December 1997).' www.cic.gc.ca (5 October 2001).

City of Toronto. 2002. *Official Plan*. Toronto: City of Toronto.

– 1998. *Smog: Make It or Break It*. Toronto: Healthy City Office, City of Toronto.

Davies, Peter. 1999. *The National Front in France: Ideology, Discourse and Power*. London: Routledge.

Dunfield, Allison. 2003. 'Urban Centres Attract Nearly Three-Quarters of New Canadians.' *Globe and Mail*, 21 January.

Durand, Géraud. 1996. *Enquête au coeur du Front national*. Paris: Jacques Grancher.

Evergreen Foundation. 2001. 'Where Edges Meet: Celebrating Cultural and Ecological Diversity.' Toronto: Evergreen Foundation.

Fincher, Ruth. 1994. 'Environmental Claims about the Impacts of Immigration.' In *Immigration and Refugee Policy: Australia and Canada Compared*. Vol. 2. Ed. Howard Adelman, Allan Borowksi, Meyer Burstein, and Lois Foster. Toronto: University of Toronto Press.

Freeman, Gary P. 1994. 'Can Liberal States Control Unwanted Migration?' *Annals of the American Academy of Political and Social Science* 534:17–30.

Ghimire, Krishna. 1994. 'Refugees and Deforestation,' *International Migration* 32(4):561–70.

Goldin, Greg. 1998. 'The Greening of Hate.' *The Nation* 266(18):7. http:// proquest.umi.com (13 January 1999).

Griffin, Roger, ed. 1995. *Fascism*. Oxford: Oxford University Press.

Hamilton, Clive, and Hal Turton. 1999. 'Population Policy and Environmental Degradation: Sources and Trends in Greenhouse Gas Emissions,' *People and Place* 7(4):42–62.

Homer-Dixon, Thomas. 1994. *Population and Conflict*. Liège, Belgium: International Union for the Scientific Study of Population.

Hugo, Graeme. 1996. 'Environmental Concerns and International Migration.' *International Migration Review* 30(1):105–31.

Jencks, Christopher. 2001. 'Who Should Get In?' *New York Review of Books*, 29 November: 57–63.

Jupp, James. 1995. 'From "White Australia" to "Part of Asia": Recent Shifts in Australian Immigration Policy Towards the Region.' *International Migration Review* 29(1):207–28.

Kanjanapan, Wilawan and Mark R. Rosenzweig. 1995. 'Introduction.' *International Migration Review* 29(1):3–6.

Knickerbocker, Brad. 1998. 'Environment vs. Immigrants: As US Population Soars, Sierra Club Votes to Stay "Neutral" on Newcomers.' *Christian Science Monitor*, 27 April: 3. http://proquest.umi.com (13 January 1999).

Laqueur, Walter. 1996. *Fascism: Past, Present, Future*. New York: Oxford University Press.

Li, Peter S. 1994. 'Unneighbourly Houses or Unwelcome Chinese: The Social Construction of Race in the Battle Over "Monster Homes" in Vancouver, Canada.' *International Journal of Comparative Race and Ethnic Studies* 1(1):14–33.

Lohrmann, Reinhard. 1996. 'Environmentally-Induced Population Displacements and Environmental Impacts from Mass Migrations.' *International Migration* 34(2):335–9.

Lonergan, Steve. 1995. 'Population Movements and the Environment.' *Refugee Participation Network* 18 (January 1995). www.fmreview.org (8 December 2000).

Lutz, Wolfgang. 1994. 'The Future of World Population.' *Population Bulletin* 49(1).

McCarthy, Shawn. 2004. 'Sierra Club Faces Rocky Future as Extremists Push Out Greens.' *Globe and Mail*, 26 January.

Mercer David. 1995. 'Australia's Population "Carrying Capacity." One Nation – Two Ecologies: A Review and Assessment.' *People and Place* 3(1):23–8.

Minister for Immigration and Multicultural Affairs. 2000. 'The Public Policy Dimensions of Population.' Speech to Australian Centre of Population Research, Australia National University, 11 October. www.minister.immi.gov.au (8 December 2000).

Mittelstaedt, Martin. 2001. 'Alberta Flayed over Gas Emissions.' *Globe and Mail*, 24 September.

Moore, Ronald F. 1990. 'Australia.' In *Handbook on International Migration*. Ed. William J. Serow et al. Westport, CT: Greenwood Press.

Morita, Kiriro, and Saskia Sassen. 1994. 'The New Illegal Immigration in Japan, 1980–1992.' *International Migration Review* 28(1):153–64.

National Population Council. 1992. *Population Issues and Australia's Future: Environment, Economy and Society.* Canberra: Australian Government Publishing Service.

National Wildlife Federation. 2003. 'Population and Environment – Consumption Patterns.' www.nwf.org (23 January 2003).

– 2000. 'Population and Environment.' www.nwf.org (13 December 2000).

Olsen, Jonathan. 1999. *Nature and Nationalism: Right-Wing Ecology and the Politics of Identity in Contemporary Germany.* New York: St Martin's Press.

Pope, Carl. 1998. 'Moving On: Lessons of the Immigration Debate.' *Sierra* 83(4):14–15. http://proquest.umi.com (January 13, 1999).

RCFTW (Royal Commission on the Future of the Toronto Waterfront). 1992. *Regeneration: Toronto's Waterfront and the Sustainable City – Final Report.* Ottawa: Minister of Supply and Services Canada.

– 1990. *Watershed (Second Interim Report).* Ottawa: Minister of Supply and Services Canada.

Rees, Tom. 1993. 'United Kingdom I: Inheriting Empire's People.' In *The Politics of Migration Policies: Settlement and Integration (The First World into the 1990s).* by Daniel Kubat. New York: Center for Migration Studies.

Regier, Henry A., and Andrew G. Bales. 1991. *Environmental Impacts of Immigration: A Preliminary Examination.* Report prepared for Employment and Immigration Canada, Ottawa.

Rybczynski, Witold. 2001. 'City Lights.' *New York Review of Books*, 21 June, 68–70.

Sainteny, Guillaume. 1999. 'Les habits verts de l'extrême droite,' *Libération*, 24 February. www.liberation.fr (30 March 1999).

Sherbinin, Alex de, and Susan Kalish. 1994. 'Population-Environment Links: Crucial, but Unwieldy.' *Population Today* 22(1):1–2.

Smith, Joseph Wayne, ed. 1991. *Immigration, Population and Sustainable Environments: The Limits to Australia's Growth.* Adelaide: Flinders Press, Flinders University of South Australia.

SOPEMI (Continuous Reporting System on Migration). 1994. *Trends in International Migration (1993).* Paris: OECD.

SPLC (Southern Poverty Law Center). 2004a. 'Hostile Takeover. ' *Intelligence Report* (Spring):55–8.

– 2004b. 'Sierra Club Rejects Anti-Immigration Candidates.' *Intelligence Report* (Summer): 4.

– 2001a. 'The Immigrants: Myths and Reality.' *Intelligence Report* (Spring):12.

– 2001b. 'Anti-Immigration Groups,' *Intelligence Report* (Spring):16–18.

Statistics Canada. 2000a. 'Migrants 5 Years and Over by Components of Migration, 1996 Census, Census Metropolitan Areas.' www.statcan.ca (8 December 2000).

– 2000b. 'Components of Population Growth.' www.statcan.ca (8 December 2000).

UNFPA (United Nations Population Fund).

– 2000. 'Population and the Environment.' www.unfpa.org (13 December).

– 1999. 'Population Issues – 1999: Population and Sustainable Development.' www.unfpa.org (13 December 2000).

– 1991. *Population and the Environment: The Challenges Ahead.* New York: United Nations.

UNHCR (United Nations High Commissioner for Refugees).

– 2000. 'Environment: Monitoring and Evaluation.' www.unhcr.ch (8 December 2000).

– 1998. *Refugee Operations and Environmental Management: Key Principles for Decision-Making.* Geneva: Engineering and Environmental Services Section, UNHCR.

Veugelers, John. 2000. 'State-Society Relations in the Making of Canadian Immigration Policy.' *Canadian Review of Sociology and Anthropology* 37(1): 95–110.

Warhurst, John. 1993. 'The Growth Lobby and Its Opponents: Business, Unions, Environmentalists and Other Interest Groups.' In *The Politics of Australian Immigration.* Ed. J. Jupp and M. Kabala. Canberra: Australian Government Publishing Service.

Warren, Robert. 1994. 'Immigration's Share of U.S. Population Growth: How We Measure It Matters.' *Population Today* 22(9):3.

Weber, Terry. 2000. 'Canada's Population Up Slightly as of July 1.' *Globe and Mail*, 26 September.

6 'Getting the Message': Effects of Canadian Law and Social Policy on Families That Immigrate to Toronto

NANCY HOWELL

Family dynamics are changing in Canada as a whole and in Toronto specifically. Statistical studies compiled by Statistics Canada confirm what we observe all around us: fertility is at a very low level among current families, and divorce is at a high level (Jones et al. 1995; Baker 1995). As sociologists and demographers, we note that Canadians are, more often than they used to be, living in common-law arrangements rather than marriages. In opinion surveys, in classroom discussions, and around family dining tables, young Canadian men and women say they are wary of marriage, and they often express some reluctance to become parents either at an early age or very often. In the courts we find new kinds of rights being asserted: grandparents suing divorcing parents for access to their children, boyfriends suing to assert their rights over the pregnancy of girlfriends they were unwilling to marry, and occasionally even children suing their parents for separate maintenance in what amounts to 'divorce' from their parents. Granted, these occurrences are few in number; even so, they contribute to the overwhelming impression that families in Canada have changed radically and rapidly in recent decades. Torontonians from a range of ethnic backgrounds discuss these cases and wonder about their families.

At the same time, Toronto (along with the other megacities in Canada: Montreal and Vancouver) has become a destination of choice for steady streams of immigrants. Since the 1970s, when Canada made a radical change in its immigration policy, immigrants to Toronto have become more cosmopolitan, better educated, and more highly skilled than those in the past. Typical immigrant neighbourhoods in Toronto have changed their ethnicity from Italian, Greek, and Portuguese to Chinese, Vietnamese, Caribbean, and Ethiopian as a result of the changing patterns of immigration. The typical immigrant-receiving housing type seems to have changed from downtown row housing to high-rise apartment complexes built along the subway system. And frank social pressure to assimilate seems to have been replaced by an official ideology of multi-culturalism and appreciation of diversity (although the extent to which this is an improvement for the immigrants is a matter for investigation). Toronto is changing its form and functions as a result of the flows of people into the city from immigration, and also as a result of their organization into ethnic groups – a primary way that people structure their experience in the new land (Breton et al. 1990). In this paper we investigate the immigration experience as reported in interviews with members of five immigrant groups in Toronto during the 1990s: Jews, Italians, Caribbeans, Ghanaians, and Sri Lankans. These groups are significant in their own right; they are also representative of other ethnic groups that are settling in Toronto. They read messages from the experiences they encounter in Toronto – in their jobs, residential arrangements, and transportation – and from their contacts with authorities and peers. By listening to their stories, perceptions, and experiences, we can understand something of the changing structure of the city.

The Role of Ethnicity in Family Studies

One vastly oversimplified model of the 'ethnic factor' in Canadian family life is that there are only three significant types of Canadians and that each type has a characteristic family structure. These types are the British and the French 'charter groups' and 'the ethnics'; all, though, are descendants of immigrants over the past few hundred years. Even stating that model points to its difficulties: it makes no mention of aboriginal Canadians, whose ancestors were in Canada long before the French and English and some of whom continue to be relatively distinct from other Canadians in family demography; it assumes that the French and English 'charter groups' are unitary and that each shares a single culture of family life; and most egregiously, it leads us to expect that all ethnics share some 'different' family patterns from the 'majority,' or that ethnic Canadians are a waste-basket category that might include any and all patterns of family life. It also seems to suggest, even if only indirectly, that each of these 'types' is unchanging. So this model of a few initially distinct categories, which over time may or will 'assimilate' to a single pattern, is more a barrier than an avenue to understanding the contributions of ethnic groups and cultural differences to family life in Canada.

The reality is far more complex: a constantly changing picture of individuals being socialized within families and investing their identities in ethnic groups, which share a heritage by virtue of having immigrated to Canada from another part of the world (Beaujot 1991, 102–51; Ishwaran 1980). Even this description is a simplification, as a single ethnic group may include people who immigrated over a long period of time and who were derived from and socialized into disparate social class, occupational, religious, and regional groups in their country of origin, so that they do not necessarily have much in common with their fellow ethnics. As diversity develops within an ethnic group, it commonly happens that members of the group increase their rate of marriages outside the group (Richard 1991); and the children of those marriages are likely to invest their identity in bases other than ethnic group membership, thereby contributing to assimilation of the ethnic group and to a lessening of the importance of ethnicity as a basis for social organization. We asked our informants in this study to tell us about their family history, how and why they came to Toronto, in what ways the experience has been stressful and surprising, and in what ways they maintain their ethnic identity. Informants were asked about their perceptions of discrimination, their hopes and fears for themselves and their children, and the activities they participate in with other members of their ethnic group in Toronto.

A second way of looking at the role of ethnicity in family studies is commonly found in census studies of ethnicity, and is often referred to as studies in 'family demography' (Bongaarts et al. 1987). In family demography studies, we look at the statistical distribution of family 'facts' (such as age at marriage for the two sexes, number of children desired and born, rate of divorce, age at divorce and childbearing, household composition over the life course, and so forth), in order to determine whether the various ethnic groups in Canada differ in these ways. For simplicity's sake, we tend to assume that ethnicity is an inherited characteristic of individuals, obtained by birth from one's parents, with 'automatic' consequences for one's beliefs and behaviour (Halli et al. 1990). In making that assumption we slide over a number of challenging questions for which we need clear answers if we are to apply the 'family demography' model rigorously. Is ethnic membership automatic, or is there a voluntary component in addition to the inherited component? If the two parents are not of the same ethnicity, do the children follow the father? The mother? The side of the family they most resemble physically? Do they choose their own ethnicity between the alternatives?

Until 1981 it was Canada's census bureau that resolved such questions by asking for the ethnicity of the father's side of the family. After that year, in response to changing public opinion, it altered the question to allow the respondents to decide for themselves which ethnicity to report, and by allowing the possibility of two (or more) ethnic choices. This seems accurate and fair to those reporting on their ethnicity, but one wonders whether permitting multiple choices will eventually lose the advantages of clarity that the family demography model encourages. In a place like Toronto, where large numbers of ethnic group members marry outside their own group, respondents could potentially claim two groups in the parent generation, four for their grandparents, eight for their great-grandparents, and so on, thus doubling the number of choices in each generation. We think of this fragmentation of ethnic membership as a modern problem, resulting from high current rates of exogamy (out-marriage); actually, though, the phenomenon of intermarriage has been fairly frequent in many periods of history. Reporting ethnicity has always involved a simplification of complex family histories, and taking account of that explicitly may make ethnicity impossible to understand (McVey and Kalbach 1995, 345–61). Studies in family demography in Canada (Halli et al. 1990) show us that ethnic groups are coming to differ relatively little among themselves in their family demography parameters, even though ethnicity continues to be an important source of social identity and differential association in Canada.

We study ethnic groups because they provide naturally occurring groups who are going through a process of adjusting to conditions in Toronto (for an alternative approach, see Salaff in this volume). Pollak and Watkins (1993, 41) stress that within complex societies ethnicity is often an identifier of cultural similarity. They cite Barth (1969, 15) to show why ethnicity is so important in understanding family behaviour:

> The identification of another person as a fellow member of an ethnic group implies a sharing of criteria for evaluation and judgment. It thus entails the assumption that the two are fundamentally 'playing the same game'... On the other hand, a dichotomisation of others as strangers, as members of another ethnic group, implies a recognition of limitations on shared understandings, differences in criteria for judgment of value and performance, and a restriction of interaction to sectors of assumed common understanding and mutual interest.

From the point of view of the 'ethnics' who label themselves in this way, the term tends to refer to the group in which they claim membership. Ethnicity as a state of identification may be a highly subjective phenomenon that varies between groups, between generations within a group, and within individuals between stages of life and over time. Census questions on ethnic identity are deliberately designed to minimize the role played by these subjective issues in order to obtain data that can be used to characterize whole groups and to make comparisons between groups, but these questions cannot be made entirely objective and still reflect the meaningful membership of individuals in groups.

And finally, we need to stress that ethnicity carries with it not only automatic membership criteria, and a self-applied subjective sense of belonging that people may or may not feel strongly about, but also a situational or circumstantial dimension that is generally experienced as a characteristic of the 'outside' society rather than the ethnic group itself. Racism and ethnic discrimination in Toronto have never been taken to the extremes found in some parts of the world, but these processes have not been absent either, as aboriginal people, blacks, Jews, Germans, Japanese, and Pakistanis can all attest from their own painful experiences. Among the groups we studied, concerns about racism and discrimination were especially important aspects of the accounts of Jews, black Caribbeans, and Sri Lankans.

In this study we allow members of some of the current ethnic groups in the local environments of Toronto to teach us what it means to be a member of their ethnic group nowadays – in particular, what it means with regard to their family behaviour and attitudes. This study falls into the 'family demography' tradition, but it takes a qualitative rather than the usual quantitative approach to the subject. Clearly, we cannot study everything about these groups. Instead, we have assembled some basic information about the numbers of people, their home locations, and their occupations, and especially we have sought information on their families and households.

These people were all asked basically the same questions, which concerned their family's composition, events of family history, their expectations for the future, and the kinds of causal factors such as employment, education, and financial goals and problems that we suspect may be related to the family composition. We asked standard questions about what people have done and expect to do, their hopes and dreams, and their friends and relatives, and we also provided them opportunities to tell the stories that people tell to illustrate their experiences. In this chapter we focus our reporting on the ways people find their family life to be different or distinctive in Toronto, relative to the places they came from. We appreciate the help our informants have given us, and we recognize that this work could not have been done without that willing cooperation.

Methods of Data Collection

The research reported here consists of the results of the data collected by fourteen graduate students in the Department of Sociology at the University of Toronto, from a number of ethnic groups. The students obtained detailed interviews with around twenty adults in each group, each informant reporting on the experiences of his or her own family, including spouse, children, parents, and siblings. In this chapter, we draw from the results of only five of these fourteen studies, to simplify the results. The study was exploratory in the sense that we were not sure what we would find or what methods would be necessary to obtain our results. For this reason, our methods were tentative and flexible.

The project started with a series of seminars led by Howell, and attended by graduate students interested in the project, to establish an outline for the topics we wanted to cover. Graduate students who wanted to continue in the project wrote research proposals describing how they planned to approach the group they knew best. Those selected for research assistantships adopted the general outline we had agreed on, but also had licence to collect the data in ways that were most appropriate to the specific group and to the individuals contacted. Our target informants were parents of young adult children, middle-aged or 'young old' people in the midst of their family life who had already made their major demographic decisions about their own marriages and fertility, and who were likely to have thought about aspects of family life as they watched their own adult children making decisions such as about marriage and children.

The nature of the history of the ethnic group determined whether that goal was achievable or even desirable. For instance, the Italian immigrants came to Canada mainly as young adults in the 1950s. Survivors of that wave of immigration are currently in their sixties and seventies, and this group had a great deal to contribute to our study, having experienced forty years of life in Canada. So they were the

primary informants in the Italian group, even though they were somewhat older than our target, and they reported on their aspirations for
their grandchildren as well as their children. In contrast, immigrants
from Ghana have been arriving mainly over the past decade, and many
of them still have small children. There are very few Ghanaians in the
older generation in Toronto to report, so the contributions of Ghanaians
to our study reflect an earlier stage of the life span than some of the
other groups. We took the opportunity whenever possible to learn as
much as we could about the families in the study, both from what they
said in formal interviews and by observation. Some of the graduate
students shared meals, family outings and celebrations, and social events
with them and had considerable informal communication with members of the family; others had more formal relations to the families they
studied.

Similarly, the exact questions asked varied across groups according
to the ethnographer's assessment as to whether the questions were
proper ones to be asked in that group. With some groups, for instance, it
was easy to ask whether they expected their children to be sexually
experienced before marriage; with other groups it would have been
offensive to ask a parent that question. Ethnographers used their own
judgment when phrasing questions for the group they belonged to, and
in some cases questions weren't asked at all. When informants were
willing to speak freely and informatively about their families and the
changes they had experienced in family life since coming to Canada, we
didn't need to ask any questions at all. Our main job as ethnographers
was to listen carefully to what our informants told us, not to probe for
information that our informants did not want to share. So we asked
questions about the first members of the family to come to Canada, and
what that was like; whom their families consist of and how often they
saw the members of their families; what occasions brought them together; and how they felt about living in Canada and whether they
could imagine living again in the country they came from. When the
ethnographers thought it best to avoid certain questions for particular
individuals or for the whole group, they were free to do so. And of
course the informants were reminded at the beginning of the interview
that their participation in the study was voluntary, and that they were
free to reject any of the questions that were asked.

The graduate-student participants in this research project were an
ethnically diverse bunch, and their ethnicity and language and cultural
skills determined the details of this research and made it possible. In

many cases they already had rapport with the families they interviewed, and in many other cases they came to interview strangers after being introduced by someone both parties knew well. They were encouraged to interview family friends, and the friends and relatives of friends, and the friends of informants who had already taken part in the study. This 'snowball' method of obtaining informants has strong advantages: it is easier for informants to establish a friendly and helpful attitude towards the interviewer when he or she can locate that person in a social world of friends and relatives. In most instances the characteristics of the interviewers were also reassuring: they were familiar with the language, the culture, the neighbourhoods, and the shared meanings of symbols and events. There are also drawbacks to using the snowball technique to obtain informants for a study like this: the informants are likely to resemble one another, and we may fail to learn about significant parts of the populations who were not reached by this method. This disadvantage was accepted from the beginning as inevitable. And so in the ensuing report we will keep in mind that a larger and more representative study would be necessary to challenge or confirm the kinds of tentative conclusions we have reached.

Typically, the interviews were conducted in the informant's home, usually with the interviewer alone with the informant. In some cases, though, other family members were present or were moving in and out of the interview situation. In a few interviews, a married couple was interviewed jointly, with the spouses responding to each other's answers as well as to the question asked. The interviews were conducted in English or in the native language of the ethnic group, or in a mixture of the two. All of the interviews were tape-recorded (with the agreement of the informant) and transcribed (and translated if necessary) by the ethnographer. During the summer of 1993, when most of the interviews were conducted, the research team of eight to fourteen members (varying as people entered and left the project) met regularly to share results and discuss the process of data collection and the results that were emerging. Our flexible method of data collection allowed us to take advantage of our learning process: some questions were modified, added, or dropped during the data collection.

Methods of Data Analysis

Interviews were typed, edited, and (if necessary) translated by the ethnographers, and a summary of the results was prepared by the ethnographer. Interviews were then pooled for further analysis by Howell, using the method of NUD*IST (Non-numerical Unstructured Data Indexing Searching and Theorizing), a qualitative data management and analysis package (QSR 1997). NUD*IST is a method that constructs a logic tree of topics and concepts out of a close study of the interviews, indexing the documents so that any passages that relate to that topic or concept can be easily retrieved. The index ends up as a summary of the contents of the documents, and the instances of reference to the topics can be counted or quoted easily. It was an ideal method for the kind of exploratory research we were conducting here, in that it produced a summary of what all our informants told us and enabled us to permit the informants to express their perceptions in their own words. Instead of summarizing what a group of people told us, often we could step aside and allow the informants to speak for themselves about the issues they felt strongly about, on the topics that emerged from the interviews as the central concerns of the informants.

Results

The 'Old Immigrants'

The Jews are a distinctive community with a long history as an ethnic group. They have a shorter history in Canada but are still one of the oldest groups of European settlers in Canada. Most of the Jewish families studied by Tracy Aaron have been in Canada for several generations. The original immigration event has become almost mythological in the family, although a minority of families have immigrated from Russia or Israel over the past twenty years. Jews have flourished in Toronto and are the ethnic group with the highest rate of education and the highest average income among those studied (Halli et al. 1990, 167). They enjoy intergenerational ties, get together to celebrate Jewish holidays, and tell us they worry about the younger generation marrying out of the group. They worry that anti-Semitism could flare up again at any time. All of the Jewish families were scarred by the Holocaust, no matter where they were living at the time, and some of the families were traumatized severely.

Italians have been arriving in Canada for a century, and came in especially large numbers in the two decades after the Second World War (see also Howell 2000). The Italians in Toronto mostly came from Southern Italy, and many or most of them came with skilled trades but little formal education. They have made a very successful adjustment to life in urban Canada despite the initial hurdles they faced, becoming prosperous businesspeople and homeowners. Ethnographer Patricia Albanese found that Toronto has several large and flourishing neighbourhoods of people of Italian descent. Most of our informants in this community are elderly, first-generation immigrants who came to Canada in the 1950s. They tell us that Italian parents worry until their adult children 'settle down' by marrying someone Italian or at least Catholic. The 'Italian wedding' seems to be the prototypical occasion for the family to display itself and for the community to get together, even if these weddings are somewhat smaller than they are reported to have been a decade or so ago. The younger generations tell us that the first generation is 'old fashioned,' always concerned about whether people are Italian, and concerned about whether both males and females are getting the respect they deserve. The younger generation differs from the older by valuing education higher (and financial success lower) and by valuing personal characteristics and Catholicism higher (and Italian background lower) in a potential spouse. Younger Italians in Toronto tend to agree with their elders about the importance of family solidarity.

The 'New Immigrants'

Our study also examines some of the more recent arrivals, from groups that are now changing the character of immigration to Toronto.

The first group of 'new immigrants,' studied by graduate student Linda Blanshay, are from the Caribbean islands of St Vincent and the Grenadines. These people came to Canada in the 1970s, 1980s, and 1990s (see also Darden, in this volume, for more discussion of Canadian immigration policy as it has affected Caribbean families in their marriage rates and economic problems). Some of these people came through the regular post-1971 immigration procedures, which are based on the 'point system,' or through family unification to follow someone who had been awarded landed immigrant status. Others – in all cases women – came under a special immigration program for home workers that was in place during the 1970s and 1980s to provide households with maids, practical nurses, and nannies. Many of the women who entered Canada under this program were overqualified for these jobs, with backgrounds as teachers, nurses, or secretaries in the Caribbean; even so, they welcomed the opportunity to obtain residence in Canada, where jobs pay much more, and to establish a basis for eventually bringing in their families. The Caribbean families in our study are notable for the presence of many strong and independent women, who are not only self-supporting (most of the new migrants share this characteristic) but who are also the mainstays of support for their families, including husbands, children, and siblings and their families.

The Caribbean workers in our study are often employed in service jobs (although rarely in home services after their initial employment), and some own their own service businesses. Many of the Caribbean adults expressed concerns about prejudice and racism in Toronto, as well as concern that their children should grow up with a positive self-image, undamaged by the negative attitudes that surround them. The parents seem little concerned that their children should marry others from the same background in Canada; at the same time, they seem to try hard to give their children some experience of the Caribbean societies they come from. In the long Toronto winters, many adults dream of retiring to the islands, where the cost of living is lower and the sun is warm, but they also agree with members of other groups that the chances their children will want to return are small, and they are likely to retain strong ties to Canada for the rest of their lives.

Ghanaians in Toronto were studied by Kwaku Obosu-Mensah (see also Howell 2000), who reports that the local society is very different from the societies the immigrants come from, where large, extended family households are common and where the sexes carry on quite segregated lives, men with men and women with women (and children). Ghanaians tell us they find it difficult to live in small apartments with just the husband and wife to care for the children, who tend to be underfoot but who are required to be extremely independent by Ghanaian standards, because often both parents are away at work until the evening. Men remark that they find themselves doing chores in Toronto that they would never be expected to do in Ghana – tasks such as washing dishes, cooking, shopping, and caring for children. Women remark that they have no sisters or cousins to help them with housework and child care and that they are expected to work all day at paid jobs as well as being solely responsible for all the housework. Both sexes report that they feel their lives are dislocated in Toronto, and they enjoy connecting with their home society through phone calls and through local community gatherings, usually around the death of senior members of the Ghanaian community. An elaborate communal life has grown up in Toronto over a short time, consisting of Ghanaian newspapers, radio programs, community halls, and churches, along with informal ties.

Sri Lankans tell our ethnographers of the bewildering process of conflict and disruption in Sri Lankan society that eventually led to their arrival in Canada. Many of the informants tell of arriving in Toronto, exhausted and nervous about the formalities, and finding other Sri Lankans at the airport, strangers but welcome reminders of home, who took them home and helped them 'get on their feet' during the first days or weeks in Toronto. The Singhalese Sri Lankans in our study, studied by Sarath Chandresekere, typically came in the late 1970s and 1980s. They had found good jobs and established comfortable homes by the time they were interviewed. Many of our informants have children of high school or university age, who are a great source of both pride and concern for their parents. They worry that their children are at risk of losing their ethnic identity as well as the respect for parental authority that is a defining characteristic of these primarily Buddhist families. The Tamil families in our study, studied by Marybeth Raddon, tend to have come to Canada later, in the 1980s and 1990s, and have younger families and smaller children. The civil war in Sri Lanka was at a more violent and depressing stage when our Tamil informants came to Canada, some of them as immigrants and others as refugees. The family stories of the Tamil Sri Lankans often focus on war atrocities, on family members who have been killed or arrested in Sri Lanka, and on the political organizations in Canada that demand support from Tamil residents for the war effort at home. The Sri Lankans seem more preoccupied with events in their home country than the members of other groups we talked to; they also seem to become involved in overtly ethnic conflicts in Canada more often than the others, in the form of political organizations and – in the case of young adult men – in street fights and the harassment of individuals and small groups.

Changes in Household Ecology: The High Cost of Living and Women in the Workforce

From a comparison of all the ethnic groups, certain themes emerge as foci of the concerns of these immigrants. Below, each of these gets its own section of discussion. These themes are, first, the intersection of opportunities for employment for women and the high cost of living in Toronto that leads to the nearly universal phenomenon of two-earner families; and second, stress and change in role relationships within families.

Immigrant families have come to Canada from around the world. They bring with them traditions relating to family size and dynamics as well as to sexual equality. When they arrive in Canada, they find they must cope with some strong pressures arising from life in Canada, which tend to change and homogenize their family norms and behaviours.

These pressures include (1) the high cost of living in Canada, (2) the opportunities (and in some cases perceived necessity) for women to earn a living by employment or self-employment, and (3) the need to provide children with sustained educational opportunities in order to help them achieve high status and a good life in Canada. For some families the standard of consumer goods consumption is much higher in Canada than in the country of origin. All of these factors together produce the phenomenon of families with women (mothers and wives as well as daughters) who are in the workforce rather than only in the home. Women who are bringing home a substantial paycheque to contribute to the family welfare have clearer claims to consideration and increased participation in decision making in the family than women have who do not hold jobs. Most husbands/fathers acknowledge that it is totally unfair to expect the wife/mother to do all the housecleaning, cooking, organizing, and chores of the family, so even when the load is not distributed equally in immigrant families (just as it is not in native-born Canadian families), adult men say they accept a larger role in housework than they ever did before.

All of this was clear to a Ghanaian man, who told us:

In this country, the women also work hard, and here people live individualistically and that has a lot of effect on people, especially stress, depression, and so forth. You are in this small apartment with your wife – only the two of you are in here – or with the children. It's not easy to communicate with a two- or a three-year-old child so that when there is a lot of work in the house, and you don't help, that means you put a lot of stress on the woman, and that means you don't love your wife.

A Jewish man reported that in his family,

because we were both working we had to have someone to take care of the children and cook and clean when they were younger. I would say now that our children are involved in the daily household duties. I do most of the cooking in the house, my wife does the laundry, and one of the kids does the ironing. Next year one of the children will be more involved in the cooking.

A particularly insightful Caribbean told us:

A woman in the workforce was never a problem in the West Indies; they've always supplemented men's income because we were always on the low end of the scale, we always needed things. You're not aware of a lot of things back home, like wage inequality ... but you don't get into things, up here you've got statistics for everything. But back home you don't need to go to the woman's shelter to be protected, the community protects you.

Virtually all of the new-immigrant families we studied had working wives as well as husbands. Many of the women had worked in some way in the country they came from, but virtually all of them took paying jobs when they arrived in Canada. They remark that jobs are more widely available for women in Canada, that the jobs pay much better than similar (or even higher-status) jobs in the country of origin, and that the family members feel they need two incomes because the cost of living is so high in Canada. Although some of the new-immigrant women took leaves of absence from work or quit for a while, intending to find another job later, when their children were born or were in the preschool years, most of the women worked full time all or nearly all of the time in Canada (Armstrong and Armstrong 1978).

The old-immigrant families – Jews and Italians – more often tell us that women took long leaves from work or stayed home with the children permanently while only the husband worked. The single-wage-earner family seems to be a rarity in today's Toronto for both immigrant and native-born Canadians (Watkins 1991).

Independence of Children

Children who grow up in households where both parents are in the workforce, and where there is no adult in the home during the daytime, have to be raised to be independent whatever the cultural standards of the ethnic group or the personal beliefs of the parents. Asian parents, in particular, often speak of their desire to keep a good sense of control over their children, of ensuring that they do all of their homework, study hard for school tests, and associate only with playmates approved by the parents. But this protective control over children is difficult or impossible to maintain when both parents are in the workforce and come home only in the evening. Children in dual-income families must learn to manage day care, after-school programs, peer-group pressures, and self-directed homework. Children with this degree of independence are not easy to control when they come to the age of dating and adolescent rebelliousness.

Empty Residences in the Daytime and the Consequences for Old Age

The Canadian pattern of the nuclear family residence – of homes that are empty during working and school hours for most families – has been widely adopted by contemporary immigrant families from all the countries of origin investigated. The consequences of the 'empty house' are pervasive: parents cannot continuously supervise and nurture small children, the elderly, and the sick in the home. These dependent members of the family have to learn to deal with and conform to institutions such as day care, homes for the aged, and hospitals and nursing homes when the family – usually meaning the adult woman or women – cannot care for them.

A Ghanaian man told the researcher:

> My wife and I will move to Ghana when we are old. In our society back home, they are very helpful to the old people, better than over here in Canada. When you are old in Canada you are isolated and it is very seldom that your family can visit you. You know, the government has to look after you. Back home we have a broad family system to take care of you.

A man from Guyana responded to a question about whether his parents would live in an old-age home: 'Definitely not. That's just not part of our values, we don't do that.' A Ghanaian man was asked: 'Suppose your parents are in Canada and they are very old. Will you like them to stay with you or will you take them to a senior people's home?' The respondent answered: 'If my parents were here I will like to be with them, because in Africa when our parents are old we live with them and help them in housework and other things. I don't want them to live alone.' Immigrants who have been in Canada longer may have different ideas about their living arrangements in old age. Jewish informants told us that they expect moral support from their adult children when they are old, but seem to dread the possibility that the children might have to provide a lot of care:

> I hope it never happens. Emotionally, in every situation, I would expect them to give me support when I get older. Financially, when I'm ninety, and if I lost all my money and I needed help, I would expect them to help me out.

An elderly Italian man told us:

> When I can't take care of myself, and if I am left alone (if his wife dies first) I would much rather go to a retirement or nursing home. I don't want to be a burden on my children or anyone else. In a Home, with my pension, I will be fine. A retirement home is fine. It all depends on if you still have your wits about you.

At the same time, employment of women changes the power structure of the household. Women command their own income. They have to make (and have the opportunity to make) independent decisions about transportation, dressing, eating at work, and association with fellow workers, male and female, inside and outside the place of work. Women tend to gain power over their own decisions, and men tend to lose power – or at least feel they have lost power – over their spouses. Children have to be encouraged to be self-reliant and independent of parents, not only for the school hours but also for the several hours daily of 'after-school' time until parents return from work. When the family comes together at the end of the day, the participants may be profoundly changed by their experiences.

Stress and Conflict between Spouses

In many immigrant families, these changes in the family lead to conflict and stress. Although it may be gratifying to live within a two-income family (or more, for families who have young adult wage-earners still living at home) because of the relatively high income and consumer possibilities, the consequences for family roles are profound. Husbands find themselves required to 'help' with housework, because of the manifest unfairness of leaving it all to the women (who are gone from the household as much as the men). For instance, a man from Ghana said:

> Even now, just before you came, I was cooking. I think back home the wife does everything – she does the cooking and things of that sort. And the role of the man is just to make provisions for the family ... We haven't made any division in the housework, but I always do try to help her wherever she falls short. She mostly does the cooking, but if I see that she is doing something else then I will do the cooking.

His wife added, 'Back home you get your sisters, your cousins, everybody is around you to help you so you won't have any difficulties [with housework and cooking].'

The forms of stress can be much more severe, of course. A number of our informants told us about family behaviour they perceived as abuse – generally of the wife by the husband, less often of the children by the parents. We found wide agreement among members of various ethnic groups that – in contrast to their countries of origin – in Canada the government sides with the oppressed and has the authority to prosecute abusers. This placed strong pressure on family dynamics in Canada. A Sri Lankan woman who had suffered greatly from her husband's inflexibility and dictatorial ways towards her and the children reported:

> He couldn't adjust. After we came here he had lots of stress, and he couldn't bear it. He has to put it on somebody else, and I am there to receive it. And the children, they didn't like it ... At one stage my children told me, 'we'll go away and live somewhere else, leaving him.' But I said to the children, 'For me, I'm happy if my children do well in life, but I have to be with my husband, whether he is good or bad. Sometimes he's a little bit dominating. But that's the way he was brought up and that's the way he is. He cannot change. A little bit he is changing. At least we should be happy for that.'

The husband in another family told of his struggles to learn new skills in dealing with his wife and other family members:

> I was just a father/husband figure in Sri Lanka. Everything was taken care of by my wife. Here I do marketing, taking children to schools, and

gardening. I still do not cook, but I help my wife cook, and I am learning cooking. Initially it was difficult to listen to everybody at home when decisions about living here were made. Now I have learned the art of joint decision-making.

A wife from Pakistan who came to Canada from the Caribbean reported that immigration had changed her husband without a struggle on her part:

> My husband is anyway my leader. However, he seems to be a different person compared to an average Pakistani male. He joins me in cooking, we share decision-making. He does not give orders to me. His living in England changed him from the very beginning of his life.

A Sri Lankan woman who had divorced an abusive husband and who was making an independent life for herself and her children was asked what she liked and disliked about Canadian society. She answered:

> I like the services here. They are very good. Wife assault is a crime in Canada. Protection and prospects for women is very good. There are ample opportunities for individual growth here in Canada. The negatives are that there is too much freedom for children. They are forced to assume too much responsibility too early.

A Ghanaian man contended that the divorce rate of Ghanaians is higher in Canada than in Ghana:

> The main reason is that here the type of life we are leading is quite different from the one we lead at home. When we come here, you know, we have to work and this thing brings a lot of differences between you and your wife. Sometimes, too, each and every one is trying to get something for him, or her, and sometimes it brings confusion between the two and it brings about divorce. Some of our women, too, they know that if they are separated from their men they can get some social benefit, so they don't care about the man.

Another Ghanaian man put it:

> Back home, it is rather difficult for a couple to get a divorce because both families set in and settle the matter amicably. Over here, it's like the

women have the upper hand in the family affairs, and one little thing happens, and the woman says 'I'm gone.'

A third Ghanaian man summarized the situation:

> When Ghanaian women come to Canada they find the freedom, the kind of freedom that this society provides to women, and they take advantage of it. OK, they are fighting for the same equality as the men, and that has a serious effect on most marriages over here. Another thing is that financial burdens also cause marriages to break down. As women become independent, as long as they can have jobs to provide for their needs, they think they are well off enough to be on their own. I'm not blaming the women – I don't want to be judgmental – but the men also have their own problems.

Stress and Conflict between Parents and Children

Attitudes towards children and what parents should aspire to give to children may also be different in Toronto from attitudes in the places these families came from. Families from all the groups we studied reported that their children needed to do well in school and have a 'good education' – which for some groups is a university education – in order to thrive. Some of the families reported that this aspiration was consistent with conditions in their country of origin; others reported that it was different; but all reported that they perceived it as very important in Toronto.

The old-immigrant families typically had higher fertility norms and aspirations than native-born Canadians. For instance, it was several decades before the Italian Canadians had a level of fertility as low as other Canadians. But regarding the new immigrants, the desired fertility level seems to be low on arrival – they are basically indistinguishable from other Canadians. Each child is difficult and expensive to raise. The parents we interviewed seemed to share the aspiration to provide their children with the best possible support and education, but they did not tell us that they wished they could have more children than the few they were having.

Immigrant children may have untraditional powers over their parents when they speak better English and can deal with the world outside the family better than their parents. This situation was common among the old immigrants but is rare in Toronto among the new immigrants, most of whom are well educated and entirely fluent in English.

However, parents may find that they cannot protect their children or influence them to the extent they have been socialized to expect, because the children are away from parental influence so much of the time. The peer group, the school, and the television have become important forces of socialization in the children's lives, along with the parents.

A Sri Lankan mother commented on these differences between Sri Lanka and Canada:

> There the parents make the decisions for the kids. Everything up to the point of marriage. Their education, extracurricular activities, where you move, practically everything. The parents are gods. They expect their kids to really perform for them, to do very well in life, to be a model to others. The main difference is in the free say that they [kids] have here. Here you don't force your kids to do something. Children have to think and decide things for themselves.

A Sri Lankan father expressed some fear when he said:

> We have given our children a lot of freedom to think and to plan their future. They can question us. They do not necessarily eat our food. However, we tend to exercise some form of control over their affairs. They are not encouraged to live separately until they get married. When my girl was schooling my wife used to escort her. Even in the university, I have paid for a parking space for her. We always hear traumatic things happen to Asian girls.

Parents commented wryly on their loss of discipline. A St Vincent man told us:

> Here the government has a lot of power over kids. They can influence kids even to avoid the authority of their parents at home. The kids tell me, 'if you hit us, we call 911.' Now I tell the kids, 'You give me any trouble I will deal with you over there' [St Vincent]. I don't hit them but somehow they get the idea here that I can't.

Some parents wanted to limit the amount they invested in their children, because the children were so independent. A Sri Lankan father said, when asked whether he expected his children to take care of him in his old age:

No. Because they are born here and raised here, I can't expect it. But my parents spent one hundred percent on us because they know we are going to support them back. In my case, I don't want to spend one hundred percent on my children: at least thirty percent I'll save for me and my wife. Because my children have their own ways, and my wife and I will have to depend upon our insurance.

A key element in relationships between children and parents in Canada is the children's sense that their parents have been legally deprived of the right to physically force them to do anything. Children believe that physical punishment of them in the form of slaps or spanking is against the law and that they can invoke police protection against their parents. Apparently, this information has become part of children's culture on the playgrounds of Canadian schools. Many respondents told us their children came home from school the first day (or at least soon after arrival) with the information that parents in Canada are not allowed to hit children. We heard a lot of nervous laughter – and some indignation – about the prospect of children calling the police (at '911') to have their abusive parents arrested.

Formation of New Families

Immigrants often change their family composition by leaving some parts of the family behind in the country of origin. Ethnic groups who live in and expect extended multinuclear families as units of production, consumption, and household composition in the old country often find themselves effectively living in a nuclear family after immigration, as a result of distance from extended kin and the high cost of the kinds of accommodations in Canada that would permit joint households. Immigrants, like other Canadians, overwhelmingly live in single-family homes and apartments. Parents of young adults or late adolescent children express considerable concern about how their children will negotiate the transfer from the family of orientation to a family of procreation of their own. The desire of parents to control the choice of spouse is a touchy issue in many immigrant families.

Parents told us they hoped their children would select a spouse from the same ethnic group but that they had to face the possibility that they might not. A Caribbean woman put it this way:

Personally I think people should not intermarry. They should marry their kind. But there are lots of people who don't believe that, you should marry who you love. It's very easy to love your kind. When you marry someone who is like you, the way you problem-solve is the same, your social life. To me, it's much better. Not only that but you lose your culture, the children are neither here nor there, neither black or white.

A Hindu woman from the Caribbean told us:

To be honest with you I would very much like my kids to get married in their own religion and their own culture because it will be a more comfortable situation in the long run. When you choose a spouse, think about everything you've learned and think about ten or twenty years down the line and how are you going to deal with this later and make your decision, just don't make the decision for today, think about the long term. Don't let your heart rule your head.

On the other hand, an Italian grandmother who had been in Canada for almost fifty years told us, when asked how she would feel if her grandchildren married non-Italians: 'Oh well, at this point, I say as long as they love each other, I'm used to it. Religion [Catholicism] is very important to me now, [not being Italian].'

The boundaries of ethnic groups are maintained or weakened through marital choices (Richard 1991). The parents in our study reported almost universally that they hoped their children would marry within their ethnic group. At the same time, parents recognized that they would have to be less selective about this than their own parents were for them, and that their children might entirely reject their preferences for the same ethnic group. The younger generation may not be rebelling against the values of their parents; it may simply be that other competing bases of identity – political orientation, religion, occupation, education, artistic affiliation, and so on – are more salient than ethnicity when it comes to choosing a spouse.

In a number of ethnic groups in Canada – the Jews are a prime case – economic success and the decline of discrimination have contributed to the opposite problem: out-marriage of the majority of young people. There has never been a time when ethnic in-marriage was 100 per cent in any group. Richard (1991, 109–10) has shown that rates of exogamy (marriage outside the group) in 1871 for husbands of various ethnic origins varied from about 25 per cent for the British-origin groups to only 3.3 per cent for French-origin husbands. In 1971 the French still had the lowest rate (13 per cent), whereas the average for all husbands was up to 37.3 per cent, and certain groups, such as the Scandinavians (79 per cent), Irish (72 per cent), and Scots (69 per cent) had substantial majorities marrying outside the group. These groups do not seem to be concerned about maintaining their ethnic group boundaries; however, the Jews – especially the religious Jews – seem to be just as concerned about the melting of the borders of their group as they are about discrimination from outside the group.

As rates of out-marriage for both husbands and wives continue to increase, as ethnic identity increasingly becomes a matter of individual choice, and as symbols of ethnicity rather than measurable differences in behaviour demarcate viable ethnic groups, it seems likely that the role of ethnicity in understanding and explaining family differences in Canada will continue to decline.

Conclusion: 'The Message' Contained in Law and Social Policy in Canada

Our informants reported that they did not experience much or any pressure to conform to the norms and values of native-born Canadians. At the same time, they often pointed to the role of law and social policy in their lives (Eichler 1988; Michelson, this volume).

The core 'message' that immigrants receive about family values from the law in Canada is that individuals are protected from assault and violence from their family members. Some of the parents expressed indignation that Canadian law does not permit them to enforce discipline and obedience of family members. Parents fear they will be unable to control their offspring, either when they are small children and are learning the important family norms and culture, or when they are adolescents and young adults and are making their own life decisions. Some of the parents are grateful for the Canadian law, and some are outraged by it, but all are influenced by its message. Of course Canadian law has not been entirely successful in stopping violence within immigrant or native-born families, but the message – that individual rights are more important than family welfare as determined by the parents – is important even when it is violated.

Rights to services in Canada are provided on an individual rather than a family basis. Thus each individual gets a health card from the provincial system of socialized medicine, and each child is entitled to a place in school no matter what the family characteristics are. Similarly, Canadian society sends a message to immigrant families through the social welfare benefits that are available. Family breakdown – by separation, by divorce, and even by the abandonment and neglect of elders or young people – is treated as an unfortunate but sometimes unavoidable 'accident' in the Canadian social welfare system, not as deliberate destruction of the authority and coherence of the family system. Social welfare payments allow unhappy and rebellious wives (and children and elders) to avoid the authority of a family head, to support themselves in a separate household. Governments, instead of forcing the family members to submit, provide welfare payments – in the form of court-ordered child support payments child allowance payments, direct benefits, and so on – to support individuals who cannot get along with a dominant family member. Canadian society has not eliminated patriarchy – far from it – but our informants tell us that Canada has changed the balance by channelling family power towards wives and children and away from husbands/fathers somewhat more than the countries they came from.

New immigrants in Canada are modifying their family structures towards a more egalitarian ethos, towards more freedom and individualism for all the members, and they are already nearly identical to other urban Canadians in their fertility and mortality rates, ages at marriage, and rates of divorce and cohabitation. It seems that Toronto is becoming a city with enormous variability in cultural and religious practices and with great diversity in symbolic consumption practices, but with very little variability with regard to the core issues of family demography.

REFERENCES

Armstrong, Pat, and Hugh Armstrong, 1978. *The Double Ghetto: Canadian Women and Their Segregated Work.* Toronto: McClelland & Stewart.
Baker, Maureen. 1995. *Family: Current Trends in Canada*, 3rd ed. Toronto: McGraw-Hill Ryerson.
Barth, Frederick A. 1969. Introduction. In *Ethnic Groups and Boundaries.* Boston: Little Brown.
Beaujot, Roderic. 1991. *Population Changes in Canada: The Challenge of Policy Adaptation.* Toronto: McClelland & Stewart.
Breton, Raymond, Wsevolod W. Isajiw, Warren E. Kalbach, and Jeffrey G.

Reitz. 1990. *Ethnic Identity and Equality: Varieties of Experience in a Canadian City*. Toronto: University of Toronto Press.

Bongaarts, John, Thomas Burch, Kenneth Wachter. 1987. *Family Demography: Methods and Their Applications. Oxford*: Clarendon Press.

Eichler, Margrit. 1988. Families in Canada Today: Recent Changes and Their Policy Consequences, 2nd ed. Toronto: Gage P.

Halli, Shiva Lingappa S., Frank Trovato, and Leo Driedger. 1990. *Ethnic Demography: Canadian Immigrant, Racial and Cultural Variations*. Ottawa: Carlton University Press.

Howell, Nancy, with Patricia Albanese and Kwaku Obosu-Mensah. 2000. 'Ethnic Families.' In *Families: Changing Trends in Canada*. 4th ed., ed. M. Baker. Toronto: McGraw-Hill Ryerson.

Ishwaran, K. 1980. *Canadian Families: Ethnic Variations*. Toronto: McGraw-Hill Ryerson.

Jones, Charles L., Lorne Tepperman, and Susannah J. Wilson. 1995. *The Futures of the Family*. Englewood Cliffs, NJ: Prentice Hall.

McVey, Wayne W., and Warren E. Kalbach. 1995. *Canadian Population*. Toronto: Nelson.

Pollak, Robert A., and Susan Cotts Watkins. 1993. 'Cultural and Economic Approaches to Fertility: Proper Marriage or Misalliance?' *Population and Development Review* 19:467–96.

QSR. 1997. *NUD*IST User Guide*. Melbourne, Australia: Qualitative Solutions and Research.

Richard, Madeleine A. 1991. *Ethnic Groups and Marital Choices: Ethnic History and Marital Assimilation in Canada, 1871 and 1971*. Vancouver: UBC Press.

Watkins, Susan Cott, with Ann Spector and Alice Goldstein. 1991. 'Demographic Patterns and Family Behavior among Jewish and Italian Women in the U.S., 1900–30.' Paper delivered at the Social Science History Association meetings, 2 November.

7 The Impact of Canadian Immigration Policy on the Structure of the Black Caribbean Family in Toronto

JOE T. DARDEN

Immigration decisions are made within existing economic, political, and social structures. Immigration policy affects these structures by influencing the size and composition of the immigrant population. In Toronto, immigration is a major component of change that works constantly on the structure and the identity of the population (Beaujot and Rappak 1986). Immigration also alters the demographic make-up of a metropolitan area by making it more diverse. Thus, immigration changes the employment and housing structures. The main thesis in this chapter is that Canadian immigration policy has clearly affected the composition of the black Caribbean immigrant population, with profound social and economic consequences for contemporary black Caribbean families.

Immigration Patterns

Toronto, like Montreal and Vancouver, is an initial destination or gateway for immigrants. The changing social and ethnocultural characteristics of the immigrant population and the extreme degree of geographic concentration – often in conjunction with the net out-migration of native-born residents – together are making the large gateway cities look very different from cities in the rest of Canada (Bourne 1999, 4). For example, between 1971 and 1996, Torontonians of African or Caribbean origin increased from 1.1 per cent of the population to 5.6 per cent. In contrast, the British-origin population declined from 60.4 per cent to 27.0 per cent (Reitz and Lum, this volume).

Toronto's 1996 metropolitan area population was 4 million; of these, more than 1.5 million had arrived over the previous six years. Clearly,

Toronto is one of the urban places in Canada that attracts large numbers of international migrants. According to Bourne (1999, 7), recent immigrants to Canada are attracted to urban places that are larger and within which there are higher incomes, service-based economies, higher educational levels, and higher average house prices.

Most recent immigrants are people of colour, and 94 per cent lived in a CMA in 1996, compared to 62 per cent of the total population. Toronto has been, and remains, the Canadian CMA of choice. The same year, it was the place of residence of 42 per cent of the total visible-minority population in Canada – the highest percentage of any CMA (Statistics Canada 1998). Visible minorities also constituted a higher share of the total population in Toronto (32 per cent) than in any other metropolitan area. As a comparison, minorities represented 11 per cent of Vancouver's population and 12 per cent of Montreal's. Of the 1.3 million visible-minority people in the Toronto CMA, about 25 per cent were Chinese; another 24.7 per cent were South Asians, and 21 per cent were blacks.

Toronto rivals New York and London as a destination for international migrants (Todd 1995). Lemon (1996, 244) has noted that even by 1975, two in five Torontonians were foreign-born (more than twice the Canadian level) – a pattern similar to that of New York at an earlier time. Toronto, Montreal, and Vancouver together accounted for 66 per cent of all immigrants who arrived between 1981 and 1991; these cities contained only 26 per cent of the Canadian-born population (Citizenship and Immigration Canada, 1997).

This increased representation of the foreign-born, who are composed largely of immigrants of colour, has heightened public awareness that discrimination against people of colour exists in Toronto and other large cities. In the 1980s the federal government became more sensitive to issues of racial equality as immigration trends altered the racial composition and structure of the Canadian population (Li 1999, 154).

Employment Structure

By the time visible minorities were allowed into Canada in larger numbers following reform of the racially restrictive immigration policies of the 1960s, economic power was shifting from Montreal, and Toronto was becoming the centre of Canadian economic power. Toronto's banks stood at the top of the Canadian financial pyramid. Toronto provided one-quarter of all jobs in finance and insurance (Lemon 1996, 249). During the 1960s, Montreal's two largest banks – the Bank of Montreal and the Royal Bank of Canada – moved their international operations to Toronto. The Toronto Stock Exchange was the largest in Canada, handling two-thirds of all trades (ibid.). Toronto also led the way in entertainment and tourism in Canada.

By the 1960s, employment opportunities were shifting away from the industrial, warehousing, and wholesaling sectors towards the white-collar, retail, and service sectors (Core Area Task Force 1974, 266–7, 281–2, 293, 319). In Toronto, service-sector growth has been driving urban economic development since the 1960s (Todd 1995).

Toronto's employment structure changed radically after 1966. The manufacturing labour force in Metro Toronto declined in relative terms between 1961 and 1971 from 30 per cent to 24 per cent of the total workforce. In the 1970s, very few manufacturing jobs were added in the metropolitan area; by the early 1980s, plant closings were creating a downward trend (Lawson 1975; Lemon 1985, 183). The Province of Ontario remained Toronto's largest employer. As Toronto's economic base came to depend less on manufacturing and more on services – especially finance – it garnered a greater share of Canada's economic influence, much of it at the expense of Montreal (Lemon 1985, 186).

By 1983, the head offices of more than two hundred of the top five hundred Canadian companies and many foreign-owned corporations were located in Toronto. By 1985, 42 per cent of Metro Toronto's workers were employed in offices and the white-collar and service sectors together accounted for almost 75 per cent of all employment (Metropolitan Toronto Planning Department 1986, 42, 60). Growth in the service sector more than compensated for losses in the manufacturing sector. Thus, total employment in the Toronto CMA increased between 1971 and 1991 (Coffey 1994). After a lingering recession in the first half of the 1990s, Toronto's employment had increased substantially by 1996, with the job increases primarily in finance, insurance, and real estate (FIRE) and in business services. These two industries accounted for 19 per cent of employment in the Toronto CMA in 1996.

Employment opportunities were increasing, but they also varied by gender. Women tended to find it harder than men to obtain good jobs and advance their careers once they found one (Oaka 2003). As we shall see later, this gender bias in the job market would have a disproportionate impact on the black population of Toronto.

Housing and Neighbourhood Structure

Immigrants who arrived in Toronto in search of affordable, decent housing and neighbourhoods found themselves in an urban environment in which residential real estate values were soaring. For example, an old downtown house in an old neighbourhood valued at $25,000 in the mid-1960s might be valued at $250,000 after the real estate boom of the 1980s (Caulfield 1994, 86).

Housing costs in Toronto were rising faster than incomes, reducing the rate of homeownership. Between 1961 and 1976 the cost of new homes increased fourfold, surpassing the residents' ability to pay. The upward spiral in real estate values caused a stampede of buyers, who were desperate to get into the real estate market before prices moved out of reach. Thus, owning a home became the investment of choice for most of the middle-class (Salter 1988, 43–5). Apartment construction increased substantially, yet at the same time, the rising prices for both new and older houses resulted in very low vacancy rates. This led to rising rents (Lemon 1996, 276). Rent review was instituted in 1975 by the province, but was lifted in the late 1990s. Many new immigrants, especially refugees, doubled up in apartments to make ends meet. Some lived in basement flats.

By the late 1980s, houses were out of reach of even the middle-class. This inspired a trend in many inner-city neighbourhoods towards the conversion of non-family middle-class household units to multi-unit use (Caulfield 1994, 87). Also, the increasing demolition of houses and the construction of apartments resulted in fewer home-owning families and increasing numbers of small-tenant households (ibid., 41).

Owing to the increased value of downtown real estate, neighbourhoods were being transformed by high-rise developments and office towers. The consequence of the rising cost of inner-city housing in Toronto has been that working-class and immigrant communities – and to some extent middle-income groups – have been displaced or effectively prevented from living in inner-city neighbourhoods (ibid., 201). Some believe that Toronto planners, backed by city policies, had decided there would simply be no room in downtown neighbourhoods for working-class or low-income residents, except in public housing projects such as Alexandra Park and Regent Park (CATF 1974, 232).

In Metro Toronto, some residents can and do choose to live in downtown developments (as opposed to the suburbs) and yet maintain their high status and neighbourhood satisfaction (Michelson 1977; Harris and Pratt, 1993). In fact, relative to other Canadian cities, Toronto has had a high percentage of high-income families living in the inner city (Ram et al. 1989). Through gentrification, downtown residents have been able to convert older structures, upgrading them to higher status (City of Toronto Planning Department 1986).

With high-income earners moving into the inner city, the poor have been pushed to outlying areas. This has eroded the stock of affordable housing and forced more poor Torontonians to rely on assisted housing, which is also limited in supply (Ley and Bourne, 1993, 22). Urban revitalization, gentrification, conversion, and renewal have all reduced housing availability in the inner city, increasing the number of homeless people (Dear and Wolch 1993).

Social polarization has become more accentuated in both the City of Toronto and the Toronto CMA (Bourne 1990). The gap between rich and poor neighbourhoods is widening. The proportion of poor people in poor neighbourhoods rose from 15 to 31 per cent between 1980 and 1995 (Philip 2000). Some of Toronto's poor are finding apartments and homes in the former suburbs of Etobicoke, East York, and North York; meanwhile, some wealthy homeowners are purchasing condominiums in the downtown core, driving up prices there. Thus, more recent immigrants to Toronto are more likely to find housing in the suburbs because of the higher rents and lower vacancy rates in the city (Bourne 1999, 4).

By 1990, according to a study by an international research firm that measured the prices of everyday consumer goods and services exclusive of housing costs, Toronto had become the most expensive city in the Western Hemisphere in which to live. In this, Toronto has surpassed New York (ranked second) and Los Angeles (fifth) (see Zarocostas 1990; Duffy 1990).

Costs notwithstanding, there is a current boom in condominium construction in downtown Toronto. At the same time, residents in other neighbourhoods are experiencing increased poverty and homelessness as a result of changes in provincial and federal housing and welfare policies (Kipfer and Keil 2000).

There are fewer neighbourhoods to which poor people can go. Waiting lists for social housing are ten years long, and almost no new housing is being constructed for the poor in the Toronto CMA. Moreover, rents have been increasing since rent controls were lifted in the late 1990s. These trends are affecting visible minorities and Native people more than whites and are creating an underclass segregated by race (Philip 2000). In Toronto, poverty afflicts people with darker skin (blacks, South Asians, Aboriginals, and so on) disproportionately. Moreover, when it comes to finding a place to live, people of colour often face discrimination from landlords, who hold unflattering stereotypes about visible minorities (Philip 2000; Novac et al. 2002).

The Black Family and Canada's Immigration Policy

The group most severely affected by Toronto's social and economic structures has been the blacks – more specifically, black single parents. Before Canada changed its racially restrictive immigration policy in 1967, many black immigrants to Canada were female domestics from the Caribbean. The Caribbean-Canadian family is the result of a female-driven immigration policy and its social and economic consequences. The structure of the black family arose not from choice, but rather from the restrictive aspects of Canadian immigration policy and its lingering effects.

Immigrants often change the form of their family composition at the point of immigration by leaving some parts of the family behind in the country of origin (Howell 2003, this volume, ch. 6). I contend that immigrants from the Caribbean to Canada and Toronto have always been disproportionately women, and that the gender imbalance has been higher than that of other immigrant groups. This overrepresentation of women in the immigration pool has influenced the contemporary composition of black families, which have a higher percentage of female-lone parents. Female-lone parents are more likely to live in poverty; it follows that the economic status of black families in Toronto has been lowered due in part to the high percentage of black female-lone parents.

Since most blacks in Toronto CMA are immigrants from the Caribbean and Bermuda, I turn now to an examination of gender imbalances in the black Caribbean immigrant population.

Black Caribbean Immigrant Gender Imbalance in Canada

Table 7.1 shows the number of male and female immigrants by place of birth for different periods up to 1996 for Canada as a whole. It indicates that black women immigrants have always outnumbered black men. For each immigration period, the gender imbalance among blacks from the Caribbean and Bermuda has been greater than for all immigrant

Table 7.1. Number and percentage of immigrants by place of birth, pre-1961 to 1996 in Canada

Country/region	Before 1961 Number M	F	Percent of Total M	F	1961–70 Number M	F	Percent of Total M	F	1971–80 Number M	F	Percent of Total M	F	1981–90 Number M	F	Percent of Total M	F	1991–96 Number M	F	Percent of Total M	F
Caribbean & Bermuda	3,810	4,575	0.74	0.85	19,825	25,445	5.12	6.34	41,550	54,475	8.64	10.58	30,810	41,590	5.81	7.40	25,530	31,785	5.17	5.83
United Kingdom	114,690	150,885	22.32	27.88	80,875	87,265	20.89	21.73	65,295	67,655	13.57	13.14	29,905	33,545	5.64	5.97	12,575	12,850	2.55	2.36
Western Europe	120,725	121,745	23.50	22.50	36,630	37,960	9.46	9.45	24,170	24,335	5.02	4.72	19,745	21,410	3.73	3.81	13,935	14,580	2.82	2.67
Eastern Europe	87,905	87,525	17.11	16.17	19,375	21,475	5.01	5.35	14,690	17,585	3.05	3.41	56,650	54,725	10.69	9.73	40,795	47,105	8.27	8.63
Southern Europe	122,580	105,565	23.86	19.51	124,865	119,515	32.26	29.77	65,305	66,320	13.57	12.88	29,975	27,805	5.65	4.94	26,410	26,040	5.35	4.77
Eastern Asia	11,880	8,675	2.31	1.60	18,200	20,670	4.70	5.15	49,870	55,065	10.37	10.69	81,130	91,590	15.31	16.29	118,525	133,815	24.02	24.53
Southeast Asia	1,200	1,285	0.23	0.24	5,190	8,850	1.34	2.20	55,650	56,055	11.57	10.88	74,280	88,210	14.01	15.69	47,105	71,160	9.55	13.04
Southern Asia	2,520	2,040	0.49	0.38	16,565	12,310	4.28	3.07	40,575	40,175	8.43	7.80	50,820	48,455	9.59	8.62	70,015	70,035	14.19	12.84
Other countries	48,425	58,895	9.43	10.88	65,530	68,035	16.93	16.94	123,990	133,400	25.77	25.90	156,750	155,005	29.57	27.56	138,545	138,185	28.08	25.33
Total	513,735	541,190	100	100	387,055	401,525	100	100	481,095	515,065	100	100	530,065	562,335	100	100	493,435	545,555	100	100

Source: The Nation Complete Edition. 1996 Census of Canada [CD-ROM]. Statistics Canada cat. no. 93F0020XCB96004. Ottawa: Minister of Industry, 1998.

groups except immigrants from Southeast Asia. However, in three of five immigration periods, the black gender imbalance surpassed that of all other immigrant groups. This imbalance is best revealed by employing sex ratios, which are provided in Table 7.2. On average, the number of black women immigrants from the Caribbean and Bermuda has exceeded the number of black men by 1.28 times for all periods of immigration up to 1996.

Black Caribbean Gender Imbalance in the Toronto CMA

When blacks from the Caribbean arrive in Canada they are most likely to settle in Toronto. Table 7.3 shows the number of male and female immigrants to Toronto for each period of immigration – before 1961 up to 1996. During all periods of immigration, black women from the Caribbean and Bermuda outnumbered black men. The ratio of female to male immigrants by place of birth is presented in table 7.4. Note that during the pre-1961 immigration period, black Caribbean women exceeded black Caribbean men by 1.64 times, whereas the ratio for total immigrants was almost balanced at 1.06. Over all the years, pre-1961 to 1996, the mean ratio for black Caribbean immigrants was 1.38 – higher than for all other immigrant groups.

I now discuss how Canadian immigration policy helped create this situation.

Impact of Canadian Immigration Policy

The gender imbalance among black immigrants from the Caribbean who entered Canada and Toronto did not occur by chance. The imbalance was related to Canadian immigration policies regulating black Caribbean immigration. Black women who came to Canada preferred Toronto as their destination (Calliste 1991, 147). Since 1955, black women from the Caribbean have entered Canada under several programs. Below, I describe each program briefly, with an emphasis on gender- and race-based characteristics. These programs were the Caribbean Domestic Scheme (introduced in 1955); the Foreign Domestic Workers Program (1981); and the Live-in Caregiver Program, a revised version of the FDW program (1992).

The Caribbean Domestic Scheme

The Caribbean Domestic Scheme was a program to import women from the Caribbean as domestic workers. This scheme was part of a

Table 7.2. Ratio of female and male immigrants by place of birth, pre-1961 to 1996 in Canada

	Caribbean and Bermuda	UK	Western European	Eastern European	Southern European	Eastern Asia	Southeast Asia	Asia	Total
Before 1961	1.32	1.30	0.97	0.97	0.85	0.79	0.94	0.85	1.04
1961–70	1.30	1.07	1.00	1.13	0.95	1.13	1.76	0.74	1.04
1971–80	1.24	1.01	0.97	1.10	0.98	1.09	1.00	0.98	1.07
1981–90	1.31	1.12	1.12	0.95	0.96	1.08	1.16	0.96	1.09
1991–96	1.25	1.02	1.05	1.15	0.99	1.13	1.51	1.00	1.15
Mean for years	1.28	1.10	1.02	1.06	0.95	1.04	1.27	0.91	1.08

Source: Computed by the author from data in Statistics Canada. *1996 Census: The Nation Complete Edition*. Ottawa: Minister of Industry, 1998.

Table 7.3. Number and percentages of immigrants by place of birth, pre-1961 to 1996 in the Toronto CMA

Country/region	Before 1961 Number M	Before 1961 Number F	Before 1961 Percent of total M	Before 1961 Percent of total F	1961–70 Number M	1961–70 Number F	1961–70 Percent of total M	1961–70 Percent of total F	1971–80 Number M	1971–80 Number F	1971–80 Percent of total M	1971–80 Percent of total F	1981–90 Number M	1981–90 Number F	1981–90 Percent of total M	1981–90 Percent of total F	1991–96 Number M	1991–96 Number F	1991–96 Percent of total M	1991–96 Percent of total F
Caribbean & Bermuda	1,620	1,980	1.27	1.45	10,565	14,625	8.07	10.53	23,215	31,625	13.61	16.67	16,275	22,680	7.66	10.10	14,590	18,550	6.99	7.98
United Kingdom	25,235	33,390	19.75	24.39	20,645	22,965	15.76	16.53	15,840	17,040	9.28	8.98	7,820	8,630	3.68	3.84	3,060	3,430	1.47	1.48
Western Europe	18,305	20,305	14.33	14.83	5,500	6,055	4.20	4.36	2,535	2,990	1.49	1.58	1,990	2,540	0.94	1.13	1,455	1,480	0.70	0.64
Eastern Europe	21,885	23,405	17.13	17.10	6,270	7,245	4.79	5.22	5,860	7,300	3.43	3.85	23,175	22,550	10.91	10.04	18,740	21,565	8.98	9.28
Southern Europe	49,255	44,515	38.55	32.52	57,630	56,810	44.01	40.90	29,125	30,675	17.07	16.17	15,760	14,690	7.42	6.54	11,345	11,275	5.44	4.85
Eastern Asia	2,685	2,165	2.10	1.58	6,470	7,265	4.94	5.23	20,660	22,655	12.11	11.94	36,945	40,955	17.40	18.23	46,305	51,985	22.20	22.36
Southeast Asia	205	285	0.16	0.21	1,645	2,985	1.26	2.15	18,900	19,805	11.08	10.44	26,730	32,325	12.59	14.39	19,550	30,200	9.37	12.99
Southern Asia	460	415	0.36	0.30	6,160	4,430	4.70	3.19	16,625	16,740	9.74	8.82	27,515	25,365	12.96	11.29	41,905	41,660	20.09	17.92
Other countries	8,105	10,415	6.34	7.61	16,070	16,535	12.27	11.90	37,855	40,920	22.19	21.57	56,160	54,900	26.44	24.44	51,640	52,295	24.76	22.50
Total	127,755	136,875	100	100	130,955	138,915	100	100	170,615	189,750	100	100	212,370	224,635	100	100	208,590	232,440	100	100

Source: The Nation Complete Edition. 1996 Census of Canada [CD-ROM]. Statistics Canada cat. no. 93F0020XCB96004. Ottawa: Minister of Industry, 1998.

Table 7.4. Ratio of female to male immigrants by place of birth, pre-1961 to 1996 in Toronto CMA

	Caribbean and Bermuda	UK	Western European	Eastern European	Southern European	Eastern Asia	Southeast Asia	Asia	Total
Before 1961	1.64	1.27	1.09	0.99	0.89	0.83	1.39	1.15	1.06
1961–70	1.40	1.07	1.10	1.23	0.98	1.12	1.70	0.74	1.07
1971–80	1.28	1.06	1.07	1.09	1.00	1.08	1.04	0.97	1.12
1981–90	1.30	1.20	1.43	0.98	0.95	1.07	1.22	0.93	1.09
1991–96	1.27	1.12	1.02	1.15	0.99	1.12	0.99	1.01	1.15
Mean for years	1.38	1.14	1.14	1.09	0.96	1.04	1.27	0.96	1.10

Source: Computed by the author from data in Statistics Canada. *1996 Census The Nation Complete Edition*. Ottawa: Minister of Industry, 1998.

gradual shift from a predominantly white European labour pool in domestic service to one in which the majority were women of colour. Canada did not have a long tradition of black enslavement; even so, the ideology of white supremacy was just as strong in Canadian society as in the United States. As Stouffer (1984, 130) reveals in his assessment of the views of Ontario journalists in the nineteenth century: 'Blacks it seemed, were fit merely to become the "good servants" of whites who were their natural leaders and guides.' The degraded status of domestic work and of people of colour proved mutually reinforcing as women of colour became identified with domestic work in Canada (Macklin 1994, 16).

The domestic scheme was virtually the only way black women could enter Canada during the mid-1950s since Caribbean women who were black were barred from entering Canada through normal channels. At this time, Canada still actively discouraged people of colour as immigrants (Daenzer 1993, 73). What was this domestic scheme, and what was the Canadian policy regulating it? First of all, it was a domestic work program. Before 1955, Canada's domestic work program recruited primarily white women. Women of colour were conspicuously absent, reflecting Canada's broader, racially exclusive immigration policies at that time (ibid., 11).

After the Second World War, fewer women from Britain (Canada's preferred choice) immigrated to Canada to work as domestics. This created a labour shortage that forced Canada to find a new source of domestic labour. It thus became difficult for Canada to continue to deny women of colour entry into the program. Hoping that it would increase trade with the West Indies, Canada entered into an agreement with the Caribbean governments of Jamaica and Barbados. Under the agreement, single healthy women between eighteen and forty with no dependents and at least an eighth-grade education would be admitted to Canada as landed immigrants on the condition that they remain in live-in domestic service for at least one year (Macklin 1994, 16). Many Canadian white women were pleased because they viewed Caribbean women as a 'cheap' source of servant labour. However, Canadian immigration officials realized that admitting Caribbean women was contrary to Canada's racially exclusive immigration policies.

In June 1955, one hundred black women from the British West Indies were approved for admission to Canada as domestics. Between 1955 and 1960, an average of three hundred black women domestics per year were admitted to Canada. Between 1960 and 1965 the number increased to one thousand black domestics per year (Bolaria and Li 1985, 178).

The formal scheme was abolished in 1966; however, certain components continued in revised form in all subsequent immigration policies.
It is important to note that the *single women only* aspect of the policy
would always remain a key feature (Daenzer 1993, 20). It was extremely
important to white households that black women be *single* and without
dependants (i.e., without family commitments). In this way, loyalty
would be to the white master. Canadian officials discouraged black
domestics from sponsoring family members (Calliste 1991, 145).

In 1961 there were 107 applications from Caribbean domestics to
sponsor their fiancés and close relatives (including five children). Since
only single black women were to be admitted into Canada, these women
required legal counsel if they hoped to have their children join them
(Calliste 1991, 145).

From the outset, Canadian immigration policy forced black families
to evolve in a way that ran counter to established norms. The nuclear
patriarchal family was regarded as the norm in Canada – men, not
women, were expected to be the primary wage earners. Yet Caribbean
black women were to be single and were not to sponsor any mates or
relatives. Because of Canadian immigration policies regarding blacks
from the Caribbean, applicants with spouses and/or children were
rejected (Petrykanyn 1989, 3). This restriction encouraged some applicants to lie about being married or having children (Macklin 1994, 19).
They did so at great risk, however. If it was discovered later that they
were indeed parents, they were subject to deportation. An example is
the case of the 'Seven Jamaican Women,' whom immigration officials
attempted to deport in 1977, after admitting them under the Caribbean
Domestic Scheme. These women had failed to list their dependent
children on their immigration applications, since doing so would have
barred them from Canada. Their omission was discovered in 1976
when they tried to sponsor their supposedly non-existent children (ibid.,
17). The campaign to fight their deportation grew into a larger struggle
over the treatment of black women workers.

Racist beliefs about the sexual promiscuity of black women motivated the Canadian government to ensure that the new arrivals were
subjected to extensive gynecological examinations for venereal disease
(Calliste 1991, 142). Furthermore, the government had the authority to
deport a black woman during the first year if she became pregnant. The
age requirement was also considered important, to ensure 'physical
suitability' to perform 'backbreaking' domestic work (Department of
Citizenship and Immigration 1966).

If black women who arrived in Canada were 'unsuitable' for domestic work, they were to be returned to their Caribbean country of origin at the expense of the Caribbean government. The word 'unsuitable' was not defined in the policy agreement. What *was* clear was that black domestics (unlike European ones) were not be given any assistance in transportation to Canada. Moreover, the Department of Citizenship and Immigration and the Department of Labor enjoyed open-ended authority to administer the program.

The Canadian government made it clear that if black women failed to complete their terms of domestic employment, the scheme would be declared a failure and cancelled. Yet European domestics were coming to Canada with an unconditional right of residency, having entered – just like other immigrants – with full landed-immigrant status and under a common-law agreement (Daenzer, 1993, 53). Thus, mobility from domestic work was restricted in principle only, not in practice. Also, when black women were admitted to the program, harsher rules were implemented to ensure that black Caribbean domestic workers did not leave household service for other occupations (ibid., 45). Whatever victimization existed for white domestic workers in Canada before 1955, Caribbean black women were doubly victimized (ibid., 52).

The only right granted to black women domestics from the Caribbean on their arrival in Canada was the right of full landed status. But this was a right in principle only. In contrast to the policy of *inclusion* for white domestics from Germany, Italy, and Greece, the Canadian government issued a carefully worded policy that set black Caribbean women apart in social status and privilege and thus redefined their citizenship (ibid., 53). The agreement with the Caribbean nations entitled the Canadian government to treat Caribbean women differently. As a consequence, they were burdened with the lowest status in the occupational hierarchy and left open to the worst exploitation. For example, domestic workers were not to be included as an insurable class of workers under the Canadian Unemployment Insurance Plan. Furthermore, black women domestics were given fewer rights and benefits than European white women domestics. And, in general, the working conditions and wages of domestic workers were inferior to those of other occupations. Domestic workers in the late 1960s were excluded from minimum-wage legislation in Ontario and other Canadian provinces (ibid., 69).

Domestic workers under the program engaged in child care, housework, and cooking. They were cheap, exploitable, and expendable

(Macklin 1994, 17). Domestic work was different from other occupations because of its dead-end nature. It involved long hours; it offered few opportunities for training and advancement, regardless of years of service; it provided little economic security for times of illness and old age; and it carried a strong social stigma (Canada Employment and Immigration, 1981).

In 1973 the Canadian government began issuing temporary work permits that would allow workers to stay in the country for only a specified period of time – usually a year – to perform a specific type of work for a specific employer. From 1973 to 1981, black domestic workers could come to Canada only as temporary guest workers, not as of immigrants (Arat-Koc 1993, 287). Canadian policy thus made a clear statement that domestics were not entitled to status as immigrants unless they earned it through service in the occupation (Daenzer 1993, 141). Overall, white British domestics were treated far better than Filipinos and Caribbean blacks.

Any domestic worker who lost her job could be deported. However, the case of the seven Jamaican women led to a change in federal policy in 1981. Foreign domestic workers could now apply for landed immigrant status under the Foreign Domestic Worker Program (Macklin 1994, 18).

The Foreign Domestic Worker Program

This program was implemented in 1981. Under it, live-in domestics who came to Canada on employment authorizations were entitled to apply for permanent resident status after they had been in the country for two years, provided they could demonstrate their capacity to settle successfully. Under the program, individuals were granted employment authorizations as live-in domestics if they had some prior experience in domestic work, had demonstrated the potential to attain financial self-sufficiency in Canada, and could show that resident Canadians were unavailable for employment (Boyd 1987, 4).

Between 1982 and 1990, the total number of women admitted as domestic workers increased by almost eleven thousand (Canada Employment and Immigration 1991). Although the total number of domestic workers had declined by 1996, Caribbean women still constituted 9.6 per cent of the total (Statistics Canada 1998). Not all black women admitted to Canada before 1961 were domestics, however; some were nurses of 'exceptional merit.' Many settled in Toronto

(Calliste 1993). From 1954 to 1960, trained or graduate nurses and 155 nursing assistants came to Canada from the Caribbean. Before 1961, 43 per cent of black women from the Caribbean and Bermuda who settled in Canada settled in Toronto. Between 1961 and 1996, the majority of immigrant women from the Caribbean chose Toronto as their destination (see Statistics Canada, 1998). Today, the Philippines surpasses all other regions as the predominant country of origin for foreign domestic workers in Canada, accounting for 68 per cent of all program participants.

The Live-In Caregiver Program

In 1992, Canada revised its Foreign Domestic Worker Program and renamed it the Live-in Caregiver Program. This program's objective is to bring workers to Canada to serve as caregivers when there are not enough Canadians to fill the available positions. A live-in caregiver provides care to children, the elderly, or the disabled in a private household. Successful applicants receive an employment authorization allowing them to work in Canada as live-in caregivers. After two years of employment, which must be completed within three years of the caregiver's arrival in Canada, program participants can apply in Canada to become permanent residents (Citizenship and Immigration Canada 1999).

Under the new policy, black women intending to do domestic work are admitted to Canada on the basis of their education and training in the care of children, seniors, and the disabled. They must have the equivalent of a Canadian grade twelve education as well as proof of six months' full-time formal training in areas such as early childhood education, geriatric care, and pediatric nursing (CEIC 1992). Live-in caregivers have the right to change jobs without their employer's permission as long as they remain live-in caregivers (Citizenship and Immigration Canada 1999).

In sum, Canadian immigration policy regulating Caribbeans' entry to Canada has been biased in favour of black women. Because of this bias, which has disproportionately restricted black men, a gender imbalance has been created whereby black women have far exceeded black men in numbers. Moreover, black women must be single. These policy restrictions have had a serious impact on the black family structure and have led to a disproportionate number of black female-headed households.

The present black family structure, with its high proportion of lone female black parents, is directly linked to Canadian immigration policies regulating Caribbean blacks' entry to Canada. These policies required black women to disconnect from their roles as mothers, partners, and caregivers in their own families and to become resources that nurtured white Canadian families (Shingadia 1975; Stasculis 1987, 5–6).

According to Henry (1994), Caribbean people in Toronto as a whole do less well than other groups on a number of economic indicators. They earn lower incomes and have a lower home-ownership rate as well as a higher poverty rate. Part of this difference is explained by a higher proportion of families headed by single females (ibid., 64).

Socio-economic Inequality between Blacks and Other Groups in Toronto

To demonstrate the inequality experienced by black families, I examined several social and economic indicators for the City of Toronto. That city is distinguished from the larger Toronto CMA. Around 4.2 million people resided in the Toronto CMA in 1996, over half or them (57.1 per cent, or 2.4 million) in the new City of Toronto. The new city is the outcome of a restructuring of governments carried out in the late 1990s by the provincial government, which eliminated the metropolitan-level government in Toronto and its six lower-tier municipalities (Boudreau 1999). The data in this section were obtained from an analysis of Toronto based on 1996 census data (Ornstein 2000).

Full-time women workers in Toronto, whatever their racial or ethnic group, have a lower median income than men ($27,000 compared to $31,000). Female lone parents, whatever their racial or ethnic group, have a lower median income, a higher incidence of poverty, and a lower homeownership rate than couples or male lone parents (ibid.). Black, African, and Caribbean women full-time workers have a lower median employment income than other women full-time workers. Black, African, and Caribbean female-lone parents with children under nineteen have the highest incidence of poverty (except for Arabs, West Asians, and Latin Americans). Finally, black, African, and Caribbean families have the lowest home ownership rate compared to other families.

The evidence comparing blacks with other racial and ethnic groups is presented in the tables that follow. Table 7.5 shows that black women's income from full-time employment is $18,000 compared to $27,000 for all women workers. That is, black women's median income is only

Table 7.5. Median income from employment by ethno-racial group in Toronto, 1996

Ethno-racial group	Women full-time workers	Percentage above or below the city median
Total groups	27,000	100
Aboriginal	24,000	88
African, black & Caribbean	18,000	66
South Asian	21,000	77
East & Southeast Asian, Pacific Islander	22,000	81
Arab & West Asian	19,200	71
Latin American origin	22,000	81
Canadian	30,000	111
Total European	30,000	111
British European	33,800	125
French European	33,000	122
American, Australian & New Zealander	40,000	148
Northern Europe & Scandinavia	34,800	128
Baltic & Eastern Europe	28,800	106
Southern Europe	26,000	96
Jewish & Israeli	36,000	133
All Other Europe only	29,000	107

Source: Percentage above or below city median computed by the author from data in Ornstein (2000).

66 per cent of the median income of all women workers – in fact, it is the lowest median income of any racial or ethnic group in Toronto.

Table 7.6 shows that among black female-lone parents with children under nineteen, the incidence of poverty was 70.8 per cent – 118 per cent higher than for all female-lone parents. Table 7.7 shows that black, African, and Caribbean families had a home ownership rate of 13.3 per cent, compared to 57.9 per cent for all families in Toronto. This was only 22 per cent of the homeownership rate for all families and the lowest rate of any racial or ethnic group.

Past research suggests, however, that the low black home ownership rate is not due to martial status alone. Racial discrimination in the housing market seems to be an important factor. A logistic regression analysis has revealed that race has a strong effect on lowering the chances of homeownership among blacks compared to whites when the two groups have similar age, marital status, immigration status, educational level, and income level (Darden and Kamel 2000).

Table 7.6. Incidence of poverty for families by ethno-racial group in Toronto, 1996

Ethno-racial group	Female lone parents*	Percentage above or below the city total
Total groups	59.7	100
Aboriginal	69.2	115
African, black & Caribbean	70.8	118
South Asian	58.7	98
East & Southeast Asian, Pacific Islander	60.2	100
Arab & West Asian	74.1	124
Latin American origin	75.4	126
Canadian	66.0	110
Total European	47.7	79
British European	46.8	78
French European	52.9	88
American, Australian & New Zealander	–	–
Northern Europe & Scandinavia	40.8	68
Baltic & Eastern Europe	59.8	100
Southern Europe	46.6	78
Jewish & Israeli	39.1	65
All Other Europe only	–	–

Source: Percentage above or below city total computed by the author from data in Ornstein, (2000), *Ethno-racial Inequality in the City of Toronto*. Toronto: Access and Equity Unit.
*Female lone parents have one or more children under nineteen.

Conclusions

This chapter has demonstrated, based on data on immigration to Canada and Toronto over time and Canada's policy towards black Caribbean immigrants, that Canadian immigration policy which encouraged the entry of black women as opposed to black men created a gender imbalance. Blacks have continued to have more female-headed households than other immigrant groups.

The gender imbalance in the black population, with its high percentage of black female-lone parents, has contributed to the overall lower socio-economic status of black families in Toronto relative to other racial and ethnic groups. Blacks in Toronto have a lower median income, a higher incidence of poverty, and a lower home ownership rate due in large part to the structure of the black family. The lower socio-

Table 7.7. Home ownership by ethno-racial group in Toronto, 1996

Ethno-racial group	Per cent home owners	Percentage above or below the city percentage
Total groups	57.9	100
Aboriginal	32.6	56
African, black & Caribbean	13.3	22
South Asian	48.9	84
East & Southeast Asian, Pacific Islander	61.3	105
Arab & West Asian	28.8	49
Latin American origin	25.0	43
Canadian	53.1	91
Total European	68.5	118
British European	64.0	110
French European	65.7	113
American, Australian & New Zealander	64.9	112
Northern Europe & Scandinavia	70.1	121
Baltic & Eastern Europe	56.5	97
Southern Europe	79.9	137
Jewish & Israeli	68.9	118
All Other Europe only	59.9	103

Source: Percentage above or below city percentage computed by the author from data in Ornstein (2000).

economic status of blacks reveals how Canadian immigration policy continues to have a negative impact on black families. These conclusions lend support to Howell's argument (chapter 6) that Canadian laws and social policies can have a negative impact on the social structure of racial and ethnic groups.

REFERENCES

Arat-Koc, S. 1993. 'The Politics of Family and Immigration in the Subordination of Domestic Workers in Canada.' Pp. 278–96 in *Family Patterns, Gender Relations*, ed. B. Fox. Toronto: Oxford University Press.

Arnopoulos, S. 1979. *Problems of Immigrant Women in the Canadian Labour Force*. Ottawa: A Report to the Canadian Advisory Council on the Status of Women.

Beaujot, R., and J.P. Rappak. 1986. 'The Role of Immigration in Changing Socio-economic Structures.' *Demographic Review*. Ottawa: Ministry of Health and Welfare.

Bolaria, B.S., and P.S. Li. 1985. *Racial Oppression in Canada*. Toronto: Garamond Press.

Boudreau, J. 1999. 'Megacity Toronto: Struggles over Differing Aspects of Middle Class Politics.' *International Journal of Urban and Regional Research* 23(4):771–81.

Bourne, L.S. 1999. *Migration, Immigration and Social Sustainability: The Recent Toronto Experience in Comparative Context*. Toronto: Joint Centre of Excellence for Research on Immigration and Settlement.

– 1990. *Worlds Apart: The Changing Geography of Income Distributions within Canadian Metropolitan Areas*. Toronto: Department of Geography, University of Toronto. Discussion Paper no. 36.

Boyd, M. 1987. *Migrant Women in Canada: Profiles and Policies*. Immigration Research Working Paper no. 2. Ottawa: Employment and Immigration Canada.

Calliste, A. 1993. 'Women of "Exceptional Merit:" Immigration of Caribbean Nurses to Canada.' *Canadian Journal of Women and the Law* 6(1):85–102.

– 1991. 'Canada's Immigration Policy and Domestics from the Caribbean: The Second Domestic Scheme.' Pp. 122–65 in *Race, Class, Gender: Bonds and Barriers*, ed. J. Vorst, et al. Toronto: Garamond Press.

Canada Employment and Immigration. 1991. *Permanent Residents Years of Schooling by Country of Last Permanent Residence for Special Programs FDM, January–December, 1989*. Unpublished. Ottawa.

– 1981. *Domestic Workers on Employment Authorizations: A Report on the Task Force on Immigration Practices and Procedures*. Ottawa: Minister of Supply and Services.

Caulfield, J. 1994. *City Form and Everyday Life: Toronto's Gentrification and Critical Social Practice*. Toronto: University of Toronto Press.

CEIC. 1992. *Immigrant Regulations, 1978*, as amended by SOR 192-214, P.C. 1992–685.

Citizenship and Immigration Canada. 1999. *The Live-in Caregiver Program*. Ottawa: Minister of Public Works and Government Services.

– 1997. *A Stronger Canada: 1998 Annual Immigration Plan*. Ottawa: Minister of Public Works and Government Services.

City of Toronto Planning Department. 1986. *Trends in Housing Occupancy*. Research Bulletin no. 26.

Coffey, W. 1994. *The Evaluation of Canada's Metropolitan Economies*. Montreal: Institute for Research on Public Policy.

Core Area Task Force (CATF). 1974. *Core Area Task Force Technical Appendix.* Toronto: City of Toronto Planning Board.

Daenzer, P. 1993. *Regulating Class Privilege: Immigrant Servants in Canada, 1940s–1990s.* Toronto: Canadian Scholars' Press.

Darden, J.T., and S. Kamel. 2000. 'Black and White Differences in Homeownership Rates in the Toronto Census Metropolitan Area: Does Race Matter?' *Review of Black Political Economy* 28(2):53–76.

Dawson, W.W. 1955. Memorandum to A.H. Brown, 'Jamaican Domestics.' 10 May. RG 76 Volume 838 File 553-36-644, part 1.

Dear, M., and J. Wolch. 1993. 'Homelessness.' Pp. 298–308 in *The Changing Social Geography of Canadian Cities*, ed. L. Bourne and D. Ley. Montreal: McGill-Queen's University Press.

Department of Citizenship and Immigration. 1966. Memorandum from T. R. Burns to Director of Planning Branch. Subject: Domestics. October 19. RG 76 Volume 992 File 5850-6-4-533, part 1.

Duffy, A. 1990. 'Hemisphere's Costliest City? Why It's Ours.' *Toronto Star*, 19 May, E1.

Harris, R. and G.J. Pratt. 1993. 'The Meaning of Home, Homeownership and Public Policy.' Pp. 281–97 in *The Changing Social Geography of Canadian Cities*, ed. L. Bourne and D. Ley. Montreal: McGill-Queen's University Press.

Henry, F. 1994. *The Caribbean Diaspora in Toronto: Learning to Live with Racism.* Toronto: University of Toronto Press.

Kipfer, S., and R. Keil. 2000. 'Still Planning to Be Different? Toronto at the Turn of the Millennium.' *DISP Journal: Network City and Landscape.* 140:28–36.

Lawson, M. 1975. *Metropolitan Jobs and the Economy: A Study of Employment and Employment Generating Activities.* Toronto. Municipality of Metropolitan Toronto Planning Department.

Lemon, J. 1996. *Liberal Drams and Nature's Limits: Great Cities of North America since 1600.* Toronto: Oxford University Press.

– 1985. *Toronto Since 1918: An Illustrated History.* Toronto: Lorimer.

Ley, D. and L. Bourne. 1993. 'Introduction: The Social Context and Diversity of Urban Canada.' Pp. 4–30 in *The Changing Social Geography of Canadian Cities*, ed. L. Bourne and D. Ley. Montreal: McGill-Queen's University Press.

Li, P. 1999. 'The Multiculturalism Debate.' Pp. 148–77 in *Race and Ethnic Relations in Canada*, ed. P. Li. Toronto: Oxford University Press.

Macklin, A. 1994. 'On the Inside Looking In: Foreign Domestic Workers in Canada.' Pp. 13–39 in *Maid in the Market: Women's Paid Domestic Labour*, ed. W. Giles and S. Arat-Koc. Halifax: Fernwood Publishing.

Metropolitan Toronto Planning Department. 1986. *Metropolitan Plan Review, Report no. 2: The Changing Metropolitan Economy.*

Michelson, W. 1977. *Environmental Choice, Human Behavior and Residential Satisfaction*. New York: Oxford University Press.

Novac, S., J.T. Darden, D. Hulchanski, and A. Seguin. 2002. *Housing Discrimination in Canada: The State of Knowledge*. Ottawa: Canada Mortgage and Housing Corporation.

Ornstein, M. 2000. *Ethno-racial Inequality in the City of Toronto: An Analysis of the 1996 Census*. Toronto: Access and Equity Unit, City of Toronto.

Petrykanyn, J. 1989. 'Foreign Domestic Workers and Misrepresentations: New Policy, Old Practices?' *Immigration and Citizenship Bulletin* 1(8):3.

Philip, M. 2000. 'Researchers Fear Segregating Rich from Poor will Bring the Ghetto to Canada: Karoline Escaped but Emmy Hasn't Been So Lucky.' *Globe and Mail*, 5 August: A13.

Ram, B., M. Norris, and R. Skof. 1989. *The Inner City in Transition*. Ottawa: Statistics Canada.

Salter, M. 1988. 'Hot, Hot Houses.' *Report on Business Magazine* 5(2):38–44.

Shingadia, A. 1975. *Non-immigrant Foreign Workers in Canada – A Preliminary Look*. A report prepared for Canada Department of Manpower and Immigration. Ottawa: Department of Manpower and Immigration.

Stasculis, D. 1987. 'Rainbow Feminism: Perspectives on Minority Women in Canada.' *Resources for Feminist Research* 16(1).

Statistics Canada. 1998. *The Profile Series Canada 1996*. Census of Canada [CD-ROM]. Ottawa: Ministry of Industry.

Stouffer, A.P. 1984. 'A Restless Child of Change and Accident: The Black Image in Nineteenth Century Ontario.' *Ontario History* 76(2): 128–50.

Todd, G. 1995. 'Going Global in the Semi-Periphery: World Cities as Political Projects: The Case of Toronto.' Pp. 192–214 in *World Cities in a World System*, ed. P. Knox and P. Taylor. Cambridge: Cambridge University Press.

Zarocostas, J. 1990. 'Toronto Ranked as Most Expensive City in Western Hemisphere, 28th in world.' *Globe and Mail*, 9 May: A1, A2.

8 Ethnoracial Differences in Mental Health in Toronto: Demographic and Historical Explanations

JACINTH TRACEY AND BLAIR WHEATON

Throughout the past half-century, a substantial body of empirical research in the social epidemiology of mental health has produced consistent findings that link position in a social structure to psychological functioning. The stress process paradigm posits that social position within a hierarchical social structure is involved both in the etiology of stress experience and in the allocation of resources across groups (Aneshensel 1992; Broman 1989; Pearlin et al. 1981; Pearlin 1989; Travis and Velasco 1994; Pettigrew 1985; Pettigrew and Martin 1987; Takeuchi and Adair 1992; Turner et al. 1995; Wheaton 1982; Ulbrich et al. 1989).

The accumulated literature on the stress process is most consistent in identifying gender, age, marital status, and social class patterns in mental health (Mirowsky and Ross 1989). These sociodemographic factors lend themselves to intensive study and replication, in part because they either entail only a few categories, and thus can be measured relatively straightforwardly, or derive from widely researched indicators of social stratification with known scale characteristics, like education and income. However, research on ethnic and racial differences in mental health has proceeded with greater difficulty, in part due to the sheer number of distinctions possible among groups, and in part due to the difficulties in classifying (and therefore measuring) ethnic and racial statuses. Despite these problems, ethnoracial group differences represent an undeniably important area of investigation in the mental health literature.

Many essential sociological questions can be asked in the context of studying ethnoracial diversity – a term used here to designate combined distinctions involving race and ethnicity. These questions touch on classic issues in sociology throughout the twentieth century, including the relationship between immigration and well-being, the fundamental role of social status in mental health differences, the possibility that ethnic cultures may cross-cut the influence of social status (Mirowksy and Ross 1980), and the experience of discrimination and prejudice resulting from minority status, especially visible minority status. From the perspective of the stress process, and the fact of greater continuous and episodic discrimination in visible minority groups, we would expect greater mental health problems among recent immigrants and especially among ethnoracial minorities.

Specifying the Source of Racial and Ethnic Differences

We do not mean to imply that research on ethnoracial differences in mental health has been ignored. A fundamental feature of this research, however, is that both reported ethnic and racial differences have not been consistent either through time or across mental health measures (Dohrenwend and Dohrenwend 1969; Williams and Harris-Reid 1999). The disparate findings on race and mental health can be attributed to a number of factors operating in conjunction, including the following: dissimilar sampling designs, with earlier findings relying primarily on treated populations (Malzberg 1940); the absence of meaningful comparison groups, making it difficult to assess differences in risk across groups (Munford 1994; Gibbs and Fuery 1994; Tran et al. 1994); difficulties in classifying or dissimilar classification of subjects into racial or ethnic groups; changes in measures of mental health over time; and research conducted in different historical periods.

For example, earlier research often focused on a single mental health outcome but studies over the past twenty years have tended to use multiple outcomes in reporting racial or ethnic differences (Robins et al. 1984; Ulbrich et al. 1989; Kessler et al. 1994). These studies have demonstrated that one outcome cannot serve as a proxy for all others and that single-outcome studies may provide biased estimates of the global effects of stress and group (e.g., racial) differences in stress reactivity (Aneshensel et al. 1991). As such, to the degree that research depends on a single outcome, such as depression, or on a specific scale, such as the CES-D, the overall picture of ethnoracial differences remains unclear.

Until the last decade, a common finding was that racial or minority group differences were largely due to social class differences across groups (Warheit et al. 1973; Weissman and Myers 1978; Mirowsky and

Ross 1980; Neff, 1984). However, the more recent findings of Kessler and colleagues (1994) from the National Comorbidity Study offer an intriguing alternative picture. Using a recently developed psychiatric diagnostic interview for general population research (the Composite International Diagnostic Interview, or CIDI), they studied more than eight thousand adult respondents in the United States and found that blacks were *not* worse off than whites in mental health terms; furthermore, they specifically reported lower lifetime rates of a range of psychiatric disorders. Unquestionably, there are numerous possible interpretations of this finding, some suggesting that such differences are artifactual. However, the fact remains that one interpretation that should be considered is that Blacks indeed have better mental health than Whites. Taking this finding at face value raises this question: How could groups that are clearly structurally disadvantaged have better mental health than dominant white groups? One potential answer is that despite greater exposure to stress in daily life, some groups may employ coping styles and responses that are particularly effective in reducing the impacts of these stresses.

Immigration Status

In any assessment of ethnic or racial differences, the possibility that differences may be due to the fact or period of immigration must be considered. This component of the social structural argument posits that differences across ethnoracial groups are due largely to differences in the patterns and history of immigration among these groups. Derived in part from stress theory, immigration theories often emphasize that populations experiencing numerous life changes (Pearlin et al. 1981), social disadvantage (Kessler 1979; Vega et al. 1987), or acculturation strain (Burnam et al. 1987) may be more vulnerable to mental health problems. Thus, this perspective has traditionally emphasized the mental health risk implied by the adjustment processes that attend migration. However, we also increasingly see in this literature a focus on the strengths and possibilities offered by immigration (Kuo and Tsai 1986; Burnam et al. 1987; Cochrane and Stopes-Roe 1977; Noh and Avison 1996). For example, Kuo and Tsai (1986) caution against treating migration as automatically detrimental to mental health. While acknowledging the predominance of theory emphasizing the stress of migration, they point out that evidence does not generally support the expectation of higher rates of mental disorders among immigrants. In fact, Harker (2001), in a study of psychological well-being among adolescents, found that first-generation immigrants demonstrated less depressive symptomatology and greater positive well-being than their native-born counterparts, and Murphy (1973) suggests that immigrants to Canada may have lower rates rather than higher rates of psychological problems. These findings provide an important context to our own findings.

Although Canada and the United States are considered two of the world's largest immigrant-receiving nations, and share some similarities in regard to immigration policies, there are important differences. First, over the course of the twentieth century, particularly after the Second World War, the rates of immigration to Canada have exceeded those of the United States (Green 1995; Greenwood and McDowell 1995). As a consequence, Canada has more immigrants per capita than the United States. Second, Canada's introduction of the point system in 1967, which gave points to applicants based on education, income, occupation, family status, and other indicators of 'social competence,' no doubt has created the possibility of a mental health selection effect among landed immigrants since that time. An example of the importance attached to the selection of immigrants based on such indicators is the fact that employment-related factors such as vocational preparation, occupation, and job experience account for approximately one-half of the total available points for independent immigrants to Canada (Aycan and Berry 1996).

At the same time, as a consequence of Canadian restructuring of immigration policy and the economic resurgence in Europe following the Second World War, which reduced European immigration, immigrants to Canada have become increasingly comprised of individuals from developing countries (e.g., the Caribbean, Africa, Asia, South and Central America – Economic Council of Canada, 1991), while immigrants to the United States are now primarily from Asia and Latin America (Massey 1995). Consequently, people who are visible minorities now comprise 60 per cent of all new immigrants to Canada (Harvey and Blakely 1993).

Neighbourhoods in large metropolitan areas are often the locations of choice for newly arrived immigrants (Frey and Liaw 1998). Immigrants to Canada settle largely in three major urban areas: Toronto, Vancouver, and Montreal. Toronto has been unique in North America over the past twenty-five years in terms of both the levels of immigration and the mix of groups immigrating. Analysis of 1991 Census data shows that almost

40 per cent of the city was foreign-born (Statistics Canada 1991). This percentage is not concentrated in a few areas of the city: 90 per cent of the census tracts in Toronto have at least a 20 per cent immigrant population. Additionally, there are more than one hundred different ethnoracial groups currently residing in Toronto (Reitz and Lum 2000), and about 35 per cent of Torontonians give a language other than English as their first language.

The mix of immigrating groups to Toronto is also unique compared to the incoming mix to most American cities. Toronto draws more heavily on Commonwealth countries such as Hong Kong, India, and various islands in the Caribbean, particularly Jamaica. The fact of a common history in the Commonwealth, and thus some degree of familiarity with the historical legacy of British culture, may be important in buffering some of the cultural dissimilarities that come with immigration. This may lead to significant differences in either the degree to which immigrant status is involved in the etiology of mental health problems in Toronto compared to American cities, or the way in which immigration status is related to mental health. For example, the effect of being black in our data may contrast with what would be observed in American data, in part because of the earlier and very different settlement history for a significant proportion of the blacks in the United States compared to the very recent settlement history of blacks in Toronto.

The overall picture of the prevalence, recency, and heterogeneity of ethnoracial groups in Toronto will be important to understanding our results. In the samples we study from the Toronto area, we find that the distribution of major ethnoracial groups is quite balanced, rather than a mix of a dominant minority with other, smaller-sized groups. This contextual reality, which contrasts clearly with patterns in many American cities, may itself alter the pattern of ethnoracial differences in mental health.

Objectives

This chapter focuses on mental health differences – as indicated by a range of mental health measures – among a set of groups classified by race and subsetted by ethnicity in the Toronto area. In our analyses we study blacks, East Asians, and South Asians in contrast to whites and to one another. These groups are formed from the data with a number of considerations in mind. First, in the samples we use from two studies in Toronto, it is necessary to have some level of aggregation of ethnoracial background into larger groups so that a minimally sufficient number of respondents can be considered in each group. Blacks include respondents primarily of Caribbean or African background; East Asians include respondents primarily of Chinese, Japanese, Vietnamese, or Korean background; South Asians include primarily respondents of East Indian, Pakistani, Sri Lankan, or Tamil background; and whites consist primarily of respondents of British, French, or other European background.

In making these classifications, we fully realize that consideration of less aggregated groups would be theoretically and empirically safer, but we also believe that the averaged differences across these larger aggregations may be important and should not be ignored, despite some internal heterogeneity. We feel that our approach balances considerations of necessity due to sample size issues with the perspectives of those who correctly point out that the collapsing of groups can mask differences in relationships between history, or stress, or resources, and mental health (Takeuchi and Adair 1992). Some of our results suggest that there may not be problems due to classification in our data as much as in other data, in part because of the similarities in the recent history of immigration across these groups. Finally, by using this classification, we are designating three groups that share visible minority status, in contrast to the dominant white group. Thus, we can test whether visible minority status per se, or differences among these groups, better represent patterns of mental health variation.

In this chapter, we consider a series of explanations for mental health variation among these groups. These explanations include, first as a baseline, demographic and compositional differences among the groups, especially age and sex differences, in order to ensure that mental health differences are not just due to differences in the proportion of young respondents in these groups or the proportion female. Next, we consider immigration status, distinguishing between the native-born and two groups of foreign-born respondents: those who immigrated before 1974, and those who immigrated after 1974. In our data, 1974 is the median year of immigration in two different studies. We make this distinction in order to allow for some variation due to stage of immigration and/or time in Canada. Finally, we consider socio-economic differences among these groups, following the emphasis in the literature on social class differences as an explanation of ethnic or racial differences. We should be clear that if we find that social class differences do account for ethnoracial differences, this may not question the fundamental importance of race and ethnicity in mental health. This is because achieved social class may in part be a mediator, an explanation, of ethnoracial differences, insofar as ethnoracial groups suffer occupational and income discrimination that results in lower social class placement.

Data and Measures

Data Sources

We use data from two sources from the Toronto area: the Work and Family Issues Study, and the Mental Health and Stress Study. Both of these data sets have been collected in Toronto since 1990 and are unique in specifying mental health as a range of outcomes, including the CIDI (Kessler et al. 1994).

The Work and Family Issues Study is a study of intact families in the Metropolitan Toronto area. The data were collected during 1992-5, and the sample size was 888 families. The study was designed to look at the effects of parental work status and work situations on the mental health of a target child between the ages of 9 and 16. In each family, three family members – the mother, the father, and a child – were interviewed. Despite the demands of the design, the response rate was 70 per cent. Because we selected census enumeration areas in which at least 25 per cent of the families were husband–wife families with children in the household, and then sampled randomly from these areas, our sample is not strictly a random sample of intact families with children in the 9-16 age range in Toronto. However, tests showed that families in these enumeration areas did not differ significantly from those in other areas in either household income or female labour force participation rates. This study includes almost 200 visible minority respondents, and fortuitously for our analyses, these respondents are divided fairly equally among black, South Asian, and East Asian groups. Thus, we have from 45 to 77 respondents in these groups, depending on whether we are analysing the husbands or the wives in this sample. We emphasize that a possible shortcoming of this study, for the assessment of ethnoracial differences in particular, derives from the fact that it is not a random sample of the Toronto adult population, since it targets intact families. Consequently, socio-economic and other social inequality indicators may be somewhat restricted in this sample.

The Mental Health and Stress Study is a study of 1,393 adults from randomly selected households in Metropolitan Toronto, with age restricted from 18 to 55 (Turner and Wheaton 1995). Sampling was based on a 1989 Statistics Canada housing enumeration. The response rate is a reasonable 77 per cent. The design of this study helps address some of the shortcomings of the Work and Family Issues Study. Because of the larger sample, we have larger numbers in each of our groups, specifically: 110 Blacks, 113 East Asians, and 63 South Asians. And since this is a random sample, we can generalize findings from the previous study beyond a certain family type.

Mental Health Measures

In our analyses we follow the general direction of research on mental health by specifying multiple outcomes (Aneshensel et al. 1991). This may be especially important with racial and/or ethnic comparisons, since trade-offs in outcomes are possible depending on cultural and historical differences across groups. Although we do not address the possibility in this chapter of differential response biases across groups, two points are worth noting. First, much of our analysis is based on measures derived from the CIDI, an instrument that was developed and has been applied across a wide array of countries, and hence has been used in culturally diverse populations. Second, consistency of differences across data sets, across different types of measures, or across groups within data sets compared to whites, may suggest that response biases are not overwhelming findings, since we would expect response biases to differ across groups and across measures that differ in content and therefore in potential cultural meaning.

Composite Distress Scale. Some of our analyses depend on a 'composite' distress scale, based on items from a number of existing distress scales, including the Langner Index, the Gurin, the CES-D, the Beck Depression Inventory, and the SCL-90 (Wheaton 1994). The purpose of this scale is to allow for comparisons of results across scales that differ somewhat in content. It is highly reliable here ($\alpha = .91$), and prior results using this scale look very much like what is usually reported in the literature for distress, except that findings are slightly stronger (ibid.).

CES-D. In some analyses, for comparative purposes, we subset items to produce results for the well-known CES-D depression scale, which is usually interpreted as measuring non-clinical and more moderate forms of depression (Radloff 1977).

Speilberger Anxiety Scale. This set of symptoms is taken from the state measure of anxiety used by Speilberger (1970). Again, it is used for contrast with more clinically specific measures in our analyses.

CIDI symptom scales. The data sets we use allow for optimal comparisons across studies in part because the CIDI, or CIDI symptoms, were administered in both data sets. Basically, scales were constructed from the eighteen generalized anxiety symptoms in the CIDI, the nine criterion-based symptom measure of depression in the CIDI, and the nineteen alcohol problems questions in the CIDI. However, our use of this information does differ somewhat in the Work and Family Issues Study compared to the Mental Health and Stress Study. In the former, symptoms were asked for all respondents; that is, no screening questions were used. In the latter, initial screening questions that led to a 'no' response precluded asking the rest of the symptoms, leading to a zero on the index. The result is that we probably have a measure of more severe depression and anxiety in the Mental Health and Stress Study than in the Work and Family Issues Study. In the end, we used a CIDI generalized anxiety symptom scale, a CIDI depression scale, and a CIDI alcohol problems scale in each study.

Controls

In addition to the previously discussed measures of immigration status, we also used measures of age (in years), respondent sex (a dummy variable for female), household income, education in years, and either a classification of occupation based on the National Occupation Coding (NOC) system in Canada or a Canadian-based prestige scale (Blishen 1987).

Results

Demographic and Psychosocial Differences across Groups

Our results begin in Table 8.1, which show comparisons of the four ethnoracial groups in immigration status, occupation, age, education, and income. This table provides a descriptive overview of essential group differences, while allowing us to compare distributions of groups on key control variables in the analysis.

The top panel shows differences across groups in the Work and Family Issues Study, separately for wives and husbands. The results in this panel reveal both the prevalence and recency of immigration to Canada among all three visible-minority groups. Generally, fewer than 10 per cent in these groups are native-born Canadians; in most cases,

Table 8.1. Differences among ethnoracial groups in immigration status and sociodemographic attributes in two studies in Toronto

A. Work and family issues study

	Wives				Husbands			
	East Asian	South Asian	Black	White	East Asian	South Asian	Black	White
Immigration status								
Native-born	10%	1%	11%	64%	7%	4%	9%	63%
Immigrant before 1974	22	11	31	18	32	36	51	23
Immigrant after 1974	68	87	58	18	61	60	40	14
Occupation								
Managerial/professional	35	13	29	31	40	44	18	51
White Collar/supervisor	13	6	14	11	12	8	0	8
White Collar/clerical	48	58	34	53	27	26	33	20
Blue collar	3	23	22	5	21	21	49	21
Age	42**	41	40	41	45**	45***	43	42
Education (in years)	16***	14	13†	14	16	16	14†	15
Household income	75K***	63K***	66K**	92K	76K**	63K***	76K*	91K

Table 8.1. (concluded)

	B. Mental health and stress study			
	East Asian	South Asian	Black	White
Immigration status				
Native-born	17%	9%	20%	76%
Immigrant before 1974	18	27	36	15
Immigrant after 1974	65	64	44	9
Education (in years)	15.3***	14.1	13.3***	14.3
Age	34	36	34	35
Household income	62K	57K	45K***	64K
SES (prestige)	47.8	45.1	40.6**	46.8

Notes: Contrasts with whites:

† p<.10
* p<.05
** p<.01
***p<.001

over 50 per cent have immigrated since 1974. South Asians and East Asians are the most recent arrivees in Toronto, with 87 per cent of the South Asian women arriving since 1974. Despite the fact that 90 or more per cent of blacks are foreign-born in this sample, they are in fact the least recently arrived group as a whole. This is especially true among husbands, with 51 per cent immigrating before 1974. Even among whites, note that more than one-third are foreign-born.

In the Mental Health and Stress general population sample – a better gauge of the overall distributions in Toronto – we see a similar relative picture, but lower percentages from foreign-born backgrounds. This is likely due to the fact that the point system counted family status as one of the qualifiers for entry. Still, about two-thirds of East Asians and South Asians have arrived since 1974, while about 44 per cent of blacks have arrived since that year. This number drops to 9 per cent of whites. Thus, differences between visible minority groups and whites on immigration status – in terms of both nativity and length of time in Canada – are striking.

We compare occupational distributions in the Work and Family Issues Study using the NOC system, which distinguishes professional and managerial occupations, supervisory white-collar, clerical white-collar, and blue-collar as collapsed sets of groups. We find that differences are especially evident among the men, with more similarity across female groups. This is as would be expected in a situation where gender itself has strong effects on occupational status. Fifty-one per cent of white men are at the professional/managerial level, only 21 per cent are in blue-collar occupations. In addition, South Asian and East Asian men show very similar distributions in this sample, with the highest percentage in managerial/professional positions (44 and 40 per cent respectively). The group with the clearest difference from all others is black men, with only 18 per cent at the professional/managerial level but 49 per cent at the blue-collar level. Thus, black men are in distinctly less favourable occupational circumstances than men in the other groups. We also note that they are in somewhat less favourable circumstances, both relatively and absolutely, compared to black women. In our sample, 29 per cent of black women are in professional/managerial positions compared to only 18 per cent of black men. This is the only group in which there are more women than men occupying professional/managerial positions. As well, black women are more prevalent at this level than South Asian women but slightly less prevalent than East Asian women.

Results show that there are few differences in age and years of education in the Work and Family Issues sample. Compared to white women, East Asian women are slightly older, on average, and men in the two Asian groups are also older, on average, than white men. In terms of educational attainment, East Asian women have more years on average and black women have fewer years on average compared to white women. Similarly, compared to white men, black men have fewer years of education, on average. Although differences in education are either small or favouring minorities, we see that all three visible minority groups have lower household incomes compared to whites. Other tests reveal that average income does not differ among the visible minority groups.

The Mental Health and Stress sample compares groups by average coded prestige of occupation instead of occupational group. In the general sample, the clearest socioeconomic disadvantage is among blacks, who have lower-prestige occupations, less education, and lower income compared to whites. East Asians have the highest level of education, and similar levels of household income compared to whites. The differences noted so far are not confounded with differences in age in the Mental Health and Stress Study, since there appear to be no differences in average ages by group.

Work and Family Issues Study

In comparing mental health across the four groups in the Work and Family Issues Study, we consider overall differences on five mental health measures. Table 8.2 shows results contrasting mental health in each of the three visible-minority groups relative to whites, first for wives and then for husbands. Each outcome measure is standardized. Table 8.2, and all following tables, show results in terms of regression coefficients. Technically, these coefficients stand for the standard deviation difference in the mental health outcome between the given group and whites. If the coefficient is positive, this means more problems compared to whites, and if negative, fewer problems than whites. However, only significant group differences (noted by asterisks) should be considered interpretable.

To provide a baseline comparison, we also estimated models for each outcome simply comparing visible minority status – an aggregation of the three groups – to the majority white group, in part to make clear what is missed by not making further distinctions among the visible minority groups. The first row of Table 8.2 gives the first clue to a

Table 8.2. Group differences in mental health in the work and family issues study

Differences with whites	Composite distress	CES-D	CIDI anxiety	CIDI depression	CIDI alcohol
Wives					
Visible minority	−.09	−.04	−.23**	−.17*	−.23**
East Asian	−.07	−.04	−.16†	−.12	−.25*
South Asian	−.07	−.07	−.22*	−.18†	−.21*
Black	−.15	−.01	−.34*	−.25†	−.25*
Husbands					
Visible minority	−.07	−.10	−.17*	−.19**	−.15*
East Asian	−.22*	−.29**	−.25*	−.35**	−.22*
South Asian	.09	.13	−.06	−.01	−.07
Black	−.13	−.17	−.23†	−.22†	−.15

Notes: † p<.10
      * p<.05
     ** p<.01
    ***p<.001

continuing theme in our results: among women, respondents of visible minority status report significantly better, not worse, mental health on three of the five mental health measures. Thus these differences are not restricted to one type of mental health problem. As well, although the coefficients for the remaining two mental health outcomes were not significant, they were in the same direction.

Differences due to visible minority status do not allow us to specify which ethnoracial groups are specifically better off than whites. In order to address this issue, the next set of results considers the four groups separately. These results reveal that blacks show the clearest advantage relative to whites, with lower levels of CIDI anxiety, depression, and alcohol problems reported among South Asians as well. Results for East Asians also follow this pattern but attain statistical significance only on measures of anxiety and alcohol problems.

The pattern among husbands, in the bottom panel of the table, shows similar differences with whites. Among husbands, respondents of visible minority status report significantly better mental health on three of the five mental health measures. When we disaggregate the visible minority category into the three ethnoracial groups, we find specifically that East Asian men report significantly better mental health than white men across all five mental health measures. Black men report lower levels of anxiety and depression than white men. South Asian men, on the other hand, show no significant differences with white men on any of the five mental health measures. Post hoc tests here actually showed no differences among the three visible minority groups on any mental health outcome, for either wives or husbands, except for specific significant differences among East Asian and South Asian men on measures of distress and depression. These data suggest that among ethnoracial groups in Toronto, either shared status as visible minorities or shared status as recent immigrants plays a role in the pattern of observed mental health differences.

One aspect of the results in this table that should be emphasized is the stronger results involving CIDI measures compared to more general measures such as the CES-D. In fact, if one were to use only the CES-D in this study – which has not been unusual in past research – one would find no differences among groups and report that ethnoracial variation has little to do with mental health. The lesson learned is that such conclusions reported earlier in the literature may be misleading, to the degree that more specific and serious measures of mental health problems may reveal important group differences.

For those mental health outcomes that emerged as significant in Table 8.2, we consider the explanation of these mental health differences across groups in tables 8.3 and 8.4, by controlling for age first, then immigration status, and finally for socio-economic differences. Table 8.3 shows results for wives, and table 8.4 shows results for husbands. These tables do not show directly how these controls predict mental health in these groups. However, it will be helpful to note relationships involving some of these control variables. In analyses not presented here, we find that among wives, more recent immigrants have significantly *higher* depression and anxiety than the native-born, but there are no differences between longer-term immigrants and the native-born. This pattern reflects what is often predicted in the literature on immigration. Recent immigration among wives is, on the other hand, related to significantly lower alcohol problems. The pattern for men is quite different. Rather than greater mental health problems, the foreign-born in general show lower anxiety and depression and alcohol problems compared to the native-born. Thus, the way in which immigration status may help explain mental health differences across groups may differ for women and men in this sample.

Table 8.3. Changes in net group differences in wives' mental health controlling for age, immigration status, and SES: Work and family issues study

| Outcome | Differences with whites | Raw | Controlling for | | |
			Age	Immigration	Education, income
CIDI anxiety	East Asian	−.14†	−.14	−.24*	−.20†
	South Asian	−.20†	−.20†	−.32**	−.30*
	Black	−.25†	−.25†	−.33*	−.32*
CIDI depression	East Asian	−.10	−.09	−.17†	−.13
	South Asian	−.14	−.14	−.24*	−.21†
	Black	−.15	−.16	−.23†	−.21
CIDI alcohol	East Asian	−.23*	−.22*	−.12	−.14
	South Asian	−.19†	−.19†	−.07	−.07
	Black	−.23†	−.24†	−.14	−.13

Notes: † p<.10
  * p<.05
 ** p<.01
*** p<.001

We also note broad differences due to education for both wives and husbands, with lower education related to poorer mental health outcomes. It should be noted that although education and income were both controlled for, our results indicated that education was more strongly related to mental health outcomes than was income. Where age is related in this age-restricted sample, it is, as expected, negatively related to mental health problems (Mirowksy and Ross 1989).

Looking at Table 8.3 first for wives, we assess changes in the coefficients showing net differences with whites across the columns, as more control variables are added to each regression model. In the first column we see that for two of the three mental health outcomes, East Asian, South Asian, and black women are advantaged relative to white women. Specifically, all three visible minority groups report lower levels of anxiety and alcohol problems compared to white women. Although there were no significant differences between visible minority women and white women with respect to depression, we should remember that these coefficients are derived from a smaller subsample, one that includes only those with values on all control variables, and thus may be attenuated. Nonetheless, the coefficients for depression are in the same direction as for the other two mental health outcomes, suggesting again that although not statistically significant, visible minority women have less, not more, depression than white women.

In controlling for age, we wish to determine whether any overall difference on these mental health outcomes may be attributed to variations in the age distribution among visible minority women relative to white women. From the table, we see that controlling for age does not explain any of the group differences in anxiety or alcohol problems, and that it does not reduce net differences for any outcome.

When we control for immigration status, we find that the coefficients for alcohol problems become non-significant for all ethnoracial groups. Results here show that from 40 to 63 per cent of alcohol problem differences across groups after controlling for age are explained by immigration status. This occurs because among these wives, recent immigration in particular is related to lower alcohol problems, and of course there is a much higher proportion of recent immigrants in the three visible-minority groups.

At the same time, we note that controlling for immigration status in the anxiety and depression models actually *increases* net group differences. In the case of depression, for example, we see that all three groups now show significantly lower levels of depression relative to whites. We also find that in the case of anxiety, net differences in favour of immigrant women increase substantially. Why would this opposite pattern of effects occur? Recall that immigration is related to *more* anxiety and depression among wives but to *lower* alcohol problems. Controlling for immigration status in the anxiety and depression models reveals a suppression effect, caused by the joint facts of higher anxiety/depression problems among immigrant wives and a higher proportion of immigrants among visible minorities. Once this influence favouring higher problems among visible minority women is controlled for (standing for a positive component linking visible minority status to mental health problems), the net mental health advantage of visible minority women is larger.

The addition of socioeconomic controls to these models fails to contribute notably to the explanation of any of these mental health differences, although a small portion of the differences in depression does seem attributable to social class, especially for East Asian and black women.

Table 8.4 shows results for the same models applied to husbands. To reiterate what was found earlier, East Asian men report better mental health than white men on all three mental health outcomes, black men

Table 8.4. Changes in net group differences in husbands' mental health
controlling for age, immigration status, and SES: Work and family issues study

| Outcome | Differences with whites | Raw | Controlling for | | |
			Age	Immigration	Education, income
CIDI anxiety	East Asian	−.27*	−.25*	−.18†	−.17
	South Asian	−.06	−.03	.06	.06
	Black	−.26†	−.25†	−.15	−.16
CIDI depression	East Asian	−.37**	−.35**	−.28*	−.27*
	South Asian	−.02	−.01	.09	.09
	Black	−.24†	−.23†	−.15	−.15
CIDI alcohol	East Asian	−.22*	−.21†	−.12	−.11
	South Asian	−.09	−.06	.02	.03
	Black	−.15	−.14	−.07	−.08

Notes: † p<.10
        * p<.05
       ** p<.01
      ***p<.001

report better health than white men on measures of anxiety and depression, and South Asian men do not differ significantly from whites. From the table we see that controlling for age does not significantly reduce the effect of ethnoracial status for any of the outcomes, suggesting that age differences do not play a role in the mental health differences between visible minority men and white men in these data.

However, controlling for immigration status leads to reductions in the effect of ethnoracial status on all three mental health outcomes. Net differences in reported mental health between both East Asian and black men compared to white men fall by 20 to 42 per cent when immigration status is controlled for. We find that controlling for socioeconomic status differences does not further reduce the size of these coefficients. As such, we can conclude that among husbands, differences between visible minority groups and the dominant white group are not due to demographic or socio-economic differences, but are due largely to immigration status.

It is clear that immigration plays a contrasting role among husbands and wives in the Work and Family Issues sample. Among husbands, the main effect of immigration on all three mental health outcomes is negative, both for newer and older immigrants, but among wives the effect is positive. The negative effect among husbands suggests that part of the reason visible minority husbands have better mental health is that a higher proportion of them are foreign-born and in turn this fact predicts better mental health.

Why would findings for husbands and wives be so different? We speculate that family immigration policy emphasizes the points attained by men in the points system, in part because they are typically more likely to be employed initially. Families are kept together and thus points are generalizable to the family level. As such, there is likely to be more of a selection effect among men than among the women they are married to. This would explain why, in this sample of married couples, the effect of immigration is in opposite directions: among men, we observe selection dominating, whereas among women we observe causation dominating (i.e., the expected effects of immigration as an inherently stressful experience).

In sum, these data most clearly suggest three things: (1) visible minority groups in Toronto demonstrate better mental health than their white counterparts; (2) immigration status plays a central role in either defining or explaining ethnoracial differences; and (3) the effects of immigration among visible minority wives are the opposite of effects among visible minority husbands.

Mental Health and Stress Study

As noted earlier, the Work and Family Issues data are somewhat limited in terms of the nature of the sample. Thus we turn to the Mental Health and Stress Study to assess the same issues in a general population sample of the Toronto area in the 18 to 55 age range. The main consequence of this broader sample is that there is more variation across social statuses, and thus a better test of the implications of demographic and socioeconomic differences.

Table 8.5 parallels Table 8.2 in that it reports raw mental health differences across groups. In this sample, sex is an additional control in the analysis. We begin with the same baseline analysis as in the earlier results, and earlier results are essentially replicated here. There are differences between visible minorities and whites on two mental health outcomes, suggesting lower levels of anxiety and alcohol problems among visible minority groups compared to whites. Additionally, although the coefficients for the remaining three mental health outcomes

Table 8.5. Group differences in mental health in the mental health and stress study

	CES–D	Speilberger anxiety	CIDI anxiety	CIDI depression	CIDI alcohol problems
Differences with whites					
Visible minority	–.08	–.21***	–.08	–.03	–.24***
East Asian	–.03	–.11	–.12	–.19*	–.25**
South Asian	–.13	–.28*	.04	.06	–.26*
Black	–.05	–.27**	–.13†	.07	–.21*
Diagnoses odds					
East Asian	–	–	.431†	.354***	.213***
South Asian	–	–	1.275†	.408**	.269**
Black	–	–	.319*	.575*	.293***

Notes: † p<.10
       * p<.05
       ** p<.01
       ***p<.001

are not statistically significant, they are in the same direction. When this visible minority–white difference is disaggregated, we see that, similar to the Work and Family Issues findings, the three visible minority groups generally report better mental health than whites. Specifically, East Asians report lower CIDI depression and alcohol problems; South Asians report lower levels of anxiety and alcohol problems; and blacks report lower levels of anxiety, in two forms, and lower levels of alcohol problems. Results for alcohol problems are somewhat stronger in these data, in part because there is much more variation in these problems in the larger general population sample, particularly among men. Again, post hoc tests reveal no differences among the three visible minority groups.

Thus, the main contrast is between visible minorities and whites, but in a direction that few would expect. Results here replicate a pattern of mental health advantage among visible minorities. We emphasize that results in this sample should also carry more weight, since sample selection was not restricted to intact couples.

It is worth noting the stronger results from the Speilberger anxiety measure here as opposed to the CIDI symptom scales for anxiety and depression. We believe the results in the Mental Health and Stress Study may be attenuated somewhat for CIDI outcomes by the screening structure of the CIDI interview in that study. In effect, if a respon-

Table 8.6. Changes in net group differences in mental health controlling for sex, age, immigration status, and SES: Mental health and stress study

Outcome	Differences with whites	Raw	Controlling for		
			Sex, Age	Immigration	Education, income
Speilberger anxiety	East Asian	−.06	−.06	.00	.00
	South Asian	−.28**	−.19	−.12	−.12
	Black	−.22*	−.23*	−.20*	−.22*
CIDI depression	East Asian	−.16*	−.16*	−.09	−.09
	South Asian	.03	.12	.20*	.20*
	Black	.08	.07	.11	.09
CIDI alcohol	East Asian	−.22**	−.27**	−.18*	−.17*
	South Asian	−.24*	−.26*	−.14	−.14
	Black	−.18*	−.19*	−.13†	−.14†

Notes: † p<.10
  * p<.05
  ** p<.01
  ***p<.001

dent said 'no' to a certain kind of question about their lifetime experience of depression or anxiety at the beginning of the interview, their score on these scales is by definition, zero. If the specific content of these questions, emphasizing worry, feeling sad or blue, or having disinterest in most things, does not equally predict answers to other anxiety or depression items across groups, observed group differences may be affected. This is not supposed to be the case for these measures, but it is clear that the CIDI scales are more skewed in this sample as a result, and this in itself could affect findings. We note that a screening structure was never used for questions about alcohol problems, and results are more similar across the two samples.

Table 8.5 also reports, for completeness, group differences in risk of lifetime DSM-III-R disorders using the CIDI. These odds ratios clearly show a pattern of lower risk for these groups in almost all cases, compared to whites. For example, East Asians have just over one-third the odds of lifetime depression compared to whites. These results are important because they stand for differences in *lifetime* risk, as opposed to differences in current symptoms. Thus, we see that all visible minorities in Toronto have significantly less mental health risk than whites, except for one case: South Asians show a slightly higher risk of lifetime diagnosis of DSM-III-R generalized anxiety.

To explain what is unexpected in the first place may be difficult, but Table 8.6 will be helpful in beginning to understand why these visible minority groups generally report better mental health than whites in these data. In this table, we control for the same factors, in the same order, as in the our earlier analyses. Results are shown for the three most distinct outcomes in the bivariate analyses reported in Table 8.5. These outcomes consist of two CIDI measures and the Speilberger anxiety scale. Beginning with anxiety, we see significant differences for blacks and South Asians as compared to whites when there are no controls in the model. Adding sex and age to assess demographic compositional differences somewhat explains the difference in anxiety reported by South Asians compared to whites – the difference is now non-significant – but does little to explain group differences between blacks and whites. Both sex and age have the usual expected effects in these models, with females and younger people reporting higher anxiety. Indeed, South Asians are slightly older on average and have a slightly higher proportion of females in this sample compared to whites. Controlling for immigration status differences does reduce group differences further although it does not completely account for differences in anxiety between blacks and whites. Adding socioeconomic controls to this model fails to add explanatory power over and above the effects of immigration status. Overall, immigration status explains 13 per cent of the net difference in anxiety between black and white men, and 37 per cent of the difference between South Asian men and white men.

Looking at results for depression, we see that age/sex differences across groups do not explain the difference between East Asians and whites. However, controlling for immigration status has clear effects on the net group difference between East Asians and whites, leaving non-significant differences between these two groups. Fully 44 per cent of the reported difference in depression between East Asians and whites is attributed to differences in immigration status. It should be noted that the coefficients for South Asians and blacks are both positive when we look at CIDI depression as an outcome. In fact, when we control for immigration, South Asians report a *higher* net level of depression than whites. This finding clearly contrasts with most of the other findings in these samples. In analyses not reported here, we find large interactions between both being South Asian and age, and being South Asian and religiosity. These interactions suggest that younger and less religious South Asians stand out as having higher levels of reported depression. We see some reflection of this in the increased effect of South Asian, controlling for age and sex, in Table 8.6 (the coefficient increases from .03 to .12). Controlling for immigration status also increases the net difference to .20. To the extent that younger and less religious South Asians comprise a disproportionate percentage of recent South Asian immigrants in our sample, recent immigration may be uniquely related to poorer mental health in this group.

Results for alcohol problems reveal significant differences for all three visible minority groups when there are no controls in the model. Controlling for sex and age fails to significantly explain group differences. However, when immigration status is added to the model, the effect of ethnoracial status on alcohol problems is completely explained in the case of South Asians, and the coefficients for East Asians and blacks and are significantly reduced. Net differences in reported alcohol problems between all three ethnoracial groups and whites are reduced by between 31 to 46 per cent when immigration status is controlled for. As such, much like the results for anxiety, results for alcohol problems show that immigration status is important in explaining mental health differences between visible minority groups and the dominant white group.

Recall that a much higher proportion of the three visible minority groups are foreign-born and, specifically, are more likely to be recent immigrants. Results not shown from the model with immigration status as a control show that both the recent foreign-born and the long-term foreign-born have lower anxiety and alcohol problems. As noted earlier, this could be due to the effect of selection. Thus, the negative effect of being in a visible minority group on anxiety and alcohol problems is explained by the joint fact that these groups are more likely to be foreign-born, and that being foreign-born is associated with lower levels of these problems.

We see from these data that controlling for socio-economic differences has little to do with group differences in mental health, despite the common finding in the literature that controlling for social class explains differences between minority groups and whites. In fact, in our data, valid differences among the ethnoracial groups still remain to be explained in some areas even after controlling for these differences. For example, in the Work and Family Issues Study, significant effects of race on anxiety and depression remain even after controlling for demographic and socio-economic status differences. Similarly, in the Mental Health and Stress Study, we find significant effects of race on mental health outcomes even after controlling for possible differences in age, sex, nativity, and socio-economic differences between visible minority and white groups. These remaining differences could be due to differences in group-specific coping resources and practices, for example.

However, the most general pattern is one in which controlling for immigration status does attenuate the effects of race on mental health outcomes. We say this remembering that the Mental Health and Stress Study is a random sample of adults in Toronto households, and thus includes never-married people, non-parents, and people from a wider range of age groups. In the case of non-marrieds and non-parents, the points system is more likely to apply individually. Among husbands in the Work and Family Issues Study and in general in the Mental Health and Stress Study, controlling for immigration status accounts for between one-quarter and almost one-half of the group differences in anxiety, depression, and alcohol problems. Given the general finding that newer immigrants have even better mental health than older immigrants, we conclude that immigration policy figures prominently in understanding mental health differences among ethnoracial groups in Toronto.

Discussion

At this point we might want to rethink our original question, and the way it is stated. As pointed out often in the literature on racial and ethnic differences, the 'standard' for comparison is usually predominantly Anglo white groups. But perhaps we are not entirely seeing a different possibility, suggested by our data – namely, that it is not immigrant groups or visible minorities who are so much better off in mental health, but whites who are specifically worse off. It is not possible to address this issue in our data without better comparative information, but we should point out that results from the National Comorbidity Study in the United States suggest similar levels of lifetime psychiatric disorders overall and often higher rates among whites (Kessler et al. 1994). Given that immigration before 1974 still sometimes predicts better mental health in our data, we wonder whether immigration or important differences in coping 'models' across groups are at issue here.

In turning our attention to the white population in Toronto, we are able to consider fundamentally important questions. It is helpful to remember that Toronto plays a comparable role in Canada as a target of internal migration as does New York and Los Angeles in the United States: it is a place of perceived opportunities, the place to go when one wants to leave economic uncertainty and poor prospects behind. Toronto draws heavily on in-migrants from the Maritime provinces, from Western Canada, and from the rural areas and small towns of Ontario. It is also true that the past twenty years have seen unprecedented growth in Toronto as a city, from 2 million in 1970 to almost 4 million in 1996. Thus, Toronto was also experiencing a simultaneous influx of white internal in-migrants over this period. This may be important to understanding our results, in that these whites are essentially facing increased competition for jobs and for education resulting from the influx of immigrants occurring at the same time. These are not necessarily the whites with the economic and political power in Toronto; typically, they form a class of hopefuls, much like the new immigrants, who have not yet made it. What may distinguish the internal migrants is higher expectations. Thus, it is possible in this group that greater expectations may breed more unrealized expectations, and that hope may be more difficult to maintain. We cannot verify this, but this reasoning deserves further consideration.

At the same time, we do not want to underemphasize the importance of immigrant status in our results. Following the discussion of Kuo and Tsai (1986), and others, we raise the possibility that the negative picture about the situation of immigrants has at times and in specific places been overstated. A more balanced picture might include a number of other factors. For example, Kobasa and colleagues (1982) have argued that immigrants may have higher levels of hardiness, which acts as a 'resistance resource' to reduce the likelihood of poor mental health functioning in the face of stressful situations. Because voluntary immigrants (unless they came to Canada as children or through family reunification or refugee policies) are screened by immigration officials for attributes that would suggest they are capable of making positive contributions to Canada (e.g., adequate level of education, good work ethic, no prior criminal convictions), selection factors may exist in the immigrant population, resulting in the most instrumental and hardy individuals being selected for entry into Canada. Thus, we see that immigrants in Toronto may in fact possess psychosocial advantages compared to the native white population.

We should note that we have not considered methodological reasons for the reported differences in this chapter. Obviously, differences in interpretation and meaning of outcome scales, for example, would clearly affect results. We have chosen not to emphasize these possibilities here because they lead to less interesting implications than interpreting the findings as substantively meaningful.

We conclude therefore by suggesting that while the literature on immigration throughout the twentieth century has specifically emphasized the stress and troubles and alienation accompanying immigrant status, it may be important to also see the other side of the coin. Immigrants, from specific places at specific points in history, may also come to a new land with hope. The ability to have and maintain hope is a major input to the maintenance of mental health, despite difficult socio-economic circumstances and a clearly stressful situation as new immigrants. It takes very little to keep hope alive, especially when that hope is invested in the future of one's children. Opportunity structures in Toronto may be just open enough that these hopes are maintained and reinforced through time.

NOTES

This research was supported in part by grants from the Social Sciences and Humanities Research Council of Canada, and in part by a grant from the National Health Research Development Program of Health Canada.

REFERENCES

Aneshensel, Carol S. 1992. 'Social Stress: Theory and Research.' *Annual Review of Sociology* 18:15–38.
Aneshensel, Carol S., Carolyn M. Rutter and Peter A. Lahenbruch. 1991. 'Social Structure, Stress and Mental Health: Competing Conceptual and Analytic Models.' *American Sociological Review* 56:166–79.
Aycan, Zeynep and John W. Berry. 1996. 'Impact of Employment-Related Experiences on Immigrants' Psychological Well-Being and Adaptation to Canada.' *Canadian Journal of Behavioral Science* 28(3):240–51.
Blishen, Bernard K., William K. Carroll, and Catherine Moore. 1987. 'The 1981 Socioeconomic Index for Occupations in Canada.' *Canadian Review of Sociology and Anthropology* 24(4):465–88.

Broman, Clifford. 1989. ' Race and Responsiveness to Life Stress.' *National Journal of Sociology* 3(1):49–64.

Burnam, M. Audrey, Richard L. Hough, Marvin Karno, Javier J. Escobar, and Cynthia A. Telles. 1987. 'Acculturation and Lifetimes Prevalence of Psychiatric Disorders among Mexican Americans in Los Angeles.' *Journal of Health and Social Behavior* 28 (March):89–102.

Cochrane, R., and M. Stopes-Roe. 1977. 'Psychological and Social Adjustment of Asian Immigrants to Britain: A Community Survey.' *Social Psychiatry* 12:195–206.

Economic Council of Canada. 1991. *Economic and Social Impacts of Immigration.* Ottawa: Supply and Services Canada.

Dohrenwend, Bruce P., and Barbara Snell Dohrenwend. 1969. *Social Status and Psychological Disorder.* New York: Wiley.

Frey, William H., and Kao-Lee Laiw. 1998. 'The Impact of Recent Immigration on Population Redistribution within the United States.' Pp. 388–448 in *The Immigration Debate: Studies on the Economic, Demographic and Fiscal Effects of Immigration*, ed. James P. Smith and Barry Edmonston. Washington, DC: National Academy Press.

Gibbs, Jewelle, and Diana Fuery. 1994. 'Mental Health and Well-Being of Black Women: Towards Strategies of Empowerment.' *American Journal of Community Psychology* 22(4):559–82.

Green, Alan. 1995. 'A Comparison of Canadian and US Immigration Policy in the Twentieth Century.' Pp. 31–64 in *Diminishing Returns: The Economics of Canada's Recent Immigration Policy*, ed. D.J. DeVoretz. Toronto: C.D. Howe Institute.

Greenwood, Michael, and John McDowell. 1991. 'Differential Economic Opportunity, Transferability of Skills, and Immigration to the United States and Canada.' *Review of Economics and Statistics* 73(4):612–23.

Harker, Kathryn. 2001. 'Immigrant Generation, Assimilation and Adolescent Psychological Well-Being.' *Social Forces* 79(3):969–1004.

Harvey, Edward, and John Blakely. 1993. 'Employment Equity in Canada.' *Policy Options*: 3–8.

Kessler, Ronald C. 1979. 'Stress, Social Status, and Psychological Distress.' *Journal of Health and Social Behavior* 20:259–72.

Kessler, Ronald C., et al. 1994. 'Lifetime and 12-Month Prevalence of DSM-III-R Psychiatric Disorders in the United States: Results from the National Comorbidity Survey.' *Archives of General Psychiatry* 51:8–19.

Kessler, Ronald C., and Harold W. Neighbors. 1986. 'A New Perspective on the Relationship among Race, Social Class, and Psychological Distress.' *Journal of Health and Social Behavior* 27(2):107–15.

Kobasa, Suzanne C., Salvatore R. Maddi and Stephen Kahn. 1982. 'Hardiness and Health: A Prospective Study.' *Journal of Personality and Social Psychology* 42(4):168–77.

Kuo, Wen H., and Yung-mei Tsai. 1986. 'Social Networking, Hardiness, and Immigrants' Mental Health.' *Journal of Health and Social Behavior* 27:133–49.

Massey, Douglas. 1995. 'The New Immigration and Ethnicity in the United States.' *Population and Development Review* 21(3):631–52.

Malzberg, Benjamin. 1940. *Social and Biological Aspects of Mental Disease.* Utica, NY: State Hospital Press.

Mirowsky, John, and Catherine Ross. 1989. *Social Causes of Psychological Distress.* Chicago: Aldine de Gruyter.

– 1980. 'Minority Status, Ethnic Culture, and Distress: A Comparison of Blacks, Whites, Mexicans, and Mexican Americans.' *American Journal of Sociology* 86:479–95.

Munford, Maria B. 1994. 'Relationship of Gender, Self-Esteem, Social Class, and Racial Identity to Depression in Blacks.' *Journal of Black Psychology* 20(2):157–74.

Murphy, H.B.M. 1973. 'The Low Rate of Hospitalization Shown by Immigrants to Canada.' Pp. 221–31 in *Uprooting and After*, ed. C. Zwingmann and M. Pfister-Ammende. New York: Springer-Verlag.

Neff, James Alan. 1984. 'Race Differences and Psychological Distress: The Effects of SES, Urbanicity and Measurement Strategy.' *American Journal of Community Psychology* 12:337–51.

Noh, Samuel, and William R. Avison. 1996. 'Asian Immigrants and the Stress Process: A Study of Koreans in Canada.' *Journal of Health and Social Behavior* 37(2):192–206.

Pearlin, Leonard I. 1989. 'The Sociological Study of Stress.' *Journal of Health and Social Behavior* 30:241–57.

Pearlin, Leonard I., M. Lieberman, E. Menaghan, and J. Mullan. 1981. 'The Stress Process.' *Journal of Health and Social Behavior* 19:2–21.

Pettigrew, Thomas. 1985. 'New Black-White Patterns: How Best to Conceptualize Them?' *Annual Review of Sociology* 11:329–46.

Pettigrew, Thomas, and Joanne Martin. 1987. 'Shaping the Organizational Context for Black American Inclusion.' *Journal of Social Issues* 43(1):1–78.

Radloff, L. 1977. 'The CES-D Scale: A Self-Report Depression Scale for Research in the General Population.' *Applied Psychological Measurement* 1:385–401.

Reitz, Jeffrey, and Janet Lum. 2000. *Immigration and Diversity in a Changing*

Canadian City: Social Bases of Inter-group Relations in Toronto (online). Available at www.utoronto.ca/ethnicstudies/Reitz-Immigration and Diversity in Toronto–Reitz and Lum.pdf.

Robins, Lee N., John E. Helzer, Myrna M. Weissman, Helen Orvaschel, Ernest Gruenberg, Jack D. Burke, and Darrel A. Reiger. 1984. 'Lifetime Prevalence of Specific Psychiatric Disorders in Three Sites.' *Archives of General Psychiatry* 41:949–58.

Spielberger, C., R. Gorsuch, and R. Lushene. 1970. *STAI Manual for the State-Trait Anxiety Inventory (Self-Evaluation Questionnaire)*. Palo Alto, CA: Consulting Psychologist Press.

Statistics Canada. 1991. *Public Use Microdata File on Individuals, Documentation and User's Guide*. Ottawa: Supply and Services Canada.

Takeuchi, David, and Russell Adair. 1992. 'The Exposure and Vulnerability of Ethnic Minorities to Life Events.' *Research in Community and Mental Health* 7:111–24.

Tran, Thanh, Roosevelt Wright, jr, and William Berg. 1994. 'The Dimensions of Subjective Well-Being among Black Americans: A Structural Model Analysis.' *Journal of Multicultural Social Work* 3(2):115–36.

Travis, Russel, and Steven Velasco. 1994. 'Social Structure and Psychological Distress among blacks and whites in America.' *Social Science Journal* 31(2):197–207.

Turner, R. Jay, and Blair Wheaton. 1995. 'Checklist Measures of Stressful Life Events.' Pp. 29–58 in *Measuring Stress: A Guide for Health and Social Scientists*, ed. S. Cohen, R. Kessler and L.G. Underwood. New York: Oxford University Press.

Turner, R. Jay, Blair Wheaton, and Donald Lloyd. 1995. 'The Epidemiology of Social Stress.' *American Sociological Review* 60:104–25.

Ulbrich, Patricia, George Warheit, and Rick Zimmerman. 1989. 'Race, Socioeconomic Status and Psychological Distress: An Examination of Differential Vulnerability.' *Journal of Health and Social Behavior* 30(1):131–46.

Vega, William, B. Kolody, and J.R. Valle. 1987. 'Migration and Mental Health: An Empirical Test of Depression Risk Factors among Mexican American Women.' *International Migration Review* 21:512–30.

Warheit, George, Charles Holzer, and John Schwab. 1973. 'An Analysis of Social Class and Racial Differences in Depressive Symptomatology: A Community Study.' *Journal of Health and Social Behavior* 14:291–9.

Weisman M.M., and J.K Myers. 1978. 'Affective Disorders in a U.S. Urban Community.' *Archives of General Psychiatry* 35:1304–11.

Williams, David R., and Michelle Harris-Reid. 1999. 'Race and Mental Health:

Emerging Patterns and Promising Approaches.' Pp. 295–314 in *A Handbook for the Study of Mental Health: Social Contexts, Theories and Systems*, ed. A. Horwitz and T. Scheid. New York: Cambridge Press.

Wheaton, Blair. 1994. 'Sampling the Stress Universe.' Pp. 77–113 in *Stress and Mental Health: Contemporary Issues and Prospects for the Future*, ed. William R. Avison and Ian H. Gotlib. New York: Plenum Publishing.

– 1982. 'A Comparison of the Moderating Effects of Personal Coping Resources on the Impact of Exposure to Stress in Two Groups.' *Journal of Community Psychology* 10:293–311.

9 Does Social Capital Pay Off More Within or Between Ethnic Groups? Analysing Job Searches in Five Toronto Ethnic Groups

EMI OOKA AND BARRY WELLMAN

In the early twenty-first century, Canada continues to receive a large share of global migrants and is facing old and new challenges of immigrant incorporation (Reitz 1998; Mercer 1995). Governmental immigration and refugee policies, the individual characteristics of immigrants, the place of settlement, and the condition of local markets determine interactively the patterns and the degree of immigrant incorporation. These, in turn, shape the long-term effects of immigration on the host society (Massey 1995).

First-generation immigrants set the stage for what is to come (Portes 1998, 814). In particular, the economic marginalization of particular groups, resulting in joblessness and spatial concentration of poverty, can disadvantage the second generation and perpetuate ethnic and racial inequality over generations (Portes and Rumbaut 2001). Sustained inequality and deprivation can be a source of social conflict and also worsen intergroup relations in the immigrant-receiving society.

In multicultural Canada, an important research agenda has been to investigate the degree to which immigrants and minority group members attain economic equality (Porter 1965; Portes and Zhou 1992; Lian and Matthews 1998; Pendakur and Pendakur 1998). Since finding a better-paying mainstream job is a first step towards economic integration into the host society, studying job searches is a strategic way to explore the social processes through which immigrants and minority members attain equality.

Social networks are an important and often successful means of searching for jobs. They provide *network capital* – a form of social capital that links people interpersonally to job opportunities. Accordingly, social contacts within and outside ethnic communities in job searches can produce, reproduce, or overcome inequalities along racial and ethnic lines. In ethnically or racially segmented labour markets, what kinds of network ties pay off, and for whom? There is a pressing need for comparative analyses of minority experiences. We tackle this issue in the present chapter.

Toronto is a city of recent immigrants from many lands and thus an excellent place to compare the job-search experiences of immigrant and ethnic groups. Therefore, in this chapter, we analyse the job searches of members of three generations of five ethnic groups in Toronto: English, German, Jewish, Ukrainian, and Italian Canadian. We focus on these two questions:

1. Which factors influence the use of intra-ethnic and inter-ethnic ties in job searches?
2. Which ethnic groups attain higher incomes when their members use job contacts within or outside their own ethnicity?

To address these research questions, we perform original analyses of data that were collected in 1978 from the 'Ethnic Pluralism in an Urban Setting' research project (Breton et al. 1981; Breton et al. 1991). They are the only data that provide information for studying in detail the kinds of job contacts that members of different ethnic groups have used in their job searches and information about income they have earned in these jobs. Because it focuses on job search experiences among the five European groups in the late 1970s, this chapter does not directly address the recent experiences of immigrants to Canada. However, our study provides a reference point for investigating the extent to which racial and ethnic segregation in the labour market can condition the structural advantages or disadvantages of intra-/inter-ethnic ties when minority members mobilize their ties for job searches. We believe our study can provide a useful perspective for understanding a socially mediated process through which varying economic opportunities are allocated along ethnic or racial lines and through which the often vertical structure of the Canadian mosaic has been sustained or altered.

Building on Previous Research

One stream of research in social network analysis has investigated which characteristics of ties and networks help people obtain information and find jobs. Mark Granovetter (1973, 1974, 1982) was the first to show that weak ties are important for obtaining professional-level jobs.

He contended that because weak ties are more likely than strong ties to connect people to different social circles, they are more likely to provide new information, including information about jobs.[1] Yet other scholars have argued that when information is scarce and valued, strong or high-status ties are key sources of information and jobs (Campbell et al. 1986; Lin and Dumin 1986; Lin 2001). For example, it is close kin and good friends who give poor Chileans information about scarce jobs (Espinoza 1999). Researchers (e.g., Stoloff et al. 1999) have since argued that it is the heterogeneous social and relational characteristics of network members and not the strength of their ties that connect people to new information. However, most discussions have continued to focus on the strength of ties rather than on the benefits of heterogeneous networks (Wellman and Frank 2000).

Another stream of research in ethnic relations has investigated how networks help immigrants or ethnic-group members obtain resources and become socially incorporated into their new host society. Researchers have shown that social networks affect the destination of migration (Boyd 1989, Koser 1997; Bauer and Zimmermann 1997), provide social capital for entrepreneurship (Light and Bonacich 1988; Zimmer and Aldrich 1987; Portes 1995; Sanders and Nee 1996; Cobas and DeOllos 1989), provide occupational niches for employment (Bailey and Waldinger 1991; Hondagnew-Sotelo 1994), and share resources that provide access to job opportunities in the new land (Anderson 1974; Fernandez-Kelly 1995). This research has focused on the benefits of densely knit, tightly bonded ethnic networks that are supported by solidarity and mutual trust (Wellman and Leighton 1979; Wellman 1988; Light and Bonacich, 1988). Yet this celebration of ethnic solidarity has overlooked the possible utility of ethnically heterogeneous ties to gain access to better opportunities (Portes and Sensenbrenner 1993; Portes 1998; Ooka 2001).

In other words, research into job searches by ethnic minorities has concentrated on comparing the benefits of social capital that the members of ethnic groups can mobilize from *within* their own groups (Granovetter 1995; Light and Bonacich 1988). Few studies have focused on comparing the benefits of using ties within one's own group with the benefits of using ties with members of other ethnic groups (intra-ethnic vs inter-ethnic ties; see the discussion in Calzavara 1982). Researchers have tended to make two assumptions.

1. Researchers have generally assumed that immigrants or members of minority groups have only one option: to rely on members of

their own ethnic group even when this can be disadvantageous (Sanders and Nee 1996). For example, because the networks of early Portuguese immigrants and job contacts were almost exclusively composed of other Portuguese Canadians, they mainly received help only from these low-status people (Anderson 1974).
2. Assimilationist analyses have also assumed that when inter-ethnic ties have become available, they are always a better means for immigrants to obtain the good jobs that exist only in mainstream milieux. Looking for jobs outside the intra-ethnic economy niche has been considered the only path for the social mobility for ethnic minorities (Wiley 1967) because intra-ethnic ties are assumed to lead to lower-status jobs in ethnic niches (Calzavara 1982, 1983).

These two assumptions should be reconsidered. The members of ethnic groups including immigrants use both intra-ethnic and inter-ethnic contacts for job searches. One study found that immigrants who work longer in ethnically mixed milieux develop more inter-ethnic ties and are less likely to rely on intra-ethnic networks for job referrals (Nee et al. 1994). Another study found that female West Indian immigrants to Toronto whose networks consisted of other West Indians depended on their co-ethnic network members for job searches and other information. They obtained jobs such as domestic cleaning for one another. In contrast, other West Indian women made and used inter-ethnic friends to move out of domestic work (Turritin 1976).

Moreover, intra-ethnic ties do not always trap workers in poor jobs. To be sure, using intra-ethnic contacts for job referrals is more likely to lead to jobs in the ethnic economy or in ethnically dominated occupations (Bailey and Waldinger 1991). Yet working in an ethnic economy can sometimes provide good returns on human capital and open up opportunities for self-employment (Wilson and Portes 1980; Portes and Jensen 1989; Zhou and Logan 1992; Cobas et al. 1993; Reitz 1991).

The advantages (or disadvantages) of working in an ethnic economy or ethnic niche depend, in part, on the resources that particular ethnic groups can mobilize through their co-ethnic networks. In particular, co-ethnic communities differ significantly in terms of the resources they can provide, depending on whether the co-ethnic group is composed mainly of working-class people or contains significant professional or entrepreneurial elements (Portes and Rumbaut 2001, 64). The resources that working-class communities can provide are limited because, regardless of the human capital newcomers bring, they can be channelled into below-average occupations as a function of co-ethnic support (Anderson 1974; Bates 1994; Waldinger 1994). In such cases, using job contacts belonging to co-ethnic groups can lead to lower-paying jobs. Conversely, more advanced ethnic communities that have professional or entrepreneurial components can provide more opportunities to translate their human capital into economic returns (Portes and Bach 1985). Thus, opportunities for mobility through co-ethnic job contacts should be more available (Portes and Rumbaut 1996). We cannot automatically assume that using intra-ethnic ties in job searches is always beneficial or disadvantageous. The advantages of using particular social contacts depend on what kinds of resources are controlled within and outside of one's own ethnic group in the particular labour market.

In studying access to varying economic opportunities among immigrant and minority groups in Toronto, it is not trivial to distinguish between searching within and outside one's own ethnic group. This is because ethnic groups have been unequally dispersed throughout the occupational structure in Toronto – and indeed, in Canada as a whole. Some ethnic groups have been concentrated in occupations with high rewards, others in occupations with lower rewards (Porter 1965, Richmond and Verma 1978). The members of the five ethnic groups we study here were overrepresented in certain jobs according to prior analyses of the data used here (Reitz et al. 1981) (see Table 9.1). When these data were collected in 1978–9, 63 per cent of the men and 40 per cent of the women worked in ethnically segregated jobs.[2]

In this ethnically segmented labour market, information about job openings is not equally accessible to all groups. Ethnic segmentation means that people may only find limited resources in ethnically homogeneous networks. They may have extensive social capital within their ethnic group, but this may not be effective social capital for getting access to resources beyond it (Gans 1962; Espinoza 1999).

To what extent do ethnic groups in Toronto use intra-ethnic and inter-ethnic ties in their job searches? Is social capital more beneficial when mobilized through intra-ethnic ties or through inter-ethnic ties? What kinds of members of an ethnic group are likely to use different kinds of ties in their job searches? Because people use what is available within their social networks as resources, we assume that the ethnic composition of their networks will affect opportunities to use intra-ethnic and inter-ethnic ties. We hypothesize that the availability of ethnically heterogeneous friendship networks decreases the use of members of one's own ethnic group for job searches (see also Calzavara 1982). Thus

Table 9.1. Typical occupations with ethnic concentration for five ethnic groups, by gender

Ethnic origin	Male	Female
English	Fire fighter Postal worker Bus driver	Postal worker Government official
German	Tool and die maker Food preparation	Electrical products Hairdresser
Jewish	Medical and health operation Textile products Lawyer	Sales supervisor Real estate sales Social work
Ukrainian	Railway work Baker Hotel management	Cleaners Food processing Hotel manager
Italian	Masons and tile setter Construction trades Barbers	Textile products Sewing Material processing

Source: Reconstructed from data on ethnic occupational concentration analysed by Reitz, et al. 1981; Reitz 1990, 166–7.

the more heterogeneous their networks, the more likely that people will use inter-ethnic ties to find jobs (hypothesis 1.1).

If being in ethnically heterogeneous networks facilitates the use of inter-ethnic ties and access to social capital located beyond ethnic boundaries, it is important to understand which kinds of people are likely to become members of such heterogeneous networks. To whom is social capital available beyond ethnic boundaries? We test the effects of generation, education, gender, and age on the ethnic heterogeneity of networks. Research into social incorporation suggests that ethnic minorities become incorporated over generations into the mainstream society and that the inter-ethnic composition of networks increases as part of this process (Isajiw 1990; Portes and Rumbaut 1996; Rose, Carrasco, and Charboneau 1999; Waldinger and Perlmann 1999). Therefore, we hypothesize that *the ethnic heterogeneity of networks becomes higher over generations* (hypothesis 1.2).

We also expect education to be positively associated with ethnic network heterogeneity because it provides social resources and opportunities to meet people from various ethnic groups. Better-educated people are more likely to form ties outside their own ethnic group

(Portes and Bach 1985; Fong and Isajiw 2000). Moreover, better-educated people of all kinds are more likely to have heterogeneous networks (Campbell et al. 1986). Thus we hypothesize that *the higher the level of education, the more likely it is that people will have ethnically heterogeneous networks* (hypothesis 1.3). Past research on friendship networks has suggested that gender and age do not affect the ethnic composition of friendship networks (Portes and Bach 1985; Fong and Isajiw 2000). Therefore, we hypothesize that *men and women do not differ in the ethnic heterogeneity of networks* (hypothesis 1.4), and that *people of different ages do not differ in the extent of their inter-ethnic ties* (hypothesis 1.5).

Comparing the Benefits of Intra- and Inter-ethnic Ties

When ethnic minority members utilize both intra-ethnic and inter-ethnic ties, which types of ties can help them access more advantageous opportunities? In a segmented labour market such as Toronto's, people may only be able to mobilize limited resources from within their own ethnic group. Inter-ethnic contacts may enable job searchers to gain access to the more diverse opportunities that lead to higher-paying jobs. Overall, we expect to find that *inter-ethnic ties help people gain access to higher-income jobs* (hypothesis 2.1).

However, the impact of inter-ethnic ties on income may not always be beneficial. It may differ depending on the position ethnic groups occupy in the social hierarchy. For example, if densely connected ethnic networks are predominantly of lower status, they may curtail social mobility. Only ethnic members who are able to reach beyond their intra-ethnic social circles will be able to locate employment opportunities. However, if job seekers belong to ethnic groups that have good job information, they do not have to move beyond their intra-ethnic networks to obtain good information.

Thus we can expect that the benefits of inter-ethnic ties in ethnically segmented markets will be conditioned by the status of job seekers' ethnic groups. Inter-ethnic ties can be a beneficial resource for people whose ethnic groups are concentrated in lower-paying jobs because such ties increase their options in the search for better information and for opportunities to act on that information. Conversely, intra-ethnic ties can be a more beneficial resource than inter-ethnic ties for people whose ethnic groups are concentrated in good jobs. Thus, the types of resources that particular ethnic groups control significantly condition the advantages of using intra- or inter-ethnic ties. We expect that *for the members of low-status ethnic groups, inter-ethnic ties are better than intra-ethnic ties for attaining higher-income jobs* (hypothesis 2.2a). Conversely, *for the members of high-status ethnic groups, intra-ethnic ties are better than inter-ethnic ties for attaining higher-income jobs* (hypothesis 2.2b).

In all ethnic groups in North America, women tend to encounter more difficulty than men in obtaining good jobs. Two phenomena are at work. Women have more difficulty in getting jobs, and more difficulty in advancing their work status once they have a job. Past research has suggested that women profit from having ties to one or more men (Calzavara 1982; Stoloff et al. 1999). By extension, we expect that *inter-ethnic ties are more rewarding for women than for men* (hypothesis 2.3). In addition to the ethnicity of job seekers, the ethnicity of job contacts may affect the usefulness of inter-ethnic ties. The use of inter-ethnic ties may be advantageous only when members of low-status groups can use members of high-status ethnic groups.[3] Therefore, we expect that *inter-ethnic ties to job contacts in higher-status ethnic groups are more rewarding than ties to contacts in lower-status groups* (hypothesis 2.4).

Methods

Sample

Analyses were conducted using data collected 1978–9 in the 'Ethnic Pluralism in an Urban Setting Research Project' (see Breton et al. 1990, 269–72, for sample details). The overall sample contains 2,338 residents between eighteen and sixty-five, belonging to one of ten ethnic groups in Toronto. Because we wanted to examine the impact of the generation of immigration, we only included in this study the five ethnic groups about whom we had generational information: English, German, Italian, Jewish, and Ukrainian.

We analyse here the 581 surveyed members of these ethnic groups who used personal contacts in searching for jobs (see Table 9.2).[4] However, when testing the strength of inter-ethnic ties on income attainment, we include only the 469 full-time workers in order to better compare differences in the income levels of ethnic groups. Job contact networks have significant implications for the niche formation and job allocation of these five ethnic groups in Toronto: more members of each ethnic group use personal contacts in getting a job than use other methods such as direct application, newspaper want ads, private employment agencies, the government-operated Canada Manpower agency,

Table 9.2. Methods of job search among five ethnic groups

	Formal method	Direct application	Personal contact
English (282)	33% (94)	23% (65)	44% (123)
German (257)	33% (84)	23% (58)	45% (115)
Italian (255)	21% (54)	28% (70)	51% (131)
Jewish (183)	27% (49)	20% (36)	54% (98)
Ukrainian (285)	32% (91)	28% (80)	40% (114)
Total (1262)	372	309	581

Source: Ethnic Pluralism in an Urban Setting data.

or union referrals. Differences in the percentage of ethnic-group members using personal contacts are not large: Jews have the highest rate of using personal contacts (54 per cent) and Ukrainians the lowest (40 per cent).

Variables

(1) Loglinear Analysis: Who Uses Inter-Ethnic Ties (N= 455)

Ethnicity of the contact used for getting a job: Respondents were asked about the person who provided help in the job search, the question being: 'Was this person also "same ethnic group"?' If the respondent answered 'yes,' the tie was coded as intra-ethnic. If the respondent answered 'no,' the tie was coded as inter-ethnic.

Generation: First-generation immigrants are coded '1,' the second generation '2,' and the third generation '3.'

Education: Years of education completed by the respondents, divided into (1) people who completed less than fourteen years of education, and (2) people who completed more than fourteen years of education.

Gender: Male = 1, female = 2.

Age: In years. Only people between eighteen and sixty-five and working in the labour market were included. For loglinear analysis, age was divided into categories spanning fifteen years.

Ethnic heterogeneity of friendship networks: Preliminary research analysed the ethnic heterogeneity of the job seekers' friendship networks. Coding of the ethnic heterogeneity of networks was based on the question that asked the ethnicity of the respondent's three closest network members.[5] If none or one of the network members was from the same ethnic group, the network was coded as heterogeneous. If two or three of the network members were from the same ethnic group, the friendship network was coded as homogeneous.

(2) Cross-tabulation Analysis: Comparing the Benefits of Intra-Ethnic and Inter-Ethnic Ties (N=331)[6]

Income: Annual job income of the respondent in 1978 (before taxes), expressed as the mean of a close-ended range (see Calzavara 1982 for details).

Ethnicity of the contact used for getting a job: Respondents were asked about the person who provided help in the job search, the question being: 'Was this person also "same ethnic group"?' If the respondent answered 'yes,' this was coded as an intra-ethnic tie. If the respondent answered 'no,' this was coded as an inter-ethnic tie and further information about the network member's ethnicity was gathered. Western and northern European ethnic groups were coded as having relatively high social status. Other ethnic groups – southern and eastern Europeans, Asians, and blacks – were coded as having relatively low social status, to reflect ethnic and racial stratification in Canada in the 1970s and early 1980s (Reitz 1990; Porter 1965; Li 1988; Lautard and Guppy 1990).

Intra-Ethnic and Inter-Ethnic Ties?

Members of the five ethnic groups studied here make use of both intra-ethnic and inter-ethnic ties for job referrals. Their use of inter-ethnic ties in job seeking is related to the ethnic heterogeneity of their friendship networks. Job seekers who have ethnically heterogeneous networks are more likely to use inter-ethnic contacts. This supports hypothesis 1.1 (Table 9.3). Almost 60 per cent of the people who have heterogeneous networks (at least two of their closest friends are of another ethnic group) have job contacts with people of other ethnic groups. In contrast, only 15 per cent of the people whose networks are homogeneous have job contacts with members of other ethnic groups. For those with heterogeneous networks, the odds of using an inter-ethnic job contact are

Table 9.3. Ethnic composition of friendship networks by ethnicity of tie used for getting current job

| | Ethnicity of job contacts (%) | | |
	Intra-ethnic	Inter-ethnic	Total (N)
Heterogeneity of friendship network	85	15	268
Homogeneous (2–3)	43	57	188
Heterogeneous (0–1)	307	149	456

x^2 = 89.22 (significance < .001)
Missing Cases = 125
Source: Ethnic Pluralism in an Urban Setting data.

1:1.35. For those with homogeneous networks it is much lower – 1:0.18. These results suggest that people who are in ethnically heterogeneous networks are more likely to have access to the diverse opportunities outside their own ethnic group.

We examined the factors influencing the ethnic heterogeneity of friendship networks – generation, education, age, and gender – since the degree of ethnic heterogeneity in friendship networks conditions the use of inter-ethnic ties for job search. The ethnic heterogeneity of friendship networks increases over generations, supporting hypothesis 1.2. The third generation has more heterogeneous ties than the second generation, which, in turn, has more heterogeneous ties than the immigrant generation. The longer people have resided in Canada, the greater the availability of heterogeneous social contacts. This result suggests that immigrants have more limited access to resources outside inner-ethnic circles of relatives and friends. The implication is that immigrants who rely on co-ethnic social networks to find work may be more likely to be in disadvantaged segments of the labour market.

Education affects the ethnic composition of friendship networks differently in each generation (Table 9.4). For the immigrant generation, education is positively related to being in heterogeneous friendship networks. About half (48 per cent) of first-generation immigrants with postsecondary education are in heterogeneous networks, compared to 26 per cent of those with less education. This supports hypothesis 1.3: the higher the level of education, the more likely people are to have ethnically heterogeneous networks. Those who lack postsecondary education are likely to lack communication skills in English and are more likely to live in ethnically homogeneous neighbourhoods (Kalbach 1990;

Table 9.4. Heterogeneous friendship (per cent) by generation and education

| Generation | Education | | | |
	High school or less	Post-secondary education	x^2	Education significance level
First	26	48	11.13	(.000)
Second	52	35	3.78	(.050)
Third	64	59	.42	(.520)
x^2	42.50	7.15		
Generation sig. level	(.000)	(.028)		

Source: Ethnic Pluralism in an Urban Setting data.

Portes 1998). These contexts tend to produce ethnically homogeneous networks (Breton 1964). Furthermore, postsecondary education can be the first generation's path to interaction with the host society. Thus, immigrants with better education may have alternatives to relying on co-ethnic ties. These alternatives allow them to avoid using co-ethnic ties when such ties are disadvantageous. In contrast, immigrants with limited education may have fewer alternatives to relying on help from co-ethnic members.

Postsecondary education has an opposite effect for the second generation. Half (52 per cent) of people with high-school level education or less have heterogeneous friendship networks; only 35 per cent of people with postsecondary education have such networks. And for the third generation, education does not have any significant effect. For example, a majority of those with less than high school education (64 per cent) or with postsecondary education (59 per cent) have heterogeneous friendship networks.

The third generation is the only generation for whom age – not education – is associated with the use of inter-ethnic ties (Table 9.5). Having lived more years in Canada, older members of the third generation are more likely than younger members to have accumulated useful job-related inter-ethnic ties and to use them in job searches. Most members of this third generation probably have developed ethnically heterogeneous networks regardless of their educational levels (Table 9.4).

The data show that each succeeding generation is more likely to be in heterogeneous networks. With the second and especially the third generations, only a minority are exclusively involved with members of their own ethnic group. At the outset, the better-educated members of

Table 9.5. Percentage using inter-ethnic ties by generation and age

Generation	Age			x^2	Age sig. level
	Younger	Middle	Older		
First	35	23	20	4.41	(.111)
Second	45	38	29	2.36	(.306)
Third	32	56	67	7.90	(.019)
x^2	3.03	9.54	9.66		
Generation significance level	(.219)	(.008)	(.008)		

Source: Ethnic Pluralism in an Urban Setting data.

the first generation are more likely to have network members outside their ethnic boundaries. But as the generations develop and as opportunities for inter-ethnic relationships become more widespread, a higher percentage of better-educated people are likely to be in ethnically homogeneous networks. This may be because they choose to make professional or business careers in niches within an ethnic community (see Portes and Jensen 1989), or it may be that they have a larger pool of people from their own ethnic group to draw on as network members.[7] Better-educated people in later generations may perceive having some knowledge of their ethnic language and enjoying ethnic activities with friends as expressions of symbolic ethnicity and as reflections of cultural capital (Alba 1990).

Overall, we have shown the following:

1. The use in job searches of intra-ethnic or inter-ethnic ties by members of specific ethnic groups is significantly conditioned by the availability of ties in their social networks.
2. The availability of such intra- and inter-ethnic ties is influenced by sociodemographic and socio-economic characteristics of job seekers such as their generational status, educational background, and variation in age.

Do Inter-ethnic Ties Pay Off in Job Searches?

How is income attainment related to the use of intra-ethnic or inter-ethnic ties? We found that both men and women who use inter-ethnic ties attain higher incomes when they use inter-ethnic job contacts. Women who use inter-ethnic ties for job searches have a 10 per cent higher mean

Table 9.6. Ethnicity of contact by mean income of males and females

	Income	
	Male (N)	Female (N)
Intra-ethnic	$16,955 (166)	$10,194 (72)
Inter-ethnic	$17,278 (54)	$11,179 (39)
Intra/inter difference	$323 (+2 per cent)	$985 (+10 per cent)

Source: Ethnic Pluralism in an Urban Setting data.
Note: Only people using personal contacts were included in the sample.

income ($11,179) than women who use intra-ethnic ties ($10,194, a difference of $985; see Table 9.6).[8] In contrast, men who use inter-ethnic contacts have only a 2 per cent higher mean income ($17,278) than men who use intra-ethnic ties ($16,955, a difference of $323). Women are more concentrated in lower-paying jobs. More women in lower-status ethnic groups work in low-paying jobs because of the double burden of paid work and domestic work (Boyd 1984). Those in lower-status groups who use intra-ethnic contacts are more likely to get low-paying jobs because their contacts (usually of the same gender) are likely to be in low-paying jobs. Hence ethnically homogeneous networks are less advantageous for women than for men. Those women who use inter-ethnic ties are more likely than men to advance beyond the lowest-income jobs their co-ethnics hold. However, we do not find any relationship between using inter-ethnic ties and income level when we analyse the sample as a whole. Thus, hypothesis 2.1 is *not* supported: inter-ethnic ties are *not* broadly beneficial for members of all ethnic groups.

Differences in ethnic groups' average socio-economic statuses are associated with the relationship between ethnic group members' use of intra-ethnic or inter-ethnic ties and the mean income that the members of this ethnic group have attained. Inter-ethnic ties are more likely to be beneficial for job seekers of low-status ethnic groups, which supports hypothesis 2.2a (Table 9.7). For example, even though the great majority (83 per cent) of Italian men and women rely on *intra*-ethnic ties, *inter*-ethnic ties provide the small minority who use them with higher-paying jobs: Italian men obtain a 15 per cent higher incomes and Italian women obtain 22 per cent higher incomes.[9] About 40 per cent of Ukrainians use inter-ethnic ties for job referral, and these ties often lead to higher-paying jobs. For Ukrainian men, the use of inter-ethnic ties is

Table 9.7. Ethnicity of contact and mean income of males and females by ethnic groups

	Males			Females		
	Intra-ethnic	Inter-ethnic	Monetary difference	Intra-ethnic	Inter-ethnic	Monetary difference
English	$20,510	$14,125	$6385	$11,038	$10,929	$109
(72)	(48)	(4)	−31	(13)	(7)	−1
German	$19.917	$17,580	$2337	$10,100	$10,300	$200
(62)	(18)	(19)	−12	(10)	(15)	+2
Italian	$15,310	$17,625	$2315	$8,789	$10,750	$1961
(83)	(50)	(8)	+15	(19)	(6)	+22
Jewish	$16,860	$20,167	$3307	$8,769	$15,000	$6211
(46)	(25)	(6)	+20	(13)	(2)	+71
Ukrainian	$11,380	$16,500	$5120	$12,265	$12, 278	$13
(68)	(25)	(17)	+45	(17)	(9)	0

Source: Ethnic Pluralism in an Urban Setting data
Note: '% Difference' describes the relative increase (decrease) in income for using interethnic ties, as compared with using intra-ethnic ties.

associated with a 45 per cent higher income; although there is no significant increase for Ukrainian women.

In contrast, *intra*-ethnic ties, and not *inter*-ethnic ties, benefit job seekers in high-status ethnic groups (table 9.7). This supports hypothesis 2.2b. The tendency for English and German Canadians to have higher-income jobs means that intra-ethnic ties provide better income opportunities for them. For example, 85 per cent of the English who use personal contacts use intra-ethnic ties. English men who use intra-ethnic ties have much higher incomes (mean = $20,510) than those who use inter-ethnic ties ($14,125). For English women, the use of intra-ethnic ties ($11,038) is somewhat better than the use of inter-ethnic ties ($10,929). A similar situation exists for German men and women (see also Reitz 1990). Thus the higher the position of the ethnic group to which the job seeker belongs, the more beneficial are intra-ethnic ties.

The situation for Jewish men is anomalous, but understandable, considering the discrimination and segregation Jews have experienced in Toronto (Porter 1965; Kelner 1969, 1970; Newman 1975–81; Reitz 1991). Although Jews have high status, nevertheless, Jewish men have 20 per cent higher incomes when they use inter-ethnic ties. We believe this is because such ties help Jewish men cross barriers of elite segregation.

There is equivocal evidence that ethnically heterogeneous networks are more beneficial for women than for men. Supporting hypothesis 2.3, inter-ethnic ties are associated with 10 per cent higher incomes for women but only 2 per cent higher increases for men (Table 9.6). More detailed analysis shows that this greater advantage for women is limited to the Jewish and Italian ethnic groups, where women's advantages in using inter-ethnic ties rather than intra-ethnic ties are 71 per cent and 22 per cent respectively (Table 9.7). There is no appreciable difference for English, German, or Ukrainian women.[10]

To this point, we have provided evidence suggesting that *intra-ethnic* contacts are good for *job seekers* who are members of high-status ethnic groups whereas *inter-ethnic* contacts are good for members of low-status ethnic groups. How is the status of *job contacts* related to income attainment? We look at the different outcomes in income attainment with regard to the status of job contacts.

The data show that people who have job contacts with members of higher-status ethnic groups (northern and western European) generally have higher incomes than those whose contacts are with members of lower-status groups (see Table 9.8).[11] This supports hypothesis 2.4. For example, Ukrainian men who received help from the members of high-status ethnic groups have attained a mean income of $17,786, as compared to a mean income of $10,500 for those who received help from lower-status inter-ethnic contacts. In general, using inter-ethnic ties with members of *high-status* groups is more closely associated with higher incomes than is using inter-ethnic ties with members of *low-status* groups. However, the intra-ethnic ties of the highest-status ethnic group (English men) with English job contacts are more beneficial ($20,510) than their contacts with other higher-status ethnic groups ($17,000) and much more beneficial than their contacts with low-status ethnic groups ($5,500).

Summary and Conclusions

In this chapter we have examined two major research questions for three generations of five ethnic groups in Toronto:

1. Which factors influence the use of intra-ethnic and inter-ethnic ties in their job searches?
2. Which ethnic groups attain higher incomes when their members use job contacts within or outside their own ethnic group?

Table 9.8. Income attainment among five Toronto ethnic groups: By ethnicity of job seeker and job contacts

	Males			Females		
		Inter-ethnic			Inter-ethnic	
	Intra-ethnic	Low status	High status	Intra-ethnic	Low status	High status
English	$20,510	$5,500	$17,000	$11,038	$8,500	$11,333
(72)	(48)	(1)	(3)	(13)	(1)	(6)
German	$19.917	$18,500	$17,333	$10,100	$10,083	$10,444
(62)	(18)	(4)	(15)	(10)	(6)	(9)
Italian	$15,310	—	$16,625	$8,789	$1,500	$12,600
(83)	(50)		(8)	(19)	(1)	(5)
Jewish	$16,860	—	$20,167	$8,769	—	$15,000
(46)	(25)		(6)	(13)		(2)
Ukrainian	$11,380	$10,500	$17,786	$12,265	$8,000	$13,500
(68)	(25)	(3)	(14)	(17)	(2)	(7)

Source: Ethnic Pluralism in an Urban Setting data.

Contrary to previous research, we found that members of all five ethnic groups, including immigrants, made use of both intra-ethnic and inter-ethnic ties. However, the composition of friendship networks is associated with the types of ties used. More than 80 per cent of those job seekers whose friendship networks were ethnically homogenous used ties within their own ethnic group. In contrast, almost 60 per cent of those job seekers whose networks were ethnically heterogeneous used ties outside their own ethnic group (see Table 9.3).

Age, generation of immigration, gender, education, and the heterogeneity of networks complexly affected the use of inter-ethnic ties in job searches. In general, the more recent the generation of immigration, the more likely people were to be in ethnically homogeneous networks and to lack access to the social capital of other, often higher-status, ethnic groups. Among immigrants, higher educational attainment was also associated with being in more ethnically heterogeneous friendship networks. Thus, better-educated immigrants had more access to social capital in the host society beyond their own ethnic circle of relatives and friends. Later post-immigrant generations were more likely to be in heterogeneous friendship networks and were more likely to use inter-ethnic ties for job searches. They were more likely to have access to social capital outside their own ethnic groups (see Table 9.4).

In contrast to the situation among the first generation, the more highly-educated members of the second and third generations were more likely to be in ethnically homogeneous networks. These people often found occupational and social niches within their ethnic groups (Merton 1957). Older members of the third generation, who had the most opportunity over the years to forge inter-ethnic ties, were more likely than younger members of their generation to use inter-ethnic ties (see Table 9.5).

What were the advantages and disadvantages of using intra-ethnic and/or inter-ethnic ties? When members of low-status ethnic groups used inter-ethnic ties in job searches, they tended to obtain higher mean incomes. Female members of low-status ethnic groups were especially likely to have higher mean incomes when they used inter-ethnic ties. Probably, this was because other women in their ethnic group (their probable intra-ethnic ties) tended to have low incomes. On the other hand, members of two high-status groups, English Canadians and German Canadians, obtained higher incomes when they used ties within their own ethnic group. Because these two groups controlled better resources within their own ethnic networks, structural opportunities accessed through inter-ethnic ties might not necessarily be as beneficial as those accessed through intra-ethnic ties.

Using inter-ethnic ties in an ethnically segmented labour market like Toronto could help people gain access to diverse resources beyond their own ethnic group. However, the advantage of using inter-ethnic ties was conditional on the positions of the ethnic groups to which job seekers and job contacts belonged. Not all inter-ethnic ties were necessarily beneficial, even for members of low-status ethnic groups. The use of inter-ethnic ties offered greater rewards when contacts were with ethnic groups of higher economic status, such as western and northern Europeans. It was less rewarding when contact was with members of lower-status groups, such as southern and eastern Europeans and non-whites.

Studies of disparities in economic integration across Canadian racial and ethnic groups have emphasized the role of discrimination in the labour market when members of different racial and ethnic groups do not receive similar returns for their human capital (Li 1988; Herberg 1990; Lautard and Guppy 1990; Pendakur and Pendakur 1998; Lian and Matthews 1998). Such sustained inequality may be partly produced and reproduced through network-mediated job searches (see also Reitz and Sklar 1997).

Job contacts are 'network capital' (Wellman and Frank 2000), a form of social capital (Borgatti et al. 1998). When co-ethnic members do not control good resources in an ethnically segregated labour market, the life chances of members of low-status ethnic groups – the job seekers themselves, their households, and their succeeding generations – depend on access to network capital through heterogeneous networks. A high-status, well-paying job provides a means to transform social capital into financial capital (earnings), human capital (skills acquisition), and further social capital (contacts with people and organizations formed on the job) over generations. It follows that, not having access to the proper social networks may set the stage for producing, reproducing, and sustaining structured inequality. This may be especially true for first-generation immigrants, who are more likely to lack other resources. Social mobility may partly depend on whether job seekers have access to network capital through heterogeneous networks.

We have found that immigrants with lower education have the fewest options in using inter-ethnic ties. We believe that this is due to the limited extent of their structural incorporation. When their co-ethnic group members do not include professional or entrepreneurial elements, they may become the most disadvantaged group in accessing better job opportunities because they are excluded from social networks that control the allocation of better-paying, mainstream jobs. Unless they form inter-ethnic ties and find access to otherwise unavailable opportunities, better-educated immigrants are not exempt from such exclusion.

For example, our findings are congruent with Salaff's demonstration (see chapter 10) that the limited networks of skilled Chinese immigrants have not led them to good mainstream jobs. Facing difficulties in locating good mainstream jobs, some have stayed in dead-end jobs, while others have returned home or became transnational 'astronauts' commuting between Canada and Hong Kong. Thus networks, as social capital, can play a significant role in structuring unequal allocation of opportunities for social mobility and in conditioning how immigrants and minority members become incorporated into the host society. Our research has shown that members of minority groups use job searches in various ways, and that in an ethnically segmented labour market, the use of inter-ethnic and intra-ethnic ties has various possible outcomes. However, there are several limitations that could be overcome in future studies of job searches among immigrants and their descendants.

First, there is a need to compare the advantages of inter-ethnic ties versus intra-ethnic ties in different urban contexts. Toronto, one of the world's supremely multiethnic cities, may not represent the dynamics of personal networks in other milieux. The resources that members of each ethnic group can mobilize surely vary by labour market. Intercity comparisons would help clarify how different social contexts can make inter-ethnic ties advantageous or disadvantageous.

Second, the limitations of our data have forced us to make the simplifying assertion that a tie to a member of a high- (or low-) status ethnic group indicates a tie to a high- (or low-) status individual. Although group context can be important, it would be desirable to know more about the socioeconomic status of the particular people in a job searcher's network.

Third, as people change their networks, the resources they can mobilize from networks also change. Analysts need to do longitudinal analyses to examine the changing dynamics of networks as resources and to see how these networks structure the incorporation of various groups into the larger structure of society.

Fourth, there is a need to examine data that are more recent and diverse than what we have presented here. Our analysis looked at the benefits of inter-ethnic and intra-ethnic ties among immigrants and later generations of white, European origin. This analysis has been based on data collected in 1978–9. Although Toronto has continued as a multiethnic city since then, there have been significant changes in the city's position in the world economy as well as in the structure of the local labour market (Richmond 1992). Radical changes in Canada's immigration law in the late 1960s have altered the composition of the immigration stream received in Toronto. Asia, Africa, and Latin America have become the leading sources of Toronto's immigrant population (Mercer 1995). East Asian ethnic groups now have higher status. Future research should focus on the consequences of these recent changes on the job search experiences of more diverse immigrant groups.

Fifth, during the 1990s and 2000s race became a more salient factor than ethnicity in structuring inequality in Canadian society (Li 1988, 1990; Pendakur and Pendakur 1998). Recent studies have shown that recent nonwhite immigrant groups are likely to be replacing previous white immigrant groups in filling less desirable jobs. Ethnic stratification has lessened among white European groups, but differences between racial groups have persisted (Lian and Matthews 1998; Ooka and Fong 2002; Hiebert 1999). When racial cleavages determine the allocation of resources, ties that connect beyond racial boundaries can become significant advantages in accessing economic opportunities. Conversely, the lack of proper social networks beyond racial boundaries can significantly harm the economic integration of racial minority groups (see also Salaff in chapter 10). Hence, future research should investigate the resources that visible minorities can mobilize within and outside their ethnic groups through the use of inter- and intra-racial ties.

To what extent do racial cleavages and the ensuing lack of appropriate social connections hinder racial minorities from accessing better-paying mainstream jobs? What are the benefits for racial minorities of using interracial ties to overcome difficulties in the Canadian labour market? It would be useful to address these questions in future studies by comparing the resources that visible minorities can mobilize within and outside their groups through the use of inter- and intra-racial ties. This research should help us understand the resources that people mobilize through network capital within and outside their ethnic groups. More broadly, such research can help us understand the socially mediated processess through which racial and ethnic inequalities in the often vertical Canadian mosaic have been substained and overcome.

NOTES

We thank Raymond Breton, Wsevolod W. Isajiw, and Jeffrey Reitz – the principal investigators of the original Ethnic Pluralism in an Urban Setting study, – for providing the data sets that we analyse here. We thank Liviana Mostacci Calzavara for advice about analysing these data, and Michael Patrick Johnson for comments on an earlier version.

1 Social network analysts describe 'strong ties' as relations characterized by feelings of social closeness, voluntary contact, and frequent contact, although not all strong ties have all of these characteristics. Ties run in a rough metaphoric continuum from strong to weak.

2 The proportion of people who are working in different occupations changes over time. As our analysis is based on data conducted in 1979, we use labour market information from the late 1970s and the early 1980s.

3 We discuss high- and low-status ethnic groups here and not individuals because we are interested in the milieux in which job seekers are located.

4 The sample includes people who used formal referrals, such as an employment agency, Canada Manpower, unions, and newspapers. It also includes those who applied directly to the employer but who also received initial help from personal contacts. Students and self-employed people are

excluded because they were not asked about job referral. Part-time work-ers (N=78), unemployed, retired, or disabled workers, and housewives (N=34) were excluded from the analysis to aid comparison of incomes.

5 The question asks: 'Think of your three closest friends who are not rela-tives. Of these three friends how many are from the same ethnic group?' The question regarding the ethnicity of the contacts used for finding jobs has a large number of missing answers, leading to a reduced sample size of 455. The first reason for this is a problem in interviewing. Some people who were approached with job offers by their prospective employers were not asked to give information about their employers' ethnicities (Calzavara 1982, 61). The second reason is that some people did not want to answer the question even if they knew their job contacts' ethnicity because ethnicity can be a sensitive and personal issue. Third, in a multi-cultural society such as Canada, it is often difficult for people to know the ethnic background of their network members. Fourth, some Canadians have multiple ethnic backgrounds.

6 For the same reason that was discussed in the previous note, a large number of missing information about the ethnicity of the contact de-creased the sample size to 331.

7 As expected, there was no significant impact of gender and age on the maintenance of ethnic friendship networks (hypotheses 1.4 and 1.5 are supported).

8 All amounts are expressed in Canadian dollars. At the time of data collec-tion, one Canadian dollar was equal to about 87 US cents.

9 For the sake of brevity, we follow the Canadian convention here of omit-ting the suffix '-Canadian'. Thus 'Italian men' are really 'Italian-Canadian men'.

10 Results from Table 9.7 should be treated with caution due to the small cell sizes.

11 The only exception is German men. Using inter-ethnic ties from lower-status ethnic groups was more rewarding for them. However, this anoma-lous result is affected by one outlying case where a person attained a very high income after using a Hungarian contact.

REFERENCES

Alba, Richard D. 1990. *Ethnic Identity: The Transformation of White America.* New Haven, CT: Yale University Press.

Anderson, Grace M. 1974. *Networks of Contact: The Portuguese and Toronto.* Waterloo, ON: Wilfrid Laurier University Press.

Bates, Timothy Mason. 1994. 'Social Resources Generated by Group Support Networks May Not Be Beneficial to Asian Immigrant-owned Small Businesses.' *Social Forces* (March): 671–89.

Bauer, Thomas, and Klaus F. Zimmermann, 1997. 'Network Migration of Ethnic Germans.' *International Migration Review* 31:143–9.

Bailey, Thomas, and Roger Waldinger. 1991. 'Primary, Secondary, and Enclave Labor Markets: A Training Systems Approach.' *American Journal of Sociology* 56: 432–5.

Becker, Gary S. 1992. 'Human Capital and the Economy.' *Proceedings of the American Philosophical Society* 136:85–92.

Borgatti, Stephen P., Candace Jones, and Martin G Everett. 1998. 'Network Measures of Social Capital.' *Connections* 21:27–36.

Boyd, Monica. 1984. 'At a Disadvantage: The Occupational Attainments of Foreign Born Women in Canada.' *International Migration Review* 18:1091–119.

– 1989. 'Family and Personal Networks in International Migration: Recent Developments and New Agendas.' *International Migration Review* 23:638–70.

Breton, Raymond. 1964. 'Institutional Completeness of Ethnic Communities and the Personal Relations of Immigrants.' *American Journal of Sociology* 70:193–205.

Breton, Raymond, Wsevolod W. Isajiw, Warren E. Kalbach, and Jeffrey G. Reitz. 1981. 'Ethnic Pluralism in an Urban Setting: Conceptual and Technical Overview of Research Project.' Research Paper no. 121. Toronto: Centre for Urban and Community Studies, University of Toronto.

– , eds. 1990. *Ethnic Identity and Equality: Varieties of Experiences in a Canadian City.* Toronto: University of Toronto Press.

Calzavara, Liviana M. 1983. 'Social Networks and Access to Jobs: A Study of Five Ethnic Groups in Toronto.' Research Paper no. 145. Toronto: Centre for Urban and Community Studies, University of Toronto.

– 1982. 'Social Networks and Access to Job Opportunities.' Doctoral dissertation, Department of Sociology, University of Toronto.

Campbell, Karen E., Peter V. Marsden, and Jeanne S. Hurlbert. 1986. 'Social Resources and Socioeconomic Status.' *Social Networks* 8:97–117.

Cobas, Jose A., Michael Aikin, and Douglas S. Jardine. 1993. 'Industrial Segmentation, the Ethnic Economy, and Job Mobility: The Case of Cuban Exiles in Florida.' *Quality and Quantity* 27:249–70.

Cobas, Jose A. and Ione DeOllos. 1989. 'Family Ties, Co-ethnic Bonds, and Ethnic Entrepreneurship.' *Sociological Perspectives* 32:403–11.

Espinoza, Vicente. 1999. 'Social Networks among the Urban Poor: Inequality and Integration in a Latin American City.' Pp. 147–184 in *Networks in the Global Village: Life in Contemporary Communities.* edited by Barry Wellman, Boulder, CO: Westview Press.

Fernandez-Kelly, M. Patricia. 1995. 'Social and Cultural Capital in the Urban Ghetto: Implications for the Economic Sociology of Immigration.' Pp. 213–247 in *The Economic Sociology of Immigration: Essays on Networks, Ethnicity and Entrepreneurship*, edited by Alejandro Portes. New York: Russell Sage Foundation.

Ferrand, Alexis, Lise Mounier, and Alain Degenne. 1999. 'The Diversity of Personal Networks in France: Social Stratification and Relational Structures.' Pp. 185–224 in *Networks in the Global Village: Life in Contemporary Communities*, edited by Barry Wellman. Boulder, CO: Westview Press.

Fong, Eric, and Wsevolod W. Isajiw. 2000. 'Determinants of Friendship Choices in Multiethnic Society.' *Sociological Forum* 15(2):249–71.

Gans, Herbert J. 1962. *The Urban Villagers: Group and Class in the Life of Italian-Americans*. New York: Free Press.

Granovetter, Mark S. 1982. 'Who Gets Ahead? The Determinants of Economic Success in America.' *Theory and Society* 11:257–62.

– 1974 [1995]. *Getting a Job: A Study of Contacts and Careers*. Cambridge, MA: Harvard University Press.

– 1973. 'The Strength of Weak Ties.' *American Journal of Sociology* 78:105–30.

Hagan, John, Ronit Dinovitzer and Patricia Parker. 1999. 'Choice and Circumstance: Social Capital and Planful Competence in the Attainments of the "One-and-a-Half" Generation.' Virtual Library Working Paper, Joint Centre of Excellence for Research on Immigration and Settlement: Toronto. July. http://ceris.metropolis.net/vl/education/hagan1.html.

Herberg, Edward N. 1990. 'The Ethno-Racial Socioeconomic Hierarchy in Canada: Theory and Analysis of the New Vertical Mosaic.' *International Journal of Comparative Sociology* 31:206–21.

Hiebert, Daniel. 1999. 'Local Geographies of Labor Market Segmentation: Montreal, Toronto, And Vancouver, 1991.' *Economic Geography* 75:339–69.

Hondagnew-Sotelo, Pierrette. 1994. 'Regulating the Unregulated? Domestic Workers and Social Networks.' *Social Problems* 41:50–63.

Isajiw, Wsevolod W. 1990. 'Ethnic Identity Retention.' Pp. 34–91 in *Ethnic Identity and Equality: Varieties of Experiences in a Canadian City*, edited by Raymond Breton, Wsevolod W. Isajiw, Warren E. Kalbach, and Jeffrey G. Reitz. Toronto: University of Toronto Press.

Kalbach, Warren E. 1990. 'Ethnic Residential Segregation and its Significance for the Individual in an Urban Setting.' Pp. 34–91 in *Ethnic Identity and Equality: Varieties of Experiences in a Canadian City*, edited by Raymond Breton, Wsevolod W. Isajiw, Warren E. Kalbach, and Jeffrey G. Reitz. Toronto: University of Toronto Press.

Kelner, Merrijoy. 1970. 'Ethnic Penetration into Toronto's Elite Structure.' *Canadian Review of Sociology and Anthropology* 7:128–37.

– 1969. 'The Elite Structure of Toronto: Ethnic Composition and Patterns of Recruitment.' Doctoral dissertation, Department of Sociology, University of Toronto.

Koser, Khalid. 1997. 'Social Networks and the Asylum Cycle: The Case of Iranians in the Netherlands.' *International Migration Review* 31:591–611.

Lautard, E.H., and L. Neil Guppy. 1990. 'The Vertical Mosaic Revisited: Occupational, Differentials among Canadian Ethnic Groups.' Pp. 189–208 in *Race and Ethnic Relations in Canada*, edited by Peter S. Li. Toronto: Oxford University Press Canada.

Li, Peter S. 1988. *Ethnic Inequality in a Class Society*. Toronto: Thompson Educational Publishing.

Lian, Jason Z., and David Ralph Matthews. 1998. 'Does the Vertical Mosaic Still Exist? Ethnicity and Income in Canada, 1991.' *Canadian Review of Sociology and Anthropology* 35:61–81.

Light, Ivan, and Edna Bonacich. 1988. *Immigrant Entrepreneurs: Koreans in Los Angeles, 1965–1982*. Berkeley: University of California Press.

Lin, Nan. 2001. *Social Capital: A Theory of Social Structure and Action*. Cambridge: Cambridge University Press.

Lin, Nan, and Mary Dumin. 1986. 'Access to Occupations through Social Ties.' *Social Networks* 8:365–85.

Mercer, John. 1995. 'Canadian Cities and Their Immigrants: New Realities.' *Annals of the American Academy of Political and Social Science* 538:169–84.

Merton, Robert K. 1957. 'Patterns of Influence: Cosmopolitans and Locals.' Pp. 387–420 in *Social Theory and Social Structure*. edited by Robert K. Merton. Glencoe, IL: Free Press.

Model, Suzanne. 1992. 'The Ethnic Economy: Cubans and Chinese Reconsidered.' *Sociological Quarterly* 33:63–82.

Nee, Victor, Jimmy M. Sanders, and Scot Sernau. 1994. 'Job Transitions in an Immigrant Metropolis: Ethnic Boundaries and the Mixed Economy.' *American Sociological Review* 59:849–72.

Newman, Peter C. 1975–81. *The Canadian Establishment*. Toronto: McClelland & Stewart.

Massey, Douglas S. 1995 'The New Immigrationand Ethnicity in the United Sates.' *Population and Development Review* 21:631–52.

Ooka, Emi. 2001. 'Social Capital and Income Attainment among Chinese Immi-grant Entrepreneurs in Toronto.' *Asian and Pacific Migration Journal* 10:123–44.

Ooka, Emi, and Eric Fong. 2002. 'Globalization and Earnings among Native-Born and Immigrant Populations of Racial and Ethnic Groups in Canada.' *Canadian Studies in Population* 29:101–22.

Pendakur, Krishna, and Ravi Pendakur. 1998. 'The Colour Of Money: Earnings Differentials Among Ethnic Groups in Canada.' *Canadian Journal of Economics* 31:518–48.

Porter, John. 1965. *The Vertical Mosaic*. Toronto: University of Toronto Press.

Portes, Alejandro. 1998. 'Social Capital: Its Origins and Applications in Modern Sociology.' *Annual Review of Sociology* 24:1–24.

– ed. 1995. *Economic Sociology of Immigrants: Essays on Networks, Ethnicity, and Entrepreneurship*. New York: Russell Sage Foundation.

Portes, Alejandro, and Robert L. Bach. 1985. *Latin Journey: Cuban and Mexican Immigrants in the United States*. Berkeley: University of California Press.

Portes, Alejandro, and Leif Jensen. 1989. 'The Enclave and the Entrants: Patterns of Ethnic Enterprise in Miami Before and After Mariel.' *American Sociological Review* 54:929–49.

Portes, Alejandro, and Rubén G. Rumbaut. 2001. *Legacies: The Story of the Immigrant Second Generation*. Berkeley: University of California Press.

– 1996. *Immigrant America: A Portrait*. Berkeley: University of California Press.

Portes, Alejandro, and Julia Sensenbrenner. 1993. 'Embeddedness and Immigration: Notes on the Social Determinants of Economic Action.' *American Journal of Sociology* 98:1320–50.

Portes, Alejandro, and Min Zhou. 1992. 'Gaining the Upper Hand: Economic Mobility among Immigrant and Domestic Minorities.' *Ethnic and Racial Studies* 15:491–522.

Putnam, Robert. 2000. *Bowling Alone*. New York: Simon & Schuster.

Reitz, Jeffrey G. 1998. *Warmth Of The Welcome: The Social Causes of Economic Success for Immigrants In Different Nations And Cities*. Boulder, Colo.: Westview Press.

– 1990. 'Ethnic Concentrations in Labour Markets and Their Implications for Ethnic Inequality.' Pp. 135–195 in *Ethnic Identity and Equality: Varieties of Experiences in a Canadian City*, edited by Raymond Breton, Wsevolod W. Isajiw, Warren E. Kalbach, and Jeffrey G. Reitz. Toronto: University of Toronto Press.

Reitz, Jeffrey G., Liviana M Calzavara, and Donna Dasko. 1981. 'Ethnic Inequality and Segregation in Jobs.' Research Paper no. 123. Toronto: Centre for Urban and Community Studies, University of Toronto.

Reitz, Jeffrey G., Joachim R. Frick, Tony Calabrese, and Gert C. Wagner. 1999. 'The Institutional Framework of Ethnic Employment Disadvantage: A Comparison of Germany and Canada.' *Journal of Ethnic and Migration Studies* 25:397–443.

Reitz, Jeffrey G., and Sherrilyn M. Sklar. 1997. 'Culture, Race, and the Economic Assimilation of Immigrants.' *Sociological Forum* 12:233–77.

Richmond, Anthony H. 1992. 'Immigration and Structural Change: The

Canadian Experience, 1971–1986.' *International Migration Review* 26: 1200–21.

Richmond, Anthony H., and R.P. Verma, 1978. 'Income Inequality in Canada: Ethnic and Generational Aspects.' *Canadian Studies in Population* 5:25–36.

Rose, Damaris, Pia Carrasco, and Johanne Charboneau. 1999. 'The Role of "Weak Ties" in the Settlement Experiences of Immigrant Women with Young Children: The Case of Central Americans in Montréal.' Working Paper, Joint Centre of Excellence for Research on Immigration and Settlement – Toronto, June. http://ceris.metropolis.net/vl/community/ rose1.html.

Rumberger, Russell, and Katherine Larson. 1998. 'Towards Explaining Differences in Educational Achievement among Mexican American Language-Minority Students.' *Sociology of Education* 71:69–93.

Salaff, Janet W., Eric Fong, and Siu-lun Wong, 1999. 'Using Social Networks to Exit Hong Kong.' Pp. 229–330 in *Networks in the Global Village: Life in Contemporary Communities*, edited by Barry Wellman. Boulder, CO: Westview Press.

Sanders, Jimmy and Victor Nee. 1996. 'Immigrant Self-Employment: The Family as Social Capital and the Value of Human Capital.' *American Sociological Review* 61:231–49.

Stoloff, Jennifer A., Jennifer L. Glanville, and Elisa Jayne Bienenstock. 1999. 'Women's Participation in the Labor Force: The Role of Social Network.' *Social Networks* 21:91–108.

Turrittin, Jane. S. 1976. 'Networks and Mobility: The Case of West Indian Domestics from Montserrat.' *Canadian Review of Sociology and Anthropology* 13:305–20.

Waldinger, Roger. 1994. 'The Making of an Immigrant Niche.' *International Migration Review* 28:3–30.

– 1993. 'The Ethnic Enclave Debate Revisited.' *International Journal of Urban and Regional Research* 17:444–52.

Waldinger, Roger and Joel Perlmann. 1999. 'Second Generations.' Pp. 240–57 in *Sociology for the Twenty-First Century*, edited by Janet Abu-Lughod. Chicago: University of Chicago Press.

Wellman, Barry. 1988. 'The Community Question Re-Evaluated.' *Comparative Urban and Community Research* 1:81–107.

Wellman, Barry, and Kenneth Frank. 2000. 'Network Capital in a Multi-Level World: Getting Support in Personal Communities.' Pp. 233–73 in *Social Capital*, edited by Nan Lin, Ronald Burt and Karen Cook. Chicago: Aldine-DeGruyter

Wellman, Barry, and Barry Leighton. 1979. 'Networks, Neighborhoods, and

Communities: Approaches to the Study of the Community Question.' *Urban Affairs Quarterly* 14:363–90.

Wellman, Barry, and Scot Wortley. 1990. 'Different Strokes from Different Folks: Community Ties and Social Support.' *American Journal of Sociology* 96:558–88.

Wiley, Norbert. 1967. 'The Ethnic Mobility Trap and Stratification Theory.' *Social Problems* 15:147–59.

Wilson, Kenneth L., and Alejandro Portes. 1980. 'Immigrant Enclaves: Analysis of the Labor Market Experiences of Cubans in Miami.' *American Journal of Sociology* 86:305–19.

Zhou, Min. 1997. 'Growing Up American.' *Annual Review of Sociology* 23:63–95.

Zhou, Min, and John Logan. 1989. 'Return on Human Capital in Ethnic Enclaves: New York City's Chinatown.' *American Sociological Review* 54:809–20.

Zimmer, Catherine, and Howard E. Aldrich, 1987. 'Resource Mobilization through Ethnic Networks: Kinship and Friendship Ties of Shopkeepers in England.' *Sociological Perspectives* 30:422–55.

10 Different Crossings: Migrants from Three Chinese Communities

JANET W. SALAFF

New skilled immigrants from Asia find it hard to get good jobs. Some may return home, while others stay. We think these decisions are not purely personal. They are shaped by structures. We need to systematically explore how social connections and political economic institutions shape the paths that international migrants take as they work out the settlement process (Basch et al. 1994; Boyd 1989; Massey and Garcia Espana 1987). In this chapter I explore some of these issues. I do so from the perspectives of three comparable individuals from three different places of origin: the People's Republic of China (henceforth PRC), Taiwan, and Hong Kong. Through their experiences, we will see some of the ways that new Chinese immigrants, who are the elite in their countries of origin, find their qualifications unrecognized in the new host society.[1]

The chapters in this book have explored a range of social structures that shape Torontonians' lives. Among these are labour force institutions, housing, and health services. This chapter looks at some of the social structures – especially labour force structures – that shape the settlement of migrants. It has long been thought that if the social structures in the sending and receiving countries are similar, and if personal social networks help people bridge the divide, movement and adjustment should be easier. However, the fit is not often there, and there is often a disjunction between social structures. People who fit into one set of labour force structures at home may move to a location where they do not. By fit, I am referring to the local recognition of human and social capital. Growing up in a place where they received a good education gave men discussed here many opportunities, as well as recognition. However, their human and social capital were not recognized abroad.

The common observation that new immigrants are downwardly mobile, and take years to recoup their wages after immigration, flows partly from this disjunction of social structures.

Another factor is the institutional decentralization of Canadian professions. The engineering profession offers few opportunities for those educated abroad to qualify easily. In Canada, entry to the professions is controlled largely by the professional associations themselves. The government vets new immigrants but cannot effect their smooth entry into a new career.

What the three engineers and their families did about their career disjunction varied according to the structures and networks they accessed from their own countries. By describing a variety of structures through the lives of these three new skilled immigrant men in Toronto, I illustrate how diverse structures in the sending countries mesh into those in the receiving country.

Background: Migration from the Pacific Region

Several explanations have been proposed for the multidirectional movements of people. Large-scale transnational corporations transfer their capital, goods, and employees (Bartlett and Goshal 1989; Fielding 1993; Findley and Li 1997; Gereffi 1998; Salt 1988). Smaller firms add density to these movements. Taiwanese firms subcontract to American firms, creating production links between Asia and the West (Gereffi 1998). For instance, in the electronics industry, Taiwanese students and employees develop commodity chains to the west coast of the United States (Ong et al. 1994; Tseng and Jou 2000). With the internationalization of educational systems, Asian managerial, technical, and professional graduates expect their credentials and experiences to qualify them for good positions in the West.

The movement of people has also reversed. As the Pacific Rim countries became the fastest-growing markets, Chinese who had lived abroad for years began returning to pursue expanding local opportunities (Lever-Tracy et al. 1996; Sung 1991). Also fostering international migration is that pioneer immigrants send back news about the standards of living abroad (Chiu 1995; Shu & Hawthorne 1996; Yoon 1993); concurrently, mass-produced consumer goods and the media stimulate imaginings of Western lifestyles (Anderson 1991). The yearnings of the Asian middle class for political security also incline them towards Western democracies.

Emigration is not a unidirectional movement. Many international migrants maintain close contact with their home countries by phone, e-mail, and frequent visits. Some have homes and jobs in two locations, going back and forth between them; this is referred to as transnational migration. By transnational migrants I refer to those who immigrate to a new country without cutting their ties to their original land. Such double lives and double identities are not simply a matter of chasing new opportunities to earn and invest. There are also many moves arising from changes of mind, mistakes, and disappointments, when access to jobs at home and abroad do not match (Wong and Salaff 1998). The professions erect barriers to new members, curtailing outsiders' entry (Collins 1979). Taken-for-granted cultural meanings become semi-permeable membranes to jobs. This incomplete globalization of institutions prompts remigration. Unable to land good mainstream jobs, many also find that the ethnic community offers little (Portes 1998; Zhou 1992). Given limited job choices, some middle-class professionals return home and even capitalize on their international experiences. Social networks that link people in many locales are the reasons for as well as the means of international migration. Networks that are so crucial in people's moves abroad can also send them back (Tilly 1990). For instance, those in the Hong Kong Chinese elite strategize familywide investment across multiple countries to spread the risks (Lever-Tracy et al. 1996; Mitchell 1995; Wong 1997). Middle-class migrants have less capital; that said, their economic transactions also rely on shared cultural ties and personal networks in different lands (Wong and Salaff 1998). However, we do not know enough about the strength, reach, or structure of the transnational links of the diasporic middle class.

Timing also affects remigration. Large, diverse, and well-placed social networks help migration and settlement (Findley 1987). If networks are new, international movements may be slow in both directions. Continuity in migrant networks eases migration, and pioneers with sparse networks may face hurdles. Early migrants may extend more support to newcomers because there are fewer of them; latecomers may face more obstacles because networks become overloaded (Manjivar 1997). Since the range of immigrant social networks expands with the entry of each new migrant into the process, networks increasingly embody more resources (Hondagneu-Sotelo 1994; Massey & España 1987; Min 1988). The numerical balance also counts. Migrants with fewer networks to link up with abroad may find it easier to return to their fully developed networks at home. Thus, in many ways the nature of people's networks on both sides of the ocean contributes both to migration and to remigration.

Not all migrants remain abroad, and not all return. Paradoxically, the easier it is to emigrate, the easier it is to return when things don't work out. To explore this paradox, we look at how networks mesh at home and abroad. At the time of our study, migrants from sending nations such as Hong Kong and Taiwan were more likely to remigrate than were those from China. And there are differences between Hong Kong and Taiwan immigrants to Canada as well. Through the lives of three middle-class Chinese families, this chapter explores the ethnic, business, and family contacts and structures that encourage migration and compares these processes across individual families from different sending and receiving populations. Through their accounts, we query how transnational institutions and networks figure in international moves.

Statistics

Middle-class immigrants from the Pacific region account for much of the immigration to Canada. Numbers differ by place of origin. Decades of immigration gave Hong Kong newcomers an edge. In 1995, 31,746 immigrants to Ontario cited Hong Kong as their last permanent residence. Taiwan lagged behind, with more following their networks to the United States; in 1995 only 7,691 came to Ontario from Taiwan. The numbers of immigrants from the PRC have recently increased, and greatly outnumber others; in 2001, 40,296 PRC immigrants arrived to Canada (Statistics Canada 2000, 2001, 8; Skeldon 1996).

Because Canada does not keep exit statistics, the numbers of returning immigrants are not known. We cannot look at the country of origin, either. For instance, since many Chinese who remigrate to Hong Kong have taken Canadian papers, they are counted as Canadians in Hong Kong. Countries that do keep exit statistics document return moves that suggest an increasing ease of 'displacement' (Ip 1997; Mak 1997).

Our Approach

The three lives we present are part of our decade-long, several-stage investigation of transnational Chinese migration. I chose these three cases from two databases. I was part of a team of researchers at the Centre of Asian Studies, University of Hong Kong, that investigated emigration from Hong Kong in the 1990s; for this study we interviewed several families who had decided to emigrate. The engineer discussed here was part of that panel study, which is now being updated for publication as a monograph.[2] I chose the PRC couple from one of fifty married PRC immigrant couples in my panel study, 'Skilled PRC Immigrants to Toronto, 1996–2003.'[3] I met the Taiwan respondent through a mutual friend. I have chosen to discuss these three men because they shared the same social class as managers, professionals, and technicians before leaving their home countries and arrived as independents based on cumulated points. All three are from the same life-cycle stage and came with their families, which included school-age children. Initially intending to remain, they could not find work as engineers and had to decide whether to return to Asia.

The qualitative method helps us distinguish the personal experiences of those from the PRC, Taiwan, and Hong Kong. These middle-class migrants had considerable choice; no catastrophe prompted their exit. The social construction approach reveals the complex ways that emigrants define options and create and change opportunities (Gold 1997; Levitt and Shaffir 1990). We used naturalistic observations and in-depth questions. Life historians study the macrostructures and social networks that aid or limit settlement choices from the bottom up (Bertaux 1997; Bertaux-Wiame 1981). Here we explore how the meanings of networks, migration, and ethnic enclaves vary with background.

Three Former Site Engineers

These technically skilled site engineers had comfortable jobs with large firms in their home country. They had experience with advanced international structures, had plenty of information about the West, and intended to use their human capital after migrating. All three families suffered a sharp decline in living standards, and when they did, they took different migration paths.

A PRC Engineer Migrates

Tom Lai felt that China's overly structured society was limiting his social contributions and advancement. Family reasons also prompted Tom to emigrate from Gwangchow, China, in early 1998, along with his pregnant wife, Siu-ying, and their daughter. Once in Toronto, his fortunes plummeted. Our story centres on why he declined to return to a good position in China (circular migration) and instead took steps to invite his relatives to Canada (chain migration). We find that recent political changes have linked the PRC's social institutions more closely than before to the international community; however, they still do not allow easy circulation.

Career Ladder

Lai's degree in mechanical engineering had prepared him to participate in China's modernization in the new liberal era. His state firm imported environmental waste machines, and he had considerable contact with the West. When the company failed to make the most use of his abilities, he quit, confident that there would be demand for his experience. A joint venture company took him on as an entry-level engineer in a small factory making electrical powder coating for medical equipment. The work was demanding. 'I had a good job but no time to spend with my family, because there's many problems in my factory ... Sometimes I received a call after ten at night.' With him at the helm, 'output improved ten times.' He was promoted to general manager's assistant. He then resigned, and in 1995 started up an import/export business, at which he worked even harder. 'I had an office, I was a boss. I earned more. But I didn't like it because it was very tiring. It may be that you've heard every Chinese wants to be boss, but I want to be an employee instead of the boss.' Siu-ying recalls: 'We were not able to have family time together since he always came home late. Back to sleep at home for several hours, and then to work again.'

The nonstop pace took a physical toll. Looking around, he noted that three colleagues had broken down. 'In China, there's no time for yourself and your family.' Besides all this, he saw an economic downturn coming and was pessimistic about the new reforms. He decided to emigrate.

Marriage and Family

Siu-ying, a former co-worker of Tom in the state firm, came from a Hong Kong family. Her father fled to China to escape the Japanese occupation and then returned much later to Hong Kong with his family. Siu-ying came back to China to marry Tom, gave birth to their first child in Hong Kong, then returned to China. She and Tom found that their marriage would be unable to mesh without a common nationality. Emigration would address this problem, but also create others.

Now in Canada and pregnant with their second child, and without a kin support system, Siu-ying has not integrated into the new society. 'I went to an English class for one night, but didn't continue after that because I didn't feel well. And it was too far away. And I can't bring my daughter to the English class.' Tom complained: 'She always depends on me.' Hondagneu-Sotelo (1994) discusses this sort of gendered division of labour, with the wife and husband integrating into the new society at different levels. After the birth of their second child, Tom hoped to sponsor his parents as dependents so that they could help with child care. Their arrival may increase Siu-ying's participation in Canadian life.

Preparing for the Move

Tom applied to enter Canada through an immigration consultant. He closed his company, sold his apartment, and waited at home for a year for his papers. He had saved C$50,000 to tide himself over until he could establish himself abroad. China does not accept dual citizenship, so on the eve of departure he turned in his residential documents and gave up the right to live and work in China. In doing so he was cutting his networks and renouncing his right to participate in civil society.

The Lais' information about the West was not too accurate. 'We were not well prepared when we came here. I just didn't want to stay in China forever, too many restrictions, and I think that the chance for me to be successful in Hong Kong may not be good either, and the life there is also full of pressures, and not suitable for me. That's why I didn't need so much information about Canada. When I studied in school, and from the books I read, I got some general ideas about life in North America. My concern was the lifestyle.'

Friends of friends recommended they come to Toronto instead of Vancouver. 'They said Vancouver's housing prices are high, but the chances for jobs are low. They know this! Many people come to Canada and then go back as new Canadians to do business in China.'

Tom was in the import/export business, so his information about consumer goods was better than about jobs. Friends had crafted for his family a one-of-a-kind Chinese dining room set. The round glass table-top sits atop legs shaped like four carved lotus flowers. Four carved chairs complete this lovely set. He shipped over his daughter's tricycle, a VCR, and a microwave oven, although on arrival he could not find a suitable adapter. The family also brought with them Chinese-made down clothing for the Canadian winter at a fraction of the Toronto prices.

Finding a Job in Canada

In the beginning, Tom worked as a labourer doing house renovations for a small Hong Kong firm. 'Nobody wants jobs like these because they're very heavy. But I don't care about that because I want to get some Canadian experience ... Many people think that it's hard to get a job in Canada. They worry about their poor living standards, but I don't! My expectations are not too high. This job only brings me money and Canadian experience, nothing else, so although I don't like it, I have to do it. I know if I want to get another job, they will ask, "Do you have any Canadian experience?" Someone once asked me what's Canadian experience, where can we buy this? At Canadian Tire?'

He had a gruelling schedule. He finished work at six o'clock six days a week, then drove home, changed, grabbed instant noodles, and went to study English. After class ended at nine at night, he returned home to have dinner. 'Even if I'm fatigued when I come back home, my brain is rested. After I sleep, I'm OK. But if your brain is tired, even sleeping can't solve the problem.

'I won't be satisfied in this position, I'll improve myself step by step. In every country, there are hard-working and lazy people, wealthy and poor people. You decide what kind of person you want to be. My ambition is not that high. I only wish to cover our living expenses and have some savings. My goal? Let's say, to support my family. I don't want to live in an apartment forever, I hope that I can have a place with trees. That's enough, why make myself so tired? Because you know there's a cost to everything. If you want to have a lot of money, you have to work very hard. And you keep on working, you earn a lot of money, but at the same time you forgo many other things. It's not worthwhile. So now I'm very happy because sometimes my family and I can do things together.'

Tom disliked the ethnic enclave. His employer took advantage of Tom's naivety and fired him when the original crew returned from their holidays in Hong Kong. Tom had no unemployment benefits, since the boss had paid him in cash. He was still optimistic. 'It's not hard to get a basic job, I got one after two weeks. I sent many résumés and seven or eight firms wanted to interview me. I took this one.' He still does manual labour, wiring office cubicles for an affiliate of a large Canadian firm. The firm is outside the ethnic enclave but scouts the ethnic job centres for new hires at the minimum wage. 'Many people have higher education than me. There's a medical doctor, and a PhD in engineering, but we only do simple jobs.' Tom's wage does not support the household; they must rely on their savings.

His job was a means for him to achieve his goals. There were other conveniences: the company did not exploit him, and they offered him parental leave. 'It's close to my home. I can reach there within five minutes by car. And I do evening shifts so I go to ESL class at nine in the morning. Then I can take care of my daughter during the day, and can go with her when she has a doctor's appointment.' The firm was large enough to offer an internal ladder, and an unexpected chance to better himself in the firm came up. 'I told the personnel manager about my professional background, and she told me in their main company they make powder coating products like I used to in China. I gave her my résumé again.' Optimistic, eager to start up the first rung of the Canadian career ladder, his eye was on his ultimate goal of re-establishing himself as a professional in Canadian society.

But this job did not last either, and he moved on to several others as a factory foreman. When I met him again in 2002, he had opened a small Chinese delicatessen, selling Hong Kong and Taiwanese appetizers. As a southern mainlander, he can speak both Cantonese and *pu tong hwa*, and his customers are from many backgrounds. His wife is working at his side – her first Canadian job. It is a seven-day-a-week responsibility for both of them. The store may be only a short-term solution. He fears it is taking too much out of his family life, because he and his wife cannot take the best care of their children when all of them are in the shop.

Future Plans

Tom had originally planned to return to engineering, by apprenticing and taking an exam or by returning to school. Before opening his deli, he hoped 'I would like to stop my job and study at U of T, because it's the only way to improve and to get a good job.' In early 2000 he considered entering the IT field but finally rejected this idea. 'I keep on researching information about how to become a professional. All the people I meet study computers.' He was wary about entering an unfamiliar field, anticipating – correctly, as it turned out – 'Too many people going to the same field. What they think about is that computer workers can earn a lot of money, but what I think is that since wages are high, and people who studied computers can get jobs easily, everyone will study in this field. Especially for new immigrants like me, we don't know what kind of labour is in demand. If you pursue a career that you're not familiar with, you'll not be able to compete with others. I think many people who studied computers won't get a job.'

He turned practical. 'If I study engineering full-time now, I have to give up my job, but I have to support my family and pay for my education. Then after several years, when I finish my studies, I would still have to look for work. Since I don't have a good background, even if I finished studying, it's still possible that I can't get a job. If I were still young and didn't have a family, I could change my career, until I find what I really like. But I'm not young now and I have to support my family, I can't afford to fail.'

He decided on a government apprenticeship program. 'Many Chinese feel ashamed to be an apprentice. But if you don't try everything, you can't do anything ... Even though I'd be an apprentice now, I can still write the exam to be an engineer and maybe I'll be an engineer some time. Since I understand this fact, my title is not important ... I can study and get professional qualifications, and at the same time I can work and don't need to look for an employer after I finish the program.' Furthermore, 'during these three years I still have plenty of time to study the Canadian labour market, what kind of workers are most wanted, so that I could change my field of study.' Later, we learned that Tom had been laid off again and had placed his career plans on hold. Lacking networks, he applied for several factory supervisor jobs through a manpower agency that he found in the phone book.

Tom accepted the menial jobs he found as the cost of being in a new environment. He was humble about his skills. 'When I came to Canada, I found I had actually few skills I can use. I was like a fool. I hardly knew how to use my hands. I cannot compete with others here, I have to learn from the beginning.' Apart from obvious language problems, his knowledge of computers – a taken-for-granted skill in his field – was weak. 'The systems are really different.' Tom accepted his career setbacks as the cost of coming from a system that was 'totally different.' His main complaint related to the disjunction between the strict point system for immigrants and Canada's refusal to recognize his personal experience. 'I just wonder why the Canadian government allows me to immigrate so easily and then after that they don't approve your educational background.' Labourer's jobs were stopgaps until he acquired more training and developed networks so that he could fit in the wider society.

Networks

At first, the Lais knew few people in Toronto. Gradually, they built a circle of Chinese friends. Former schoolmates surfaced, and friends introduced others. They got their first apartment and chose a Chinese doctor from the Chinese press. A friend introduced the Lais to a Chinese lawyer, who would help Tom apply for his parents to enter Canada. Their world is now peopled with new Chinese acquaintances. I asked him how many friends he now had in Canada. 'Many. Two friends from high school, one in Richmond Hill and one in Scarborough. I didn't know that another friend was here, I just realized that when I came ... We met another Hong Kong couple here. And then some ESL classmates. Newcomers who just arrived from China contacted us a few days ago. Also, you're my friend in Canada!' All of these people have formed a mutual support network. 'Sometimes I fax my friends useful information, like about the apprenticeship program ... Because you know we have to support each other in a new country and new environment.'

Immigration was supposed to solve some problems. In doing so, it created others. Coming from a 'totally different' system, he had few credentials to succeed in Canada and few alternatives to low-paid work. His solution to this was to import relatives to help with child care, so that he could retrain and his wife could get a job. 'If I could bring my parents over, my plans could proceed right away.' Yet another solution was remigration. So far he has rejected the idea of returning to China, having left it so long ago and cut himself loose from his contacts there. Returning would now be difficult.

A Taiwanese Engineer Migrates

The Chius, Bob and Rosa, a forty-three-year-old former site engineer from Taiwan married to a securities officer in a bank, were part of the global labour force before migrating. A technical-college graduate in computer engineering, Bob had worked for fifteen years on the computer team of a large oil company in Taiwan. This firm had links to companies in Asia and the Middle East, not North America. The Taiwanese community in Toronto is small, which limited his contacts further. His networks in Taiwan were more active, which suggested remigration as a solution to his job problems in Canada.

Deciding to Emigrate

Bob is part of the flow of people looking for new opportunities and a better lifestyle. He had no pressing personal reason to emigrate. The Chius had no relatives abroad when they applied. 'It was the political uncertainty – when will China take back Taiwan? – and secondly the kids' education. Why not the States? It cost less to come here. I paid six thousand dollars to agents, but to go to the United States we'd have to pay twenty thousand. Also, the wait is very long.'

His company's strong links to Asia and the Middle East had given him a sense of life outside his home country. 'Our company constructed most of the engineering factories in Taiwan. We create a factory from the initial design to construction, and it's a big job: a hundred people and one engineer go to gear up and build it. About ten years ago, my company sent me to Saudi Arabia, Thailand, and Singapore.' Working abroad was lucrative. It did not occur to the Chius that he would not be able to prosper equally well in Canada.

Bob and Rosa thought they knew enough about Canada to make a decision. 'We saw a movie on Prince Edward Island. I thought, that place is very nice. Anything is possible there. We also went to New Zealand to sightsee. We liked it, but to immigrate, your specialty must match what they want. We didn't consider Singapore. Australia is near Taiwan, and people who came back told us a lot of things about the poor economy – more racism than here.'

They left behind both sets of parents, Bob's brother, and Rosa's siblings. Bob had already secured his parents' living standards. From his Middle Eastern earnings, he had bought them a house with two apartments, in one of which he had lived. (It is now rented out.)

Finding a Job in Canada

In Toronto, Bob sought to follow his original profession, becoming a partner with other Chinese in a computer sales and repair company. All were qualified in the field and had earned college or graduate degrees in their home countries. The Taiwanese partner had organized the store as a business investment to meet the requirements of the immigration authorities. However, the line of products was not profitable. 'The usual thing when you do business is the first year you put in money, the second year you don't put in, but don't earn anything either, and the third year you begin to earn. But that computer store has been going five years and doesn't earn. A few years ago, you could sell one computer and get 20 per cent profit, now it's only 7 per cent. In one month how many can you sell? At most, forty to fifty systems. The information they collect is not very good. You must keep up to date. We have "just in time" and don't stock any inventory. For instance, it takes only two weeks to get a card to install for a Sun [Sun Microsystems makes servers and other proprietary hardware]. The customer orders the system, we pay for it, yet in only two weeks the price drops from $300 to $200. So we lose. The customer is very smart. They know the prices, they check everything in *Toronto Computes* ... That store doesn't earn. The boss is waiting to sell to some business immigrant who needs it for a visa.'

Bob next opened a boutique, which he called Biza, and began importing hand-crafted Taiwanese garments that joined folk themes with high-quality materials. This was in a poor part of the city, where Caribbean newcomers were joining more established Polish residents and a dozen other immigrant cultures. The rent was low, and artists were moving into the area. The street had a greengrocer selling mangos, avocados, and West Indian foods, next to a Polish sausage shop and a Korean store with fresh flowers. A European designer clothing store had brought its established clientele from more trendy Yorkville. But the area itself was not known for au courant shopping, and dollar stores outnumbered those with labels. Bob could not draw customers for his one-of-a-kind garments.

Connections from home supported this enterprise. Another Taiwanese immigrant backed the store; his niece shared the rent and upkeep and helped the Chius run the store. Tom explained: 'I asked my good friend in Taiwan to sell me these clothes at cost. We worked together in the same factory for four years. His wife set up this clothing business ten years ago, and my friend quit to help her ... Because the market is not so good in Taiwan, he knows that he cannot sell so much there, and wants to try abroad.'

Bob was thinking ahead. He considered marketing children's clothing. 'I have a cousin who makes children's sports clothing in Taiwan. I first thought I'd import his clothes. But I thought, you can get those things in Canada. It was better to do this line which is high quality and value added and unusual.' He deliberately chose a concept that was rooted in Taiwanese culture. 'These are handicrafts, special to Taiwan. Wearing these kinds of clothes is a "special taste" even there. That's why my prices are high.' However, he lacked local information and networks and was again frustrated at being unable to earn a living. New immigrants try hard to fit into Canadian lifestyle, because they need Canadian experience for their résumés. This means they must try to interpret local culture every day. My conversations with Bob revealed the subtlety of cultural meanings that natives take for granted.

The experience with the boutique taught Bob that he was a retailing neophyte. For one thing, the store's name did not convey any information about the product. 'What does "Biza" mean?' I asked. Clicking on his electronic dictionary to 'bizarre,' he explained: 'I'm thinking of a strange thing, a wonderful, wondrous thing.' I suggested: 'In English, "bizarre" means bad strange things, not good strange things ... Maybe you want "Bazaar." Except that a bazaar in Turkey is a happening place where many cultures gather, but here it has a "flea market" sense ... How about, "East meets West?"' Rosa conceded that name recognition was a problem: 'We placed our flyer in different stores and people took it and didn't know what kind of thing we were selling. Some called here to reserve a table for dinner!' Bob later changed the sign to 'Biza, the clothing shop where Eastern meets Western.'

The clothes were jammed together on narrow clothing racks, with house dresses next to party clothes, leaving a hodgepodge impression. Understandably, passers-by entered looking for bargains. The décor was more suited to low-cost products. Albums of three-by-five photographs of Chinese models in front of typical Chinese scenes, and young Western girls wearing the long dresses in Toronto, showed how people would look in the frocks. An unframed Taiwanese tourist poster hung on a wall; artificial flowers on the table suggested cheap clothing. Colour was another cultural difference: pink walls and a green door gave off a juvenile impression. Bob justified the colour scheme he had chosen: 'Before we moved in, it was very dirty and dark. I did a lot of renovating and had in mind pink and green as the colours of the lotus flower. We have them in Buddhist temples.' Rosa said plaintively: 'We didn't know. We take the Chinese ideas and come here, but after just two-and-a-half years, we don't know anything. We think of moving the counter to the front, then my husband says, "It's not good for fung shui!"' 'Better not move it.' I advised, 'Someone can rob you easily if you put it near the front door.' Discussions about how to import the products pointed to an ad hoc business plan. 'My wife can bring 200 dresses in a suitcase, without any customs. You go to Terminal 2 and 3 – not Terminal 1, where Hong Kong people go, because customs know that they bring in a lot.' Rosa: 'If you go with children, they don't check you.' Bob seized a chance to improve sales. Another immigrant, in exchange for placing his elaborate Japanese silk wedding kimonos in the store, changed the interior design to a sharp black-and-white motif, to appeal to the avant-garde. But a marketing plan was missing.

Still trying, Bob spun another hope. 'I prefer to do wholesale business, not for retail. To retail clothes is very difficult. You spend all day standing inside. If you're a small store you can't earn too much, because customers walk in and don't buy. But if you're big everybody knows you. The more people come in and understand our things, the better. You can earn more than this. I just want to try, but you know I'm not a businessman.' In the end, time ran out. The backer passed his citizenship test and lost interest in the boutique. Bob, who wanted the store to secure his family's living in Canada, felt betrayed. 'He used me!'

Rosa had opposed the whole venture. 'Immigration was his idea. I didn't agree much but also was not very much against it either.' But the store was worse. 'My husband and investors decided what kind of product to have on their own. I wasn't here, I was in Taiwan with my daughters, I didn't know anything, and when I came back, I said, "Oh my God!" I didn't agree. Because I know sales in Canada are not very good, especially for clothing. It's not necessary to buy new clothing. It's not like eating – every day you have to eat. Buying clothing is different. But when I came back he had already done a lot of things and had it all prepared. He always does what he wants.' Meanwhile, Rosa attended evening college to earn an accounting diploma.

Bob had lost his backing, and the store was not making money. While family savings paid for overhead, he beat the bushes for other jobs. 'In only two years here I dropped ten kilos from worrying, and going here and there. I went to volunteer, to help seniors shop, things like that, for Canadian experience.' When he looked for work, he confronted preconceptions of Taiwanese. 'I'd do anything, I even applied to be a security guard, but they don't want me. I say I'm from Taiwan, and they say "It's not possible you want this job"! The definition of Taiwan is "rich." Even if I meet an ordinary person like a carpenter, when I say, "I come from Taiwan," they say, "Oh, you are rich. I just built three big houses, for just one Taiwanese!" They forget there are working Chinese too. They think the Canadian dollar is supported by Asia. The reality is different!'

He also faced discrimination. 'When I first came here I had to have an interview. I met three persons – one in human resources, and others are technical. When you pass the first human resources, you don't feel discrimination. With the next interview, you feel it is beginning, and the last, oh my God! You're finished!' He is critical of the demand for Canadian experience and doubts there is such a thing as 'Canadian.' 'One thing is mixture. Here you have Indians, Pakistanis, people of many countries, who can trust only people from their own country. You say "Taiwan," but maybe he had a bad experience, like a Taiwanese has cheated him, and he thinks you will too.' Canadian experience was mainly a matter of cultural understanding. 'You feel you are dumb! Every three months, the Raddison Hotel has job interviews. I've been there two or three times, for technical interviews. Some managers take your résumé and just throw it away.' I asked him who got those jobs. 'I think it must be Canadians. They are educated here and have Canadian experience.' What did they mean by Canadian experience? 'More knowledge – you know, the news, the concepts. Somebody can ask a small question, but you don't understand what it is. There's also technical problems. Even when someone from the agency has a conversation with you, he doesn't know anything technical, he just looks for an equal match, point by point. Suppose they need a [computer] network person. He asks you about networks. Even if your résumé is equal to his technique, if the résumé doesn't say it, he doesn't understand it ... My friend a technician did that – he said he was suited for the company, gets the job, and goes to the company next day, but they only use him as a technician 10 per cent of his time. If we work like that, we waste our technique.'

Future Plans

Bob's next step is to return to Taiwan. 'I could go back to the same company, because my supervisor likes me. I was a team leader with eight people and I treated them very well. His son is studying in a visa school in Hamilton and wants to go to college here. That supervisor visits his son more than once a year. When he comes, he meets me and understands. He said, "Okay, I'll tell the boss and you can come back immediately." I wish to go back by myself because the Taiwan money is good, I can support them here.'

Networks: Being a Taiwanese without Money

The Chius' Canadian-based networks were limited. They were the 'pioneers' in their family to go abroad. Nor did Bob have organizational contacts with Canadian enterprises. Furthermore, the few Taiwanese immigrants to Canada they knew had either applied in the investment category or had retired. The information they passed on was inapplicable to the Chius. Rosa: 'Our neighbour's daughter lives in North York. It's the "Taiwanese area." Before we left Taiwan, she showed us a newspaper with a lot of computer jobs, and we were confident ... We didn't know you needed Canadian experience and a lot of references, because my friend never applied for a job and neither had her husband.'

The Chius preferred not to have dealings with those better-off Taiwanese because Bob's earnings could not match theirs. To save money, the Chius rented a basement in Toronto's east end some distance from the better-off Taiwanese area. They knew a few middle-class Taiwanese like themselves before arriving. 'One was my mentor in the petroleum company, but six months after I joined his team, he said he wanted to emigrate ... He's in an insurance company here, and I think he knows I don't have work, but probably they don't have any high positions to give out. Maybe if I came fifteen years ago, like my mentor, I ... could have made it.' Also, being Taiwanese is a minority position. 'Here people say Cantonese is the real Chinese language. I say it's a local language! We are Minnan, from Fukien. I teach both Mandarin and *minnan hua* to my children.' His Chinese minority status and lack of English and Cantonese language skills excludes him from useful Chinese networks. 'The Hong Kongers say "slap this cheek, slap the other, slap both cheeks." You come here and can't get a job, and you lose your money and go back to Hong Kong and the Hong Kong economy drops, so you get hit twice. You're a double loser. Life is not fair.'

Soon after, the Chius closed the boutique and sold off the stock, and Bob returned to Taiwan to support his family. Rosa will soon complete her accounting course and look for a job in Canada. Bob hopes they will join him to Taiwan after they get citizenship. However, the children are closer to Canada than to Taiwan. The 'ultimate' location of the family is being negotiated spatially.

A Site Engineer in Hong Kong

The Luks bitterly recalled their parent families' heavy business losses in China. Mr Luk was senior project engineer in a Hong Kong firm that built high-rise buildings, with a side-business in interior design. Mrs Luk built networks, oversaw family relations, managed her husband's business, and worked short hours as a salesperson. Through hard work, they overcame their families' setbacks; even so, their collective memories shaped many of their important decisions and drove them to emigrate early. The Luks applied to immigrate in 1989, became landed immigrants in 1996, and then returned to Hong Kong. They planned to complete their immigration 'project' in 2001. The wave of migration from Hong Kong in the decade before them meant they already had strong collegial contacts in Canada. But these social networks could not match those in Hong Kong, nor could they solve the Luks' job problems. Their experiences illustrate how the slight social distance between Hong Kong and Canada nevertheless eases transnational migration.

Family Background

Mr Luks' parents had owned goldsmith and shipping firms, a cinema, and garment factories in China. These were confiscated in 1953, four years after the family fled to Hong Kong. Expecting the Communist takeover to be brief, Mr Luk's father did not try to adapt. 'My father had his lands and his property taken away. He waited for years to have this rescinded and didn't take a job. Because of that, I didn't go to school until I was ten. Then when I was finished, I had to go to work, and gave half my earnings to my younger brothers to go to school. I never had a chance to finish college.' Mr Luk's late start inspired him to study hard. It was his dream to finish college in Canada.

Mrs Luk's family also fled the Communist takeover. She is proud that she has overcome her family's hardships, and she seizes the chance to learn at every turn. After secretarial school, she took evening courses in management, English translation, and computer software. After graduating from high school, she travelled to Canada, having saved enough for a ticket. 'I survived because my classmate in Calgary had opened a luncheon counter. I worked and earned $200 so I could travel more.' She still keeps in touch with friends she met during that trip.

As the best off in his family, Mr Luk has taken economic responsibility for his mother; Mrs Luk sees to the social and emotional needs of three parents. She organizes outings, shops for them, sends their granddaughter to visit, and arranges family dinners. Because of kin reciprocity and Mr Luk's projects, they had delayed emigration. While pregnant with their daughter, Mrs Luk joined protests in Hong Kong against the 4 June Tiananmen Square massacre. Starting a new family spurred them to move sooner than they might have.

WORK NETWORKS
Construction jobs are often found through colleagues. Mr Luk built his earliest networks while in school, and these were job linked. After

secondary school, while working as a clerk in a property firm, he studied building trades for six years at night. Those who completed this gruelling stint continue to help each other. 'We all have good jobs, in government or large firms. We're too busy for reunions, but we know where the others work. We look each other up when we need a job done.' After working for the government housing department and for architectural, construction, and engineering firms, he gained a reputation in the architectural and construction fields.

'Networks are important in this field. Work has always come to me. People know if I'm dissatisfied with my job and call me up. I don't have to look in the want ads.' An ex-colleague had returned to Hong Knog from Sydney, Australia, and now invited him to join his group. Four schoolmates staffed his interior design firm. But he felt that 'running your own business is not worth it. It's better to be an employee and buy stocks ... At least, I pay lots of tax that will show the Canadian government my worth!' He sold his small interior design business to start an immigration fund. A PRC firm was the purchaser. 'To do business in Hong Kong, to get a licence, you need to be known, have a reputation and track record. So the firm bought an "empty name." They didn't want the furnishings or even the office.'

He foresaw that Hong Kong's pending return to China would bring problems to his field.' Once in China, I visited a site in Shanghai, where we're building a large hotel, and talked to the engineer about his training. He said he was trained as a chemist and assigned to this architectural job! ... The Chinese government may ask our firm to take one hundred of their workers, who don't have the training, and we won't be able to refuse!' He anticipated a recession, and this fuelled his desire to leave before conditions grew worse. 'If they begin to welcome people from China to Hong Kong, and if foreign companies invest elsewhere, we'll have fewer large projects.' He was proud of his accomplishments. His dream was to rebuild his family's fortunes, and retire in Canada where the pace of work was slower.

HOME IS AN INVESTMENT TOO

The Luks' housing situation attests to the success of their hard work and planning. The Luks have bought two apartments for both sets of parents and two for themselves; they moved so that their daughter could go to a better school.

Their lifestyle requires a car, and they can easily afford one. Mr Luk needs a car for his work. They also drive their daughter to visit her grandparents. They change cars to mesh with tax laws.

The Luks have planned for their financial security. Mr Luk married late. They had intended to have children after emigrating and to have only one child. Mrs Luk limited her career, while Mr. Luk planned to retire early and complete his higher education in Canada. Mr Luk saves a considerable sum every year in foreign currencies for his daughter's education fund. 'Every three to five years, I change my plan. It's true I have a serious life with a tight schedule, but it's a must. When the world changes so fast, we can't wait.' They did not buy any goods that might encumber their plans to emigrate. They did not repair their stereo equipment, and they maintained their VCR solely for their daughter's education. For recreation, Mr Luk plays mah-jong and follows horse racing: his wife has built her own networks while swimming, dancing, doing aerobics, playing golf, and visiting relatives and friends.

INFORMATION ABOUT THE WEST

Friends who had already immigrated helped them formulate their views on Canada. Colleagues phoned them from Canada and told them the economy was weak. Mr Luk could not understand how a country so rich in natural resources was doing so poorly. 'In Hong Kong, you have to struggle, and be commercial minded, keep up and go out with your friends ... It is said that Canadians do not like to work.'

Others influenced them through negative example. They visited a friend in Vancouver who had become like the Canadians. 'He was very active in Hong Kong, bought houses and made lots of money. In Vancouver, he changed 100 per cent. He says, 'Why bother?' He even returned to Hong Kong and married an unattractive woman in an arranged match. He doesn't care anymore. The local environment did it.' Another friend gave them advice on how to answer the Canadian High Commission's immigration questions.

Mrs Luk asked about our research project: 'Any feedback from your respondents? Any letters back about life in the West?' She tried to help our research. We were invited to meet her astronaut friends. We enjoyed a barbecue in a mixed Chinese-expatriate community. Our host, a construction engineer, had gone to middle school with Mr Luk. On their large patio, on long tables, the hosts had laid out two Mongolian fire pots on gas burners. We dipped in sweet shrimp, crab, scallops, chunks of fresh fish, meatballs, and marinated pork. While two maids cared for the tiniest charges, the adults chatted and their teenagers served the guests. Three of the four families had papers to leave, and talk revolved around the personal cost of emigration. The host maintained: '"One country two systems" is impossible ... Originally we thought Hong Kong and South China would become similar, and that Hong Kong would lead South China. But Hong Kong is so small, all of China can integrate Hong Kong. Nevertheless, we still think China will want Hong Kong to make money.' He contended that getting papers for Canada was too expensive. 'There's no reason to emigrate,' he insisted. 'It is a crisis of confidence. If you get a passport to leave and then return it's a waste of time. You might as well stay here. It's not necessary to have a passport. I can send my children to England to study without one. If things are really bad, you can go as a refugee.' However, this man had the British Right of Abode. 'It was the cheapest way – only cost us $2,000.'

Another guest was introduced as a 'typical case': he had gone to Canada in 1989, remained the three years necessary to acquire citizenship, and then returned to Hong Kong. His wife, who had found a good engineering job and who had relatives in Canada, remained behind. He had not tried to find work while in Toronto. 'Hong Kong people build tall buildings, and they are quite complex, but Toronto builds mostly low buildings. All construction is in the hands of Italians, and they are very skilful. I didn't even send out résumés.' Instead he developed a computer software package that tracked shifts in FOREX money-market trends, and he practised martial arts. On his return, he had little problem finding contract work, but he took a cut in pay. 'I'd read up on all the changes in Hong Kong statutes. No, there wasn't much I could learn from Canada. In fact in Canada, the rules are so cumbersome, you take three years to apply for all the paperwork. Within that time, here the building would have been finished.'

Preparing for the Move

The Luks' strong family ties and working commitments delayed their plan; finally, though, they made their move. They applied in the skilled worker category. 'I don't want to tie up half a million Canadian dollars in a business,' Mr Luk explained.

Before they left, from friends, they learned what they could about the immigration scene. Mr Luk knew which items – taxes, housing, and electric appliances –were cheaper in Canada. They brought with them a rice cooker, an electric Thermos, and warm clothing. They did not bring their car, refrigerator, or stove. But the information they had gathered was faulty when it came to jobs.

Having learned from his father's experience, Mr Luk hoped to involve himself in Canadian society, even to start a joint venture with 'locals.' But to fund a firm would require more local connections than he had. He tried his hand at business in Canada, but the culture was different and he lost money. With colleagues, he bought a home-maintenance service company in Montreal in 1987; he was forced to sell it to cover a debt left by the previous owner.

After that company folded, he joined four former co-workers and opened a window-frame factory to get enough points to immigrate and to earn a living. Business picked up when new immigrants from Hong Kong, who were used to having steel bars outside their windows, bought these from the company while renovating their Canadian homes, which came with wooden frames. The company expanded. The investors now investigated molding machines to make plastic frames. 'Canada makes machines that mold egg cartons. We're hoping to sell them to China.' However, they did not entirely commit themselves to Canada, and kept up their interests in Hong Kong. The five partners rotated in order to maintain their dual positions in Hong Kong and Canada. When one partner met his six-months-per-year Canadian residence requirement, he returned to Hong Kong to be replaced by another. Those who became citizens returned to Hong Kong permanently. Bedevilled by lack of both management skills and commitment, and unable to develop markets, they found themselves stuck with inventory. The company began to lose money and eventually folded.

The Luks also invested in real estate. They bought a house in Vancouver but spent more on upkeep than they received in rent. 'In Hong Kong it's always better to buy – you never lose out. At least you'll earn it back and have a free place to live. In North America, it's different!' Immigrant friends from Hong Kong helped them navigate the Toronto housing market. 'I was going to buy three apartments in Mississauga. My friend faxed me details. They were reasonable, but I knew I could get them cheaper. I looked up the construction costs and figured they should cost 120 dollars a square foot to build, and I thought I could get them for 86 a square foot, but someone got there first. Friends suggested, "rent and live here for a year before you buy, see the market and where you want to live" ... You need people to care for you. Or we may even get a place for free. Our friend will return to Hong Kong and he offered to let us live in his place.' They perused slick advertisements, whose names – for example, Pacific Place – borrow the aura of well-situated Hong Kong developments. Finally, they bought a flat in Richmond Hill, and maintained it during remigrations.

Mr Luk now hired an immigration adviser, who applied for them to delay settling without jeopardizing their landed status. The Luks had been eager to settle permanently in Canada; now they drew back, and Mr Luk decided not to quit his Hong Kong job. His wife and daughter moved to Canada, and Mr Luk visited them during vacations. Mrs Luk put in the months necessary for them to qualify for their citizenship hearing, then rejoined her husband in Hong Kong. She was reluctant to keep their daughter out of the Chinese system for more than a year. Initially, they expected to postpone a final move to 2002, when their daughter would be in secondary school and the husband could afford to retire. They then rethought their plans, and have remained past that date. Having invested so much of their lives in Hong Kong, they found that the more experience they had, the more returns they could get from their personal networks.

Remigrant Friends in Canada

The Luks had taken advantage of Hong Kong's investment climate but lacked the channels to do the same in Canada. They initially planned to fully embrace Canada, but their failure to rebuild the family fortunes here undermined this resolve and led them to keep their home in Asia. Having set up a transitional life abroad, they deferred the move. For this middle-class Hong Kong family and their emigrant colleagues, chain migration combined with circular migration. They were not alone in their renewed commitment to Hong Kong. More than half a dozen families in their circles had quit engineering, architecture, and other construction-related jobs in order to come to Canada. Mr Luk, whose company was under great pressure to complete key construction jobs, arranged work in Hong Kong for them. Within a few years, not many remained in Toronto.

Summary: Different Crossings

None of these three Chinese families planned transnational careers, but when they could not find good jobs, two became astronauts. The transnational framework directs us to explore the social structures that ease ocean crossings in order to understand why some remigrate and others do not.

The three men grew up in different Chinese societies. They were trained in fairly similar institutions as engineers, and they worked under similar conditions. In their home countries, all participated in the technically advanced sector of the global economy. Their education was recognized by their employers, they found work easily, and they gradually built careers and reputations. Their jobs included work in leading-edge companies that took on large projects and gave them opportunities to travel and work outside their country. In the society in which they developed their careers, they met colleagues who sought them out for projects. They developed rich networks of contacts, with whom they exchanged tips and help.

This background did not follow them abroad. At home, they were part of the modern labour force; once they left, they could not find jobs. Local institutions in Toronto did not recognize their credentials or assume their knowledge could be useful. Their personal networks did not connect them to good jobs outside the home context. All had to find work to support their families, but they found it in different places. Tom Lai, an engineer from the PRC, had few personal contacts in Canada. When his family immigrated, they severed their contacts with organizations and networks at home. Tom gave up his business, as well as his links with former colleagues, which he could not rebuild. He has not thought of remigrating and remains in Canada with his family, going from job to job.

In contrast, immigration to Canada did not break the ties that the engineers from Hong Kong and Taiwan had with their colleagues. Before immigrating, Mr Luk had enjoyed many collegial exchanges with large numbers of Hong Kong immigrants. He decided not to sever his employment contract, but began a period of transmigration. Ultimately his family returned to Hong Kong, with little overall disruption. Although Mr Chiu, the engineer from Taiwan, had quit his job, he kept up with his former employer as well, and ultimately returned to work there, similarly crossing the seas to visit his family.

These stories suggest that the more structurally similar local institutions are to those abroad, the easier it is to immigrate, and the easier it is to remigrate to solve settlement problems. For the two astronaut families, personal networks spanning the seas were central to transnational migration. The Taiwanese and Hong Kong structures were more like those abroad, so they could be residents in two locales. Their dense international networks eased initial immigration and also suggested remigration to work out the settlement process. The Chius and Luks did not cut their ties with home, which were stronger than those they developed in Toronto. Furthermore, their migrant networks were connected on both sides of the ocean. When their networks did not lead to jobs as good as the ones they had left, these networks worked in their favour when it came to finding jobs back home.

These strong personal connections suggested remigration as a solution rather than settlement in Toronto. This being so, can we expect similar transnational migration patterns to emerge in the PRC in the future? PRC institutions are changing, and PRC citizens are becoming increasingly mobile. Immigrants will become Canadian citizens and then return; along the way, new immigrants will begin maintaining contacts with those remaining behind. All of this will contribute to the ongoing remigration of Asian families.

Over the past decades, many Chinese professionals have immigrated to Canada as 'skilled workers' from Hong Kong, Taiwan, and the PRC. Like other scholars who have examined recent emigration, we expected immigrants to follow a dense stream of networks leading out of their Asian homeland. Who comprised these networks? What were these immigrants' goals, and where did these networks lead? (Wong and Salaff 1998; Salaff et al. 1999). The PRC diaspora that emerged in the mid-1990s is encountering few networks in Canada. Yet people who leave Mainland China are apparently less likely to return, despite their poor economic reception abroad, although no exit figures exist. Why is this?

What explains the diverse migration patterns we have discussed in this chapter? These three men and their families represent the differential impact of global institutions on their countries. They are similar, however, in that all three, as professional engineers, are familiar with an international profession. Professional institutions have a global reach. All three engineers have worked in companies with international links and have even worked abroad. They have up-to-date training and have travelled as part of their work. They think of themselves as engineers beyond borders: they have assumed that they can work in their field outside their homeland. However, the Canadian professional associations do not accept their credentials. Canada has not restructured its entry requirements to ease the way for the many skilled workers who immigrate. The experiences of the three men discussed in this chapter reflect this.

They have reacted by flowing with their networks. International institutions have given rise to immigrant networks in Taiwan and Hong Kong. Those from Hong Kong and Taiwan come from a dense migration stream, one that is decades long. They have rich sets of contacts abroad. They know many returned migrants back home. They are intermeshed with co-migrants. They are part of a flow that has already left or could leave at any time. This flow returns readily and often, and thus there is a circulation of migrants from Hong Kong and Taiwan abroad and back. Mr Chiu and Mr Luk returned to jobs in their Asian homeland, leaving their settled families in Toronto. In contrast, immigrants from the PRC are pioneers. Not being part of a migration system, they know few migrants abroad and few at home. They cannot easily draw on a community of settled recent PRC migrants as their social capital. This community is just now being formed and is not equipped to provide much help. The recency of the migration flow has also left these immigrants unable to return easily. When a person leaves the PRC, he does not expect to return. He does not maintain contacts. His home social structure does not easily retain a place for him, and it is hard to create a place. Having immigrated, Mr Lai has remained in Canada; in part, this reflects the fact that a return flow of migration networks has yet to be created.

Migration networks have to be built. Flows of people from different places have their own histories; they do not inevitably create the same dense fabrics that link them back home. Once migration starts, it becomes supported by social structures and networks begin to develop. In comparing the three individuals from the three aforementioned locations, we find that global institutions have found their way into all three places of origin. The engineering profession in Canada remains parochial and outside those forces. Similarly, immigrant networks are not well developed in China. The result of the uneven institutional penetration can be seen in the diverse choices the three cases have made.

NOTES

1 The Hong Kong research on which this paper is based was funded generously by the Hong Kong Universities Grants Association, administered by the Centre for Asian Studies, University of Hong Kong. We gratefully acknowledge the support for this research on PRC immigrants by the Social Sciences and Humanities Council of Canada. We wish to thank the people who shared their views and experiences with us.
2 For further details of the sampling procedure, see Salaff, Fong, and Wong 1999.

3 I chose the PRC engineer from the roster of a Toronto settlement agency with Chinese clients. Further information on the source of selection can be found in Salaff, Greve, and Xu 2002.

REFERENCES

Anderson, Benedict. (1983/1991). *Imagined Communities: Reflections on the Origin and Spread of Nationalism.* New York: Verso.

Bartlett, C.A., and Goshal, S. 1989. *Managing Across Borders: The Transnational Solution.* Boston: Harvard Business School Press.

Basch, Linda, Nina Glick Schiller, and Cristina Blanc-Szanton. 1994. *Nations Unbound: Transnational Projects, Postcolonial Predicaments, and Deterritoralized National States.* Basel: Gordon and Breach.

Bertaux, Daniel. 1997. 'Transmission in Extreme Situations: Russian Families Expropriated by the October Revolution.' Pp. 230–57 in *Pathways to Social Class: A Qualitative Approach to Social Mobility*, ed. Daniel Bertaux and Paul Thompson. Oxford: Clarendon Press.

Bertaux-Wiame, Isabelle. 1981. 'The life-history approach to the study of internal migration.' Pp. 249–65 in *Biography and Society*, ed. Daniel B. Bertaux. Thousand Oaks, CA.: Sage.

Boyd, Monica. 1989. 'Family and Personal Networks in International Migration: Recent Developments and New Agendas.' *International Migration Review*, 23(2):638–71.

Chiu, Shyh-jer. 1995. 'Migrant Selectivity and Returns to Skills: The Case of Taiwanese Immigrants in the United States.' *International Migration* 33(2):251–71.

Collins, Randall. 1979. *The Credential Society.* New York: Academic Press.

Fielding, A.1993. 'Mass Migration and Economic Restructuring.' Pp. 7–18 in *Mass Migration in Europe*, ed. R. King. London: Belhaven.

Findley, Sally E. 1987. 'An Interactive Contextual Model of Migration in Ilocos Norte, the Philippines.' *Demography* 24(2):163–90.

Findley, A.M., and F.L.N. Li. 1997. Economic Restructuring, Flexibility, and Migration: Hong Kong's Electronics Industry in the Global Economy. *CAPR Research Paper.* Department of Geography, University of Dundee, Centre for Applied Population Research.

Gereffi, Gary. 1998. 'Commodity Chains and Regional Divisions of Labor: Comparing East Asia and North America.' Paper delivered at International Sociological Association (ISA) (Montreal).

Gold, Stephen J. 1997. 'Transnationalism and Vocabularies of Motive in Inter-
    national Migration: The Case of Israelis in the United States.' *Sociological
    Research* 40(3):409–27.
Hondagneu-Sotelo, Perrette. 1994. *Gendered Transitions: Mexican Experiences of
    Immigration.* Berkeley: University of California Press.
Ip, Manying. 1997. 'The Successful Settlement of Migrants and Relevant
    Factors for Setting Immigration Targets.' Paper delivered at the Population
    Conference, 12–14 November. Wellington, Australia. Typescript.
Lever-Tracy, Constance, David Ip, and Noel Tracy. 1996. *The Chinese Diaspora
    and Mainland China: An Emerging Economic Synergy.* London: Macmillan.
Levitt, Cyril, and William Shaffir. 1990. 'Aliyah and Return Migration of
    Canadian Jews: Personal Accounts of Incentives and of Disappointed
    Hopes.' *Jewish Journal of Sociology* 32(2): 95–106.
Li, F.L.N., A.J. Jowett, A.M. Findlay, R. Skeldon. 1994. 'Talking Migration: An
    Interpretation of the Migration Intentions of Hong Kong Engineers and
    Doctors. Applied Population Research Unit Discussion Paper 94/1. Univer-
    sity of Dundee.
Mak, Anita S. 1997. 'Skilled Hong Kong Immigrants' Intention to Repatriate.'
    Asian and Pacific Migration Journal 6(2):169–84.
Manjivar, Cecilia. 1997. 'Immigrant Kinship Networks: Vietnamese, Salvad-
    oreans and Mexicans in Comparative Perspective.' *Journal of Comparative
    Family Studies* 28(1)(Spring):1–24.
Massey, Douglas S., and Felipe Garcia España. 1987. 'The Social Process of
    International Migration.' *Science* 237:733–38.
Min, Pyong Gap.1988. *Ethnic Business Enterprise: Korean Small Business in
    Atlanta.* New York: Center for Migration Studies.
Mitchell, K. 1995. 'Flexible Circulation in the Pacific Rim: Capitalisms in
    Cultural Context.' *Economic Geography* 71:364–82.
Ong, Paul, Edna Bonacich, and Lucie Cheng, eds. 1994. *The New Asian Immi-
    gration in Los Angeles and Global Restructuring.* Philadelphia: Temple Univer-
    sity Press.
Portes, Alejandro. 1998. 'Social Capital: Its Origins and Applications in Mod-
    ern Sociology.' *Annual Review of Sociology* 24:1–24.
Salaff, Janet W., Eric Fong, and Wong Siu-lun, 1999. 'Paths out of Hong Kong:
    Social Class and Contacts of Emigrant and Nonemigrant Families.' Pp. 299–
    330 in *Networks in the Global Village: Life in Contemporary Communities*, ed.
    Barry Wellman. Boulder: Westview Press,
Salaff, Janet W., Arent Greve, and Lynn Xu Li Ping. 2002. 'Paths into the
    Economy: Structural Barriers and the Job Hunt for Skilled PRC Migrants

in Canada.' *International Journal of Human Resource Management*. Special Issue on Globalization and HRM in Asia Pacific. 13(3):450–64.

Salt, J. 1988. 'Highly Skilled International Migrants, Careers and International Labour Markets.' *Geoforum* 19:387–99.

Shu, Jing, and Lesleyanne Hawthorne. 1996. 'Asian Student Migration to Australia. *International Migration/Migrations Internationales/Migraciones Internationales* 34(1):65–95.

Skeldon, Ronald. 1996. 'Migration from China: Contemporary China: The Consequences of Change.' *Journal of International Affairs* 49(2):434–55.

Statistics Canada. 2000, 2001. *Citizenship and Immigration Canada, Publications, Facts and Figures, Immigration Overview*, http://www.cic.gc.ca/english/pub/facts2000/3tor-02.html

Sung, Y.W. 1991. *The China-Hong Kong Connection: The Key to China's Open-Door Policy*. Cambridge: Cambridge University Press.

Tilly, Charles. 1990. 'Transplanted Networks.' Pp. 79–95 in *Immigration Reconsidered: History, Sociology and Politics*, ed. E. Yans-McLaughlin. New York: Oxford University Press.

Tseng, Yen-Fen, and Su-ching Jou. 2000. 'Taiwan-Taiwanese American Linkages: A Transnationalism Approach to Return Migration.' Paper presented at the 95th annual meeting of the American Sociological Association, Washington, D.C. 14 August.

Wong, Lloyd L. 1997. 'Globalization and Transnational Migration: A Study of Recent Chinese Capitalist Migration from the Asian Pacific to Canada.' *International Sociology* 12(3):329–51.

Wong Siu-lun, and Janet W. Salaff. 1998. 'Network capital: Emigration from Hong Kong.' *British Journal of Sociology* 49.3:258–74.

Yoon, In-Jin. 1993. 'The Social Origins of Korean Immigration to the United States from 1965 to the present.' Papers of the Program on Population 121. Honolulu, East-West Center, University of Hawaii.

Zhou, Min. 1992. *Chinatown: The Socioeconomic Potential of an Urban Enclave*. Philadelphia: Temple University Press.

Contributors

Joe T. Darden is a professor of geography at Michigan State University and was former dean of Urban Affairs Programs from 1984 to 1997. He is a former Fulbright Scholar, Department of Geography, University of Toronto, 1997–8. His research interests are urban social geography, residential segregation, and socio-economic neighbourhood inequality in multiracial societies. His books include *Afro-Americans in Pittsburgh: The Residential Segregation of a People* (1973) and *Detroit: Race and Uneven Development* (1987). He is co-author of the report *Housing Discrimination in Canada: The State of Knowledge* (2002). His most recent book is *The Significance of White Supremacy in the Canadian Metropolis of Toronto* (2004).

Eric Fong is a professor of sociology at the University of Toronto. His research interests include racial and ethnic residential patterns and ethnic economy. He is currently writing a book on the social consequences of participating in the ethnic economy.

Nancy Howell is a professor emerita of sociology at the University of Toronto. Her work includes a network analysis, *The Search for an Abortionist* (1969); a study about the demographic functioning of a hunting and gathering people, *The Demography of Dobe !kung* (1979 and 2000); and a study of the dangers and diseases associated with anthropological fieldwork, *Surviving Fieldwork* (1989).

Janet M. Lum is an associate professor and co-director in the Graduate Program in Public Policy and Administration, Ryerson University. She is also a research associate at the Joint Centre of Exellence for Research in Immigration and Settlement. Dr Lum's areas of research and teaching focus on health, aging, equity, and human rights.

William Michelson is the first S.D. Clark Professor of Sociology at the University of Toronto. His special interests in the fields of urban sociology and social ecology focus on people's everyday behaviours and the social and physical contexts in which they occur. His most current book is *Time Use: Expanding Explanation in the Social Sciences* (2005). Previous sole-authored volumes include *From Sun to Sun: Daily Obligations and Community Structure in the Lives of Employed Women and Their Families* (1985); *Environmental Choice, Human Behavior, and Residential Satisfaction* (1977); and *Man and His Urban Environment: A Sociological Approach* (1970, rev. 1976). He was elected to the Royal Society of Canada in 1994 and to the Sociological Research Association in 1998.

Emi Ooka is a research fellow at the Japan Society for the Promotion of Science and an adjunct lecturer at Meiji Gakuin University in Japan. Her research interests include race and ethnicity and social networks. She has published her work in both North America and Japan, and is currently working on a study of differential second-generation incorporation processes among visible minority high school students in Toronto.

Jeffrey G. Reitz is a professor of sociology, R.F. Harney Professor, and Director of Ethnic, Immigration and Pluralism Studies at the University of Toronto, and research associate at the university's Munk Centre for International Studies. His books include *Warmth of the Welcome* (1998) and *The Illusion of Difference* (with Raymond Breton, 1994). He is also editor of *Host Societies and the Reception of Immigrants* (2003), and co-editor of *Canadian Immigration Policy for the 21st Century* (2003) and *Globalization and Society* (2003). Recent articles include 'Canada: Immigration and Nation-Building in the Transition to the Knowledge Economy,' 'Immigration, Race and Labor: Unionization and Wages in the Canadian Labor Market,' and 'Tapping Immigrants' Skills: New Directions for Canadian Immigration Policy in the Knowledge Economy.'

Janet W. Salaff is a professor of sociology at the University of Toronto and a member of the Munk Centre for International Studies. Her research has focused on Chinese society in the Pacific Rim nations. Based on in-depth interviews in Hong Kong between 1971 and 1976, her study of the effects of labour force participation of unmarried women on family status and influence has been published as *Working Daughters of Hong Kong* (1981). Her other publications include *Lives: Chinese Working Women* (with Mary Sheridan, 1984), *State and Family in Singapore* (1988), and *Cowboys and Cultivators* (with Burton Pasternak, 1993). She is currently studying international migration of Hong Kong and PRC Chinese to Canada.

Jacinth Tracey is a doctoral candidate in the Department of Sociology at the University of Toronto. Her doctoral thesis explores the relationship between neighbourhood context and ethnoracial differences in mental health. Other research interests include the unique impact of cultural coping mechanisms in mediating stress outcomes. She is currently employed as a manager at the Canadian Institute for Health Information in the Research and Analysis Division.

John Veugelers is an associate professor of sociology at the University of Toronto. The focus of his research has been right-wing extremism and the politics of immigration in Canada and Europe. A chapter on immigration politics in Italy and France (written with R. Chiarini) has been published in *Shadows over Europe: The Development and Impact of the Extreme Right in Western Europe* (M. Schain, A. Zolberg, and P. Hossay, eds.). Another comparative work – 'Conditions of Far-Right Strength in Contemporary Western Europe: An Application of Kitschelt's Theory' (written with A. Magnan) – has recently appeared in the *European Journal of Political Research*. His current research (supported by SSHRC) examines the connection between colonialism in Algeria and right-wing extremism in contemporary France.

Barry Wellman received his PhD from Harvard in 1969. At the University of Toronto, he directs NetLab at the Department of Sociology and the Centre for Urban and Community Studies. He edited *Networks in the Global Village* (1998), and co-edited *Social Structures: A Network Approach* (1988) and *The Internet in Everyday Life* (2002). He founded the International Network for Social Network Analysis in 1976 and is chair emeritus of the Community and Urban Sociology and the Communication and Information Technologies sections of the American Sociological Association.

Blair Wheaton is a professor and chair in the Department of Sociology at the University of Toronto. He was recently director of the Institute for Human Development, Life Course, and Aging at the University of Toronto (1999–2003), as well as academic director of the Statistics Canada Research Data Centre in the Toronto Region (2001–4). He also was chair of the Mental Health section of the American Sociological Association for 2002–4, and a keynote speaker at the Eighth International Conference on Social Stress in April 2002. He was co-author of a paper that won the best publication award from the Mental Health section of the American Sociological Association in 1997, and was the first recipient of the Leonard I. Pearlin Award for Distinguished Contributions to the Sociology of Mental Health in 2000. His current research is on temporal and spatial influences on mental health in individual lives over time, with an emphasis on past living and working environments as formative influences in the determination of mental health across adulthood. He is also involved in research on the implications of childhood adversity for long-term adult socio-economic achievements, on the nature of the joint effects of mother's and father's mental health on children in intact families, on the mental health consequences of divorce, and on the mental health adjustment of immigrant children in Toronto.